HOPE IN ACTION

SOLUTION-FOCUSED CONVERSATIONS
ABOUT SUICIDE

HEATHER FISKE

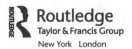

Routledge
Taylor & Francis Group
New York London

Routledge
Taylor & Francis Group
270 Madison Avenue
New York, NY 10016

Routledge
Taylor & Francis Group
2 Park Square
Milton Park, Abingdon
Oxon OX14 4RN

© 2008 by Taylor & Francis Group, LLC
Routledge is an imprint of Taylor & Francis Group, an Informa business

Printed in the United States of America on acid-free paper
10 9 8 7 6 5 4 3 2 1

International Standard Book Number-13: 978-0-7890-3394-9 (Softcover) 978-0-7890-3393-2 (Hardcover)

Library of Congress Cataloging-in-Publication Data

Fiske, Heather.
  Hope in action : solution-focused conversations about suicide / Heather Fiske.
      p. ; cm.
  Includes bibliographical references and index.
  ISBN: 978-0-7890-3393-2 (hard : alk. paper)
  ISBN: 978-0-7890-3394-9 (soft : alk. paper)
    1. Suicide--Prevention. 2. Solution-focused brief therapy. 3. Suicidal
behavior--Prevention. I. Title.
    [DNLM: 1. Suicide--prevention & control. 2. Psychotherapy--methods. WM 165
F541h 2007]

  RC569.F573 2007
  362.28--dc22

                                                                    2007046192

Visit the Taylor & Francis Web site at
http://www.taylorandfrancis.com

and the Routledge Web site at
http://www.routledge.com

To my grandmothers,
Florence Irvine Longley and Jean Sutherland Fiske,
two women who *lived* "hope in action"

ABOUT THE AUTHOR

Heather Fiske, PhD, is a licensed psychologist with over thirty years of clinical experience. She has worked in hospitals, community clinics, schools, and correctional facilities. Currently, Dr. Fiske is in private practice. She is one of the founders of the Solution-Focused Brief Therapy Association, and teaches a postgraduate program in solution-focused therapy at the University of Toronto. She also trains service providers 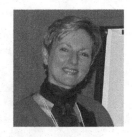 to the homeless. Dr. Fiske is an active volunteer and frequent speaker for provincial, national, and international suicide prevention advocacy organizations. She is a member of the Provincial Advisory Board of the Ontario Suicide Prevention Network, a past director of the Canadian Association of Suicide Prevention (CASP), and a recipient of the CASP National Service Award.

CONTENTS

PART II: APPLICATIONS

Foreword

When meeting people who are contemplating suicide, risk assessment is the current norm. As a psychiatrist seeing a patient who has talked about suicide, you have to follow a protocol to evaluate the seriousness of the situation: Do you think about killing yourself? Have you made any previous attempts? How did you do them? Have you started making plans? Have you started preparing? How depressed are you? Do you use drugs/alcohol? etc.

Challenging these protocols, as Heather does by suggesting that one can do something different, is a risky business. I am sure that some people working in the field of suicide risk and prevention will find the thoughts and ideas expressed in this book absurd and perhaps outrageous. This will be a good sign: "All evolution in thought and conduct must at first appear as heresy and misconduct" (George Bernard Shaw). "If at first the idea is not absurd then there is no hope for it" (Albert Einstein).

Heather makes the case for a very different way of talking with suicidal patients, and she is quite convincing. Building on extensive research and enormous personal experience, she emphasizes the usefulness of a focus on life—what there is to live for—and of assessing the risk of suicide indirectly through the lens of hope and chances of survival, as the therapist actively builds hope and desire for life in dialogue with the client. She says it simply, and it is self-evident when you think about it: "Working to increase or reinforce reasons for living is generally easier than trying to destroy or weaken reasons for dying."

This book advocates meeting clients with the idea that if they are there with us, there is hope somewhere: the client or someone in the client's network has hope that life can get better. However, it is not enough to have this idea; therapists need tools to facilitate a conversation that can tap into hope. Heather has provided just such a tool in this book, through writing about how solution-focused interviewing can be used to tap into hope and make it grow into action, while also doing what needs to be done around safety and protection.

This book is an addition both to the field of solution-focused therapy and the field of suicide prevention. It transforms the world of suicide risk assessment into a world of survival chance assessment. At its heart lie the very simple principles of solution-focused brief therapy, compassionately described not only as techniques but as a worldview and philosophy.

This book contains so many gems and moving stories: Heather talking about "resistance"; the story of the shift in her work with parent groups, "Getting to what parents can do"; Ashley's story; and more. The book also covers many practical situations. Whether practitioners are working with acute or chronic crisis, there is something in this book for everyone.

Heather has found a way to work with some of the most difficult situations that mental health professionals face. I think *Hope in Action* is a truly great book. It breathes hope and breeds it. Buy it and use it.

Harry Korman, MD
Private Practice, Malmö, Sweden
Author of Snacka om mirakel *(1994)*
Co-Author of More Than Miracles:
State of the Art of Solution-Focused Brief Therapy *(2007)*

Preface

Stories of Hope and Healing

There's a story I know. It's about the earth and how it floats in space on the back of a turtle. I've heard this story many times, and each time someone tells the story, it changes. Sometimes the change is simply in the voice of the storyteller. Sometimes the change is in the details. Sometimes in the order of events. Other times it's the dialogue or the response of the audience. But in all the tellings of all the tellers, the world never leaves the turtle's back. And the turtle never swims away.

Thomas King (2003)
The Truth About Stories: A Native Narrative

There's a story I know. I've heard the story many times, and each time someone tells it, it changes. It is a story about suicide. In all of the versions of this story, there is always pain and fear, and someone always feels alone. *But,* for some tellers, and some listeners, this is also a story about the strength to endure, the courage to go on, the warmth of connection, the light of hope, the power of healing.

Fifteen years ago I began to hear a new way of telling the story of the work that I do; this way was called solution-focused brief therapy (SFBT). It is not the only story about how to do useful work with people troubled by thoughts or plans or actions related to suicide, or with those bereaved by suicide death. It is not magic. Freud said, "There are many ways and means of practicing psychotherapy. All that lead to recovery are good" (1904/1959, p. 252). I agree.

And, solution-focused practice helps me to hear and to tell a story about a person in pain that may be unheard or unacknowledged in some of our professional conversations about suicide. Tellers of this story include—even favor—past and current strengths, resources, and successes; they wonder about possibilities for a better future; they find unique ways to utilize and celebrate unique capacities.

I am an apprentice storyteller (in other storytelling traditions sometimes called a "therapist"). Fortunately, in solution-focused work the apprentice is always teamed with an expert or master (in other traditions sometimes called a "patient" or "client"). If apprentices practice with respect and curiosity, and are willing to learn from the real experts, these collaborations can shape our capacity to listen for the hope-full story, and to retell it together.

In this book I will use the language of many traditions to talk about helping desperate people make changes. My aim is to utilize whatever ways of knowing are helpful. In the language of solution-focused practice, I will focus on what already works, and how to put that to use in our helping conversations. I hope also to suggest some ways of conversing differently when what we are already doing *doesn't* work, or could work better, or more simply.

Inevitably, I will misunderstand some of the stories that I hear or misconstrue other tellers' meanings. I hope that some of my misunderstandings are useful ones.

Acknowledgments

Thank you to my mentors: to the clients who teach me every day how to live with hope, dignity, and humor; to Steve de Shazer and Insoo Kim Berg, whose being and doing and thinking have profoundly changed my work and my life; and to Brenda Zalter, whose professional example and friendship have been shaping and sustaining influences. Thank you to my "homies," the wonderful humans who make up the assemblies of world-changers prosaically known as the Ontario Suicide Prevention Network, the Canadian Association for Suicide Prevention, and the Solution-Focused Brief Therapy Association (SFBTA) Founders Group. In particular I want to thank the members of the SFBTA Summer Clinical Intensive Faculty, whose work has inspired whatever clinical acumen there is in this book. Thank you to the students at Toronto Advanced Professional Education and elsewhere who have asked the great questions that helped me put what I do into words.

For help with particular aspects of the book, thank you to Thorana Nelson for volunteering her vast editorial expertise; to Peter Froehlich and Buzz for assiduously chasing down my most outrageously obscure references; to Jan Bavelas for restoring my perspective when I needed it; to Madelaine Hill for helping out with library research; to Dave Masecar for northern stories; to Beatrice Traub-Werner and Shirley Bergman for taking the time to read parts of the manuscript and give cogent feedback and kindly encouragement; and especially to "James" for his valuable editorial suggestions.

I want to thank Terry Trepper, Senior Editor, and Yvonne Dolan, Series Editor, for giving me the opportunity to write this book. Yvonne has been the most supportive, encouraging, and interested presence imaginable throughout this process. Working with her has been an absolute delight.

Thank you to the friends who have been patient and kindly about this project (although they did give me an "F" on vacation last summer). With their support and good example, I hope to do better.

Thank you to my immediate family—Maddy, Mike, Nelly, Claire, Ralph, Shari, Devon, Casey, Ceilidh—and especially to my husband, Adrian. I am a lucky woman.

Introduction

How to Use This Book

Please read this book in whatever way is useful to you.

Chapter 1 offers a set of practice principles for solution-focused therapy in cases involving suicide risk. Chapter 2 describes how these principles can be applied in therapeutic conversation using solution-focused tools. Subsequent chapters provide examples and stories of specific applications.

If you are most interested in hands-on relevance, you might begin with Chapter 3, which consists of three case examples with partial session transcripts, or you could go to one of the later chapters that deals with an application that interests you. Check out the contents of the book to find something that seems practical for your own work before you begin to read through the general framework in Chapter 1 and review of strategies in Chapter 2.

If you are research-phobic, skip over the parts with lots of references in them (much of the first chapter, for example). If you rely on research data to evaluate or understand things, look for those same parts and read Appendix B on "evidence."

If you have never encountered solution-focused brief therapy (SFBT) before, you might look at Appendix A on the basics of that approach early on in your reading. If you want the most user-friendly introduction to solution-focused practice imaginable, read *Interviewing for Solutions,* Third Edition, by Peter De Jong and Insoo Kim Berg (2007).

If you like to understand philosophical bases, try reading some of Steve de Shazer's work, especially *Words Were Originally Magic* (1994) or his last (co-authored) book (de Shazer et al., 2007), *More Than Miracles.* Steve himself might have suggested reading Wittgenstein (e.g., 1968, 1980). For a solution-focused approach to understanding the beliefs and assumptions inherent in SFBT, you could watch some therapy sessions or read some case transcripts and see what you can observe (not infer, *observe*).

If you want to know the theory behind the model, well . . . I could talk about postmodernism and social constructivism and other "-isms," but really this is a model based on practice and on careful evaluation of *the client's response* to differences in practice.

If you are a practitioner, and especially if you learn experientially, try reading some of the case transcripts aloud with your colleagues to see how the dramatization works for you, as therapist or client. Consider how some of the questions used here would work with your own clients. Try them out and come back to the book with your own perspective on their usefulness. As Insoo Kim Berg (and my grandmothers) said, the proof of the pudding is in the eating. Read selectively. Read skeptically. Look for the plums in this pudding. I invite you to seek out whatever bits and pieces may fit with and add to what you already do that is useful for your particular clients, in your particular setting.

Many important applications and settings are either not represented or are underrepresented in this book. The reason for this is simply that I chose to write about applications and settings with which I have reasonable familiarity, experience, and access. I must leave to you the task of translating and adapting what I have written so that it fits the specific work you do and the needs of your clients.

If you would like to learn more and to hear about solution-focused work in action through many applications, try logging on to www .sfbta.org and consider attending one of the annual conferences of the SFBTA. I will be there and would love to meet you.

If you want to know more about the communities of survivors, researchers, practitioners, and first voices who are working together to prevent suicide, you could begin at www.suicideprevention.ca (site of the Canadian Association for Suicide Prevention) or at www. suicidology.org (site of the American Association of Suicidology).

I would appreciate hearing what you think about the ideas and practices described in this book. I am especially curious about how you might make use of some of these in your own work—or how you do things differently. I can be reached at heatherfiske@yahoo.ca.

PART I:
FOUNDATIONS

Chapter 1

What Works? Building on What We Know to Develop Practice Principles

In this chapter, I propose a series of practice principles for therapeutic talk about suicide. These principles are based on several ways of knowing:

1. The context of clinical experience—what clients teach us about what works
2. The hard-earned wisdom of survivors (people who have been bereaved by suicide) and first voices (people who have lived and struggled with their own suicidal thoughts and actions)
3. The application of solution-focused brief therapy (SFBT) methods, as developed by Insoo Kim Berg, Steve de Shazer, and their colleagues at the Brief Family Therapy Center in Milwaukee (e.g., Berg & de Shazer, 1994; Berg & Dolan, 2001; De Jong & Berg, 2002; de Shazer, 1985, 1988a, 1991a, 1994; de Shazer et al., 2007)
4. What the available literature tells us about what works (see Appendix B for a discussion of the evidence base)

These principles are not rules, guidelines, theories, or "best practices." "Best practice" in solution-focused therapy is simply *what works* for a particular client-therapist system. And the current state of empirical knowledge about helpful treatment in suicide intervention is still so limited (Comtois & Linehan, 2006; Hawton, 2000; Heard, 2000; Linehan, 1999a, 2004; Rudd, Joiner, & Rajab, 2001) that our best practice guidelines or standards of care must be regarded as highly tentative works-in-progress. We must be prepared to "take action with imperfect knowledge" (White, 2004). These practice princi-

Practice Principles for Suicide Intervention

Utilize what the client brings.
Focus on *reasons for living.*
Make *every encounter therapeutic.*
Contain crisis.
Tap into *hope.*
Help the client set *constructive goals.*
Collaborate with clients *and* with colleagues.
Work with *systems.*
Be *mindful.*
Watch your *language!*
Evaluate effectiveness.
Do what you can do.

ples are a description of how I take action—how I approach and work with the most critical resources for helping clients who are struggling with suicidal thoughts or behaviors: their own knowledge, capacities, and communications.

UTILIZE WHAT THE CLIENT BRINGS

The concept and practice of *utilization* is one of Milton Erickson's many gifts to the helping field (de Shazer, 1988b). Erickson utilized capacities and beliefs already within the client's repertoire to build helping interventions. This practice is supported by over forty years of convergent research findings showing that "client factors" make the single most important contribution to positive treatment outcomes, accounting for 40 percent of the variance, compared to only 15 percent accounted for by therapeutic model or technique (Asay & Lambert, 1999; Lambert, 1992; Tallman & Bohart, 1999).

One of my favorite Erickson stories concerns his meeting with an elderly woman (as with any good story, there are numerous versions of this one, e.g., Bertolino & O'Hanlon, 2002, and Gordon & Meyers-Anderson, 1981). This woman lived by herself in an old house. She was in poor health and confined to a wheelchair. Her social world had become increasingly limited, and she seemed despondent and uninterested in life. A relative who lived in another state, concerned about her decline, asked Dr. Erickson to consult, and he made a house call. The woman was polite but clearly reluctant to speak with him, and he resorted to asking for a tour of her home. Their tour was quick: the house was dreary and crumbling, the only signs of life a collection of African violet plants in the back. Dr. Erickson suggested to the woman that if she would agree to do just one thing—something easy for her to do—he would in turn promise to leave and never come back. When she agreed to the bargain, he asked her to find out which families in her community had recently experienced important events—births, deaths, engagements, weddings—and to take such families a small African violet plant. He left and never saw the woman again.

There is, of course, a punch line to this story, a newspaper clipping with the headline "African violet queen dies. Thousands mourn."

I love the simplicity and richness of this story, how it demonstrates Erickson's capacity to pay attention to what got the client's attention, and to utilize what mattered to her. He helped her to take a small step that (1) was within her existing repertoire and (2) made a difference in her life—a difference that made a difference.

Fortunately, in our day-to-day work we rarely have to match Milton Erickson's perceptive gifts to help people to utilize what they have. People tell us quite openly what is important to them (where they keep their own African violets). Often, they also tell us how to make use of these gifts: how to help them reconnect, or stay connected, with life. Our task, then, is to watch and listen for the African violets. It doesn't matter where we start, as long as we start with something—*anything*—that is live and real and meaningful for the individual.

Tips for Utilizing What the Client Brings

- Remember: "If you are going to help people change, *first you have to get their attention.*" (Berg, 1989; emphasis added)
- To get their attention, focus on whatever is *salient, relevant*, and *important* to them.
- Look for ways that you and your clients can
  — increase utilization that is already occurring
    (what they are already doing that works) and
  — further utilize whatever matters to them.

FOCUS ON REASONS FOR LIVING

As our grandmothers could have told us, reasons for living are highly potent African violets. Identifying, highlighting, and reinforcing reasons for living is key to engaging in helpful conversations with individuals who are viewing suicide as a solution to their problems. Therefore, "as clinicians we should be unabashed in our active pursuit of reasons for living in the patient's life" (Jobes, 2006, p. 87).

Ambivalence has long been viewed as a significant aspect of the phenomenology and behavior associated with suicide (e.g., Shneidman, 1993). The person both wants to die and, at the same time, in at least some small, real way, wants to live. Much of our suicide intervention practice has dealt with the wanting-to-die side of this ambivalence, "unpacking" the individual's views chiefly in terms of achieving a better understanding of reasons for dying. I suggest that we redress this imbalance by allocating at least as much air time to reasons for living.

Research findings support the importance of this shift in balance. For example, "attraction to life" has been shown to be an important variable in suicide risk, adding unique information to that provided by assessing "repulsion toward life" and "attraction toward death" (Muehlenkamp, 2003). Heisel and his colleagues have demonstrated that meaning in life and satisfaction with life are preventive factors for suicidal ideation (e.g., Heisel & Flett, 2000).

In validation work with the Reasons for Living Scale developed by Marsha Linehan and her colleagues, predictive accuracy improved significantly when reasons for living were included in suicide risk evaluation (Linehan, Goodstein, Nielsen, & Chiles, 1983; Strosahl, Chiles, & Linehan, 1992). In addition, just completing Reasons for Living questionnaires stimulated new and useful conversations in the subjects' therapy relationships, providing new direction and a different kind of "grist for the mill" (Linehan, 1999a).

In practice, taking an interest in the client's reasons for living means attending to whatever is *salient, relevant, and important* to the client. Beginning with whatever is "live" for the client, and then following those leads, is the simplest and usually the fastest route to understanding real or potential reasons for living. I try to remember one of my grandmother's lessons: that African violets can survive even in dark places.

Tip for Focusing on Reasons for Living

Ask yourself:

- Am I spending at least as much of the time I have with this person focusing on reasons for living as on reasons for dying?
- What is relevant, salient, and important to this person?
- Where are the African violets?

MAKE EVERY ENCOUNTER THERAPEUTIC

The modal (most common) number of sessions in any kind of psychotherapy is one (Talmon, 1990). Furthermore, "because of the nature of this [suicidal and self-harming] client group, the likelihood that the first session will also be the last is even greater than across psychotherapy in general" (Callcott, 2003, p. 76). Therefore, we need to maximize the helpful impact of any conversation with a person involved in suicidal thinking, planning, or behavior—that conversation may be our one opportunity to make a difference.

In virtually any text or professional journal article on clinical work with individuals struggling with suicide, the predominant emphasis is on risk assessment. This emphasis reflects suicidology research, which is heavily weighted toward studies of epidemiology and risk factors and, at the practice level, toward risk assessment and prediction.

The plethora of quantitative research findings on hundreds of significant predictors of risk, from gender to family history of depression, can certainly offer some information about where we should direct primary prevention efforts (e.g., Jenkins & Singh, 2000; White & Jodoin, 1998). However, risk prediction research has yet to provide an inventory of useful tools for clinical use with a troubled person (Chiles & Strohsal, 1995; Goldney, 2000; Rudd et al., 2002; Sakinofsky, 2000). "Suicide is notoriously difficult to predict at the level of the individual" (Sakinofsky, 2000, pp. 393-394). The most valid and reliable assessments on two critical dimensions of suicidality, *intent* (to die) and *lethality* (of plan and method), are those made by the individuals being evaluated. Professionals can neither agree among themselves nor match the validity and reliability of self-assessment (Furst & Huffine, 1991; Joiner, Rudd, & Rajab, 1999).

Nor is a typical risk assessment interview likely to encourage kindling of the "single molecule of hope" (Quinnett, 2000, p. 205), or of the life-saving curiosity about possible change, that can encourage a desperate person to hold on for just a little longer. Furthermore, a "question and answer interview" may "cover our organizational agenda, but risk antagonizing the patient" (Callcott, 2003, p. 76). Chiles and Strosahl (2005) caution:

> Going through textbook suicide risk factors for their own sake can be a futile exercise and can be antitherapeutic if the exercise leaves your patient with a sense of not being understood. *Be sure to collect information that can be used in a positive set of interventions.* (p. 74; emphasis added)

If we spend our precious time with a despairing person conducting a thorough risk assessment—and doing *only* that—we may miss a valuable and perhaps unique opportunity to be helpful.

My colleague Michael Kennedy is an experienced solution-focused practitioner and teacher who for many years directed a crisis intervention program in the emergency service of a large Toronto teaching hospital. He and his staff often had very limited time (perhaps twenty minutes) in which to meet with a person in crisis, sometimes following a suicide attempt. In that time, they had to collect the information on history, symptoms, mental status, etc., which was required for hospital records, *and* to decide on diagnostic, referral, and treatment recommendations. Despite these pressures and demands, Kennedy insisted that "every contact can and should be a therapeutic one" (personal communication, October 3, 2002). His message seems critically important to me.

I am also struck by Kennedy's report that when he approaches clients in a solution-focused way, he typically ends up with all the information about their problems and histories that he needs, but without having subjected his clients to a "problem-saturated" interview. Instead, the data are obtained in the context of a conversation about what changes would be useful, and what strengths and resources of the individual may be helpful in achieving such changes (Michael Kennedy, personal communication, October 3, 2002).

Kennedy's experience mirrors my own and that of other solution-focused practitioners who are also familiar with risk assessment procedures. For example, Swedish psychiatrist Harry Korman conducts "survival assessments" rather than risk assessments, emphasizing information that is relevant to the client's possibilities for living (personal communication, April 24, 2006). His approach might be seen as analogous to searching for "signs of safety" in child welfare work (Turnell & Edwards, 1999).

Thomas Joiner's interpersonal-psychological theory offers a persuasive retelling of suicide risk factors that integrates many lines of research data within a compelling and coherent model (Joiner, 2005; Stellrecht et al., 2006). The first of three primary factors he proposes is the *acquired ability* to die by suicide. He refers here to the sum of experiences that can allow an individual to overcome human beings' instinctual aversion to fatal self-harm. These experiences include all of the self-destructive thoughts, feelings, and behaviors that over time constitute both desensitization to painful self-harm and "rehearsal" for death by suicide. Suicide prevention researcher and advocate DeQuincy Lezine, who lives with bipolar disorder and has survived three suicide attempts, puts "acquired ability" into everyday terms:

> It's incredibly scary to think about ending your life. When people get past that, they may practice or go over it in their mind until it feels more comfortable. Some people decide it's easier if they drink (alcohol) to facilitate it. (Bright Mind, 2006, p. 14)

Joiner's (2005) articulation of the acquired ability factor highlights the importance of attending therapeutically to *every level* of self-harming cognition and behavior. This is in direct contrast to an assessment approach that, at its worst, focuses on "canned" triage interviews to select only the most imminent-danger individuals for help and effectively dismisses the rest—often without follow-up.

Joiner's (2005) second and third factors contribute to the individual's desire for death. The second factor is a *thwarted sense of belonging* ("I don't fit in"); the third, *perceived burdensomeness* ("They'll be better off without me"). These two factors sing to me of implications for immediate helpful action. Clinicians need not know an entire history nor have completed an hours-long comprehensive assessment in order to respond helpfully. We can identify, highlight, and reinforce evidence contradictory to negative beliefs about belonging and burdensomeness; support alternative views and possibilities; and begin to establish an alternative experience "on the spot" through the style and content of our own interactions with the person at risk.

I wonder, however, about the impact of routine, repeated risk assessments, a practice frequently recommended for clients perceived to be at risk. I accept the oft-repeated suicide prevention wisdom, recently upheld in research (Gould et al., 2005), that asking an individual about suicide will not make them more likely to think about it or to behave in suicidal ways. However, Joiner (2005) describes repeated cognitive rehearsals of suicide plans as desensitizing, in fact, as "mental practice" for suicide. In that sense, might asking clients to talk about these plans in every therapy session contribute to the capacity to die by suicide? What about clients in hospital settings, or those involved with several helping agencies, who sometimes describe responding to the same set of questions about suicide risk several times in a single day? How much helping time is lost to such assessments? Are we assessing and reassessing risk when we could be changing it?

I wonder how much context and balance matter. Does it make a difference if the questions are asked in the context of a relationship—however new, however brief—that is perceived to be genuine, caring, and respectful? Certainly the therapeutic outcome literature—and our clinical experience—would suggest that it might. Does it make a difference if the client perceives the focus of the conversation to be "what is helping me to stay alive"? Alternative foci would be "what is driving me to suicide"—or even "questions about suicide that they have to ask me to cover their butts" (a description I have heard far too many times). We have more work to do, both as researchers and as clinicians, in considering the nature and impact of the take-home messages we leave with clients.

I suggest that it is feasible to put the need for immediate, personalized help first—and still be attuned to issues of risk. As a solution-focused practitioner, I try to engage in active treatment from my first contact. For practitioners who believe in, or are required to do, formal risk assessment, I propose a revision of current procedures to allow for

1. a primary focus on what will be of immediate help;
2. a more individualized or client-centered approach;
3. assessment of protective as well as risk factors; and
4. taking histories of overcoming, coping, and resisting rather than solely those of deficit, pathology, and injury. (It is almost impossible to describe one's coping without describing the prob-

lems that necessitate it—but the conversation in which the problem descriptions are embedded is then very different.)

Tips for Making Every Encounter Therapeutic

Ask yourself:

- Am I spending at least as much time on *seeking possibilities for helpful change* as on understanding the problem?
- What does this person want?
- *What change will make a difference* for this person?
- What is the take-home message?

CONTAIN CRISIS

Recent, well-publicized concerns about potential suicidogenic side effects of antidepressant medication have reminded us that treatment can sometimes *increase* the risk of suicide (Montgomery, 1997). While these concerns may have been exaggerated (Beautrais, 2004; Bostwick, 2006), there is no doubt that medications can increase risk for certain individuals. More commonly, iatrogenic effects may be likely in situations where well-intentioned therapists exacerbate the experience of what Shneidman (1993) calls "pain, perturbation, and press" (p. 42) by insistent focus on the intensely painful details of negative emotions, thoughts, and experiences. This is particularly true in crisis situations, during which the person's imminent danger for suicidal behavior is high. Imminent danger of suicide, being in suicidal crisis or "suicide mode," is associated with physiological arousal, that is, with increased activation of autonomic, motor, and sensory systems (Rudd, Joiner, & Rajab, 2001, p. 24). Shneidman's (1985, 1993) early and continuing focus on calming such perturbation is well-founded (Allgulander, 2000; Jobes & Nelson, 2006; Rudd, Joiner, & Rajab, 2001).

Thus, while physical safety is paramount in a suicide crisis, the person's *sense* of safety, or "emotional safety," should also be of concern. Fear of being pushed to confront and "deal with" their most overwhelmingly painful emotions, especially when combined with a conviction that such confrontation is required in therapy, may be one

of the factors that keeps people in distress from seeking help. A suicide crisis is an occasion when attending to the "surface of the problem" (de Shazer, 1994, p. 29) may be the most sensible course.
Yvonne Dolan's (1991) position, often articulated directly to her
traumatized clients, is that she will ask them to uncover "only what is
necessary for healing" (p. 142). We can communicate to our clients,
both implicitly and explicitly, that they retain considerable control
over the content of our conversations and that we are interested in
what may be of immediate benefit to them, rather than on uncovering
the roots or causes of their problems. When helpers do this, clients
may be more likely (1) to open up freely—an apparent paradox that is
very common in practice; (2) to engage in the treatment process; and
(3) to return for help when they need it. This last consideration is important in that those who are assessed as most in need of therapeutic
help because of suicide risk are often least likely to follow through
("comply") with referrals and further treatment (Berman, 2005;
Appleby, Amos, Doyle, Tomenson, & Woodman, 1996).

Suicide has been described as a "multidimensional malaise"
(Leenaars et al., 1998, p. xix). Almost always, overlapping "layers"
of factors combine to contribute to a perception of suicide as the preferred solution. The good news about this is that when we look at the
list of problems affecting the person, there is almost always *some* aspect that can be addressed immediately. Helpers may not be able to
quickly "fix" patterns of self-hatred, loneliness, or drug abuse, cure
chronic illness, or get the person a job, but, perhaps they can do something that changes just one of the items on the person's particular
"problem list" in a positive way: offer comfort, acknowledgment, and
respect; admire the person's efforts to carry on under difficult conditions; get the person a cup of tea, a burger, or a toy; remind the person
of one good relationship, or help to contact that support; teach breathing exercises; ask a doctor or massage therapist for help with sleep or
pain management; or make a telephone call to find out about retrain-
ing programs.

To summarize: in suicide crisis situations, therapeutic "uncovering" work is best omitted in favor of efforts to (1) establish safety
(emotional as well as physical) and (2) relieve or at least *contain* pain
and agitation. In practical terms, containment may mean using soothing tones of voice, eliciting and reinforcing calmer aspects of the individual, asking closed- rather than open-ended questions, focusing

Tips for Helping to Contain Crisis

- Focus on *whatever* can relieve the person's pain and perturbation— even a little bit—as soon as possible.
- Remember the first rule of brief therapy: *Go slow.*
- *Respect and acknowledge* the person's efforts to withstand pain and perturbation.
- *Consider your questions and their wording seriously.*

on resources and possible change, and careful attention to anything— however "trivial" through outside eyes—that for this individual would constitute some immediate relief. When effective, contain- ment may bring the beginning of hope that at least some of one's suf- fering can be avoided, will eventually end, and, in the meantime, can be borne. Such hope counteracts the belief that one's problems are *in- escapable, interminable, and intolerable*—a triad of perceptions associated with death by suicide (Chiles & Strohsahl 1995, 2005; Strosahl, 1999).

HELP THE CLIENT SET CONSTRUCTIVE GOALS

Treatment goals can be "constructive" in several ways. Solutions can be put together or "constructed" from many small parts or pieces. Such an approach is consistent with the understanding of suicide as a "multidimensional malaise." The approach is also a pragmatic one, allowing for utilization of whatever resources exist and for interven- tion at whatever points of access are available.

Goals can be built around clients' resources, strengths, successes, and *reasons for living,* rather than focused exclusively on remedia- tion of deficits or treatment of underlying pathology.

Goals can aim to build client capacity to cope or solve problems. Skill building has been an effective tactic for reducing suicide risk factors and/or suicidal behavior in vulnerable groups. Strategies shown to be helpful include skills to tolerate emotional intensity (e.g., self-soothing, improving the moment; Linehan, 1993a, 1993b); challenging negative cognitions and encouraging positive self-talk (Brown et al., 2005).

Tips for Setting Constructive Goals

Develop goals with the following qualities:

- *Mutual* (therapist and client can collaborate)
- *Achievable*
- *Concrete and observable* (what will be present rather than what will be absent)
- *Incremental,* or addressing one aspect of the problems at a time
- Meaningful and important to the client

Goals can be chosen to be possible, *achievable*. This process is typically constructive in its impact. A despairing view of one's problems as inescapable, intolerable, and interminable may be altered by small positive changes in a desired direction, or even by focusing in concrete detail on the possibility of such change.

The process of goal setting in and of itself can help to build a positive working relationship between client and therapist. This is not automatic; it can occur as a result of the therapist listening well, showing interest in what is important to the client, and actively seeking something that will make a difference. Setting goals can contribute to, uncover, or reinforce clients' hope.

TAP INTO HOPE

The patient needs to experience herself or himself as being more than the sum of the problems. Only then will the patient be motivated to deal with his or her problematic sides. (Gassmann & Grawe, 2006, p. 2)

Michael Kennedy describes his interactions with individuals brought to the emergency room for suicidal statements or actions as "interviewing for hope" (personal communication, October 3, 2003). Until recently, hope as a protective factor was rarely considered in research. *Hopelessness,* on the other hand, has been extensively researched as a risk factor in suicidal behavior and death by suicide (e.g., Abramson, Metalsky, & Alloy, 1989; Beck, Brown, Berchik,

Stewart, & Steer, 1990; Beck, Kovacs, & Weissman, 1975; Rudd, 2004).

Hope is potent. Many grandmothers, most hands-on workers in suicide prevention (e.g., Ackerman, 1997; Quinnett, 2000), and especially the real experts—our clients—have always known that even a "single molecule of hope" (Quinnett, 2000, p. 205) could make a real difference. When we ask our clients what was helpful about our work together, they often describe the first faint glimmerings of hope. They may talk about discovering "enough" hope to help them to "wait out" a painful process of recovery, or to try something different. Often they tell us directly that seeing that "little bit of hope" (as one of my clients put it, "some light at the end of the tunnel that isn't a train") is something that will help them to carry on with life a little longer.

Research, catching up with our grandmothers, shows that hope is a foundation for therapeutic change regardless of therapeutic modality—that is, one of the most powerful common factors in successful treatments (Snyder, Michael, & Cheavens, 2000). Findings from studies of positive emotion, including hope, suggest that the experience of positive emotion—even if transitory, and even during times of great pain and despair—predicts recovery and is also associated with the capacity for learning new behaviors, skills, or ways of thinking (Frederickson, 2000; Frederickson and Joiner, 2002). "Patients' positive emotional states should render them more open to considering, learning, practicing and implementing the skills presented in therapy, thus maximizing the likelihood of the patients' acquiring these skills and obtaining benefits from treatment" (Wingate et al., 2006, p. 270). The beneficial effects of positive emotional states have been shown to apply in individuals with suicidal thoughts and behaviors (Joiner et al., 2001).

Hope is based on particular ways of thinking. Snyder (2000) describes two essential components underlying hopeful cognitions: (1) "pathways" thinking (p. 130), that is, seeing a way of getting from where one is now to a better place; and (2) "agency" thinking (p. 130), believing that one is able to take actions that will constitute steps on such a pathway. This framework seems to suggest that inviting clients to consider the possibility of a different and better future, and then helping them to construct achievable goals for moving toward that future—key aspects of solution-focused practice—may be especially useful. And as Yvonne Dolan has pointed out, there are also implicit effects of *not* asking clients about the future: we may be communicating that we do not believe they have one (Cooper, Darmody, & Dolan, 2003).

Hope is contagious:

> Many [suicidal] patients report that . . . the single most important thing that kept them going was their therapist's faith in them. . . . As perceived and remembered by the patients, it was the therapists' tenacious belief in a positive outcome that led to the ultimate victory over despair and the undoing of the forever decision. (Quinnett, 2000, p. 204)

Positive treatment outcomes are more likely when clients perceive that their counselors have hope for them (Bachelor, 1991). This finding does not mean that we should greet every new client with a hearty "I'm hopeful about you!" It does suggest, however, that we have an explicit responsibility as helpers to do whatever is necessary to keep our own hopes alive. Furthermore, it indicates that therapists should consider what practices and attitudes are likely to convey implicit messages of hope to clients. Snyder and his colleagues cite the review of positive experiences and life successes as explicitly hope engendering for clients (Snyder, Michael, & Cheavens, 2000). This finding seems to align with Gassmann and Grawe's (2006) research on the importance of "resource activation" in successful therapeutic interacations (p. 1). "It seems that the prerequisite for successful work on a patient's problems is an atmosphere of activated resources" (Gassmann & Grawe, 2006, p. 10). I suspect that helping to create "an atmosphere of activated client resources" also serves a useful function for therapists, in providing concrete reasons to be hopeful about clients. Asking about, noticing, "unpacking," and reinforcing clients" positive experiences and successes may both convey and strengthen therapists' hope.

Hope alone is not enough; a person has to do something. MacLeod's research (MacLeod, Pankhania, Lee, & Mitchell, 1997; MacLeod, Rose, & Williams, 1993) suggests that people who are driven toward suicide by hopelessness may be able to identify future goals but have very low expectations of being able to achieve those goals. For such individuals, a pragmatic focus on active change is especially important. "Hope is reciprocal with action: it can both initiate, and be initiated by, taking just one small step in a positive direc-

Tips for Tapping into Hope

- Look and listen for *reasons to be hopeful* about this client.
- Use "hope-friendly" practices, including
  — highlighting clients' *resources and resource utilization,*
  — asking about clients' *desired futures,* and
  — *reviewing strengths and successes.*

tion: feel more hope ↔ do something better" (Taylor & Fiske, 2005, p. 82). One of our helping tasks is to collaborate with our clients to initiate and maintain these constructive cycles.

Hope exists. As a solution-focused therapist, I assume that hope is available; that my task is not to somehow *create* hope, but rather to "tap into" an existing, if hidden, resource.

BE MINDFUL

Mindfulness . . . [is] the aware, balanced acceptance of present experience. (Boorstein, 1995, p. 4)

There is no beyond, there is only here, the infinitely small, infinitely great and utterly demanding present. (Iris Murdoch, in Eisen, 1995, p. 179)

If I were to be "thinking," i.e., talking to myself about what to do next, then I would be unable to hear what the client was saying. I would be much too busy listening to myself and thus unable to respond in useful ways. (de Shazer et al., 2007, p. 141)

Mindfulness is a term imported from Eastern traditions, especially Buddhism (Langer, 1989). When I first heard it used in the context of its application to therapy, by Insoo Kim Berg (1989), I thought that it meant concentrating really hard. I had the wrong end of the stick, of course: mindfulness as a therapist is closer to having an empty or quiet mind—or at least an open one.

This seems like a reasonable notion: therapists from many kinds of backgrounds strive to be "nonjudgmental," and this mindfulness idea appears to fit rather well with that. The problem I had in applying it was that my own mind was trained to be busy most of the time, and *especially* when I was with clients. After all, I had DSM decision trees in there, and lists of possible dispositions and referrals, and ideas about how I would word the report on this case, and all the many levels at which I was interpreting what my clients were saying so that I could remain one step ahead, and . . ., and . . ., and . . . Even supposing that I had the total professional discipline never to stray into any personal realms of thought during therapy sessions, my head was a noisy place.

The challenge of practicing with all this mental racket is that it interferes with the capacity to be present with another person, to do perhaps the most essential part of our jobs: to appreciate, as best we can, that person's views and experience. Practicing mindfully brings us closer to the here and now and helps us to stay with clients, rather than bringing in and following an agenda of our own that may be both entirely foreign and not at all useful to them. Mindfulness is critical in order to appreciate and practice "leading from one step behind," where we have the opportunity to see what clients see (Cantwell & Holmes, 1994, p. 18). We can then base our work together on what the clients know, rather than on what we know or on the assumptions (or presumptions) that we make about them as we busily file, slot, and categorize—instead of listening.

Mindfulness is a platform for listening with a "beginner's mind" (Duncan, Hubble, & Miller, 1997, p. 45), which is related to the Chinese concept of *wu wei,* the "continuous letting go of expectations" that can allow us to be "alert but not tense, non active but not passive, and relaxed yet intensely concentrated" (La Cerva, 1999, p. February 9). Mindfulness frees us to practice *ting. Ting* is the transliteration of a Chinese word that means "to listen with the heart, eyes, ears, and mind" (La Cerva, 1999, p. September 17).

Note that being mindful as a therapist, or taking a "not knowing" position in relation to clients, does not mean that the therapist does not know anything: "What comes with me into the room, all of my experiences, book knowledge, values, are always there. But I don't want it to be at the forefront filtering or leading" (Harlene Anderson, in Malinen, 2004, p. 73).

A mindful approach to learning supports the acquisition of skills in ways that enhance the capacity to make small adjustments in response to changed circumstances, rather than learning by rote to do things one right way (Langer, 1997). Such learning seems eminently practical for therapists.

I observe the power of mindful practice when I watch colleagues (e.g., de Shazer, 2004) who appear to need a minimum of time and verbalization to engage meaningfully with clients. Clients know when we are present with them; mindful listening seems to enhance the impact of reflective attention. One of the side effects is that there may be less need for an extended problem story.

As practitioners, it is useful for us to find ways to be more mindful with our clients. For some of us, this may mean incorporating formal mindfulness practice, such as meditation, into our everyday lives as well as our work. For others, it simply means finding effective ways to regularly experience and access a quiet mind, and enacting that skill as a routine part of our practices.

> Teach us to care and not to care
> Teach us to sit still (Eliot, 1930/1969, p. 90)

Tips for Being Mindful

- Cultivate the experience of a *quiet mind.*
- *Practice* in therapy.
- *Notice* the results
  — for you and
  — for your clients.

WATCH YOUR LANGUAGE!

> You never can tell about a person by guessing. . . . That's why language was invented. (Hoffman, 1995, p. 290)

Part of solution-focused practice is careful attention to how the language that we use helps or hinders positive outcomes for clients. Language is not the only means that therapists use to facilitate change. For most of us, however, it is a primary tool. Therefore, it behooves us to consider carefully how the language we use can make a difference.

Language Issues Specific to Suicide and Suicide Prevention

Clear, consensual definition of terms is a perennial challenge in suicidology (Dear, 2001; DeLeo, Burgis, Bertolote, Kerkhof, & Bille-Brahe, 2004; Egel, 1999; O'Carroll et al., 1996; Rudd, 1997). My specific interest here, however, is in terms that are likely to affect clients' perceptions and progress.

In its *Blueprint for a National Strategy,* the Canadian Association for Suicide Prevention (2005) uses the phrase "died by suicide." This phrase is considered relatively clear and neutral and is used in preference to other common terms:

1. *Committed suicide,* which is offensive to many survivors in that it suggests that their loved ones "committed" a crime (Sommer-Rotenberg, 2005)
2. *Successful suicide,* which might mean that staying alive would be a failure
3. *Completed suicide,* which could imply that deciding to live leaves a task "incomplete"

Just this one example illustrates some of the potenial linguistic pitfalls and sensitivities.

I have tried in writing this book to avoid *suicidal person* and similar terms. As in so many areas, it is important not to identify and label a human being only by way of a particular illness, disability, or problem. We have learned to say *a person with AIDS* or *a woman living with schizophrenia,* instead of *an AIDS patient* or *a schizophrenic.* We can learn to say *a person struggling with suicide,* or *a person affected by suicide,* or even *a person dancing with suicide,* or perhaps, if it fits and the people involved agree, *consumer, first voice,* or *survivor.*

Many suicidologists and practitioners use the term *suicide attempt* to denote behavior that is fully intended to result in death, and *suicidal gesture* to describe behavior that may "look" similar but is undertaken without the intention of dying—for example, as a "cry for help." A task force of the Suicide Prevention Resource Center (SPRC; www.sprc.org) has recently recommended just such a distinction (What's in a Name? 2006). However, in many years of practice I have come to regard *suicidal gesture* as an imprecise, illogical, and potentially dangerous term.

As noted earlier, clinicians are not reliably able to distinguish suicidal intent. Specifically, the lethality of suicidal methods, which is often used as part of the discrimination, is not reliably related to intent. People may choose highly lethal methods without understanding or believing that they are in fact likely to be fatal. Conversely, people may die from methods chosen with no intent to die, or with the firm belief that the methods selected would not kill them, or with the clear expectation of timely rescue.

In spite of these facts, I perceive that the use of the word *gesture* often has the impact of minimizing, discounting, or negating the seriousness of the behavior and the person's very real pain and distress. Such effects can sabotage therapeutic efforts to build positive relationships with clients and may undermine any positive take-home message.

One effect of this apparent minimizing is frequently to short-circuit the process of getting help, since the apparent suicidal act was "merely" a *gesture*. This effect may be particularly common—and dangerous—for individuals diagnosed with borderline personality disorder (Joiner, 2005).

Another effect of saying *gesture* is to reduce the concern and anxiety of significant others as to the person's health and well-being. However, that very concern and anxiety may in fact facilitate helpful involvement, such as family members' willingness to support or participate in the person's treatment—and I have seen concern quickly replaced by frustration or anger at the disruption and worry caused by a mere *gesture*. I suggest that, rather than minimizing the dangers, we can utilize suicidal crisis to promote needed treatment and ease painful anxieties, with clear information about what has happened and what can be done to help (e.g., Fiske, 1992, 1998b; Zimmerman, Asnis, & Schwartz, 1995).

Calling some self-destructive acts *gestures* may also reduce our anxiety as helpers. I submit, however, that we can sleep better, and our clients be much better served, if we find more useful ways to deal with our own anxieties about suicidal behavior. We might, for example, begin an active helping process, or activate our own support and consultation networks, or learn more about effective intervention, or attend more responsibly to our own self-care.

Last—in this discussion, not in importance—even the most apparently benign, "token" act of self-destruction may, as Joiner (2005)

warns, constitute practice and desensitization and thereby contribute
to the person's increasing capacity for eventual death by suicide. Every such act should be taken seriously as an indication of pain, risk,
and need for help. The bottom line: Be wary of using *gesture* in conversations about self-destructive behavior.

In fact, in working with people who are thinking about, planning,
or engaging in suicidal behaviors, be wary of any terminology that
begins with or implies *just*. One common example is *just looking for
attention*. As Harvard suicidologist Dr. Pam Cantor notes, "If people
are going to these lengths to get attention—let's pay attention!"
(*Young People in Crisis,* 1990). *Just manipulation* may be a hot-but-
ton signal for resentment and rejection of the person who has attempted suicide, among professional or volunteer helpers as well as
friends and family members. Another example is *just a cry for help*.
If the need for help is so exigent that this dangerous means has been
chosen to communicate it, help should be provided. (Of course, we
may also want to help the person establish a more nuanced and fac-
eted warning system. Nor should we ignore the fact that a cry for help
is *good news*.) Similarly, explaining suicidal behavior away as *just
habitual behavior* or *just learned behavior* may normalize and re-
assure—while leaving individuals in acute distress without the help
they need to develop new habits or learn alternative coping methods.

It is important to acknowledge that language is a living process.
Our efforts to grapple with the language reflect our efforts to grapple
with the problem—and vice versa. Because today's neutral term can
become tomorrow's negative euphemism, consideration and refinement of the connotations of suicide-related language should be
ongoing.

Solution-Focused Language Practice

SFBT has sometimes been mistakenly described as based on "positive reframing," or even "turning negatives into positives." This mis-
conception informs some of the objections I have heard to its application in suicide prevention—and rightly so. "Reframing" the level of
pain and distress that sets people on a path toward suicide seems to
me profoundly disrespectful. Solution-focused language is not
geared toward introducing facile "positives" into a problem-saturated
story. Instead, we try to honor the *whole* story: discovering, highlight-

ing, and reinforcing real strengths and possibilities that have been overshadowed by real difficulties. "The therapist . . . listens to the whole story: the confusion and the clarity; the suffering and the endurance; the pain and the coping; the desperation and the desire" (Duncan & Miller, 2000, p. 70). Much of this shift occurs in our use of language, and will be considered more specifically in Chapter 2, as well as demonstrated in case examples in succeeding chapters.

Briefly, solution-focused language acknowledges the individual's real pain and distress, while opening the door to consideration of other, more constructive aspects of the person's experience and capacities. Much solution-focused conversation consists of the client talking while the therapist listens and asks questions. The basic stance is one of respect and curiosity (Berg, 1992). Curiosity, put into action in asking questions, is an articulation of respect for the client: I don't presume to know about the client's experience, views, or desires; I have to ask. Nothing that I know from other clients—or even from the same client on a different day—can be assumed to fit for *this* client on *this* day. The client is the expert; the therapist asks questions in order to learn from the client how to be helpful.

Another critical feature of solution-focused language is the extent to which it mirrors or actively borrows from the client's language. This is a departure from many other methods in which clients are in effect trained to speak in therapeutic languages.

"Brief counselors avoid becoming language teachers" (Littrell, 1998, p. 19). Our efforts to learn and use the language of the client have several aims. First, it is a fundamental assumption of SFBT that we must work with clients where they are, focusing on what is important, salient, and relevant to them. "Our narratives are only therapeutic when they snugly fit the client's contours and are closely molded to the client's needs" (Omer, 1998, p. 425). Attending to clients' specific words and phrases helps us to understand where clients are in their views of their problems and possible solutions. More generally, what clients say offers us a glimpse of their ways of looking at the world and themselves.

Second, carefully using clients' own language to reflect our understanding of their positions typically enhances clients' perceptions that we hear them, and their satisfaction with the treatment they receive (Patton & Meara, 1982). It is helpful in building a collaborative basis for change that clients perceive us as acknowledging their pain and

Tips for Helpful Use of Language

- *Avoid pejorative terms.*
- Use *diagnostic language with caution.*
- Use *language that will fit* with clients' views, make sense in their terms, and facilitate helpful action.
- Choose terms that imply *hope and possibility.*

difficulty and appreciating the impact that their problems have on their lives. These are important factors in any successful treatment; in suicide intervention, they are critical. Clients need to tell us their stories, and to know that we have heard them.

Third, our use of clients' language in the therapeutic conversation makes the shift from problem to possibility more palatable, and clients' acceptance of specific therapist suggestions more likely. This is true both in the specific sense of using their actual words and phrases, and in the more general meaning of utilizing ideas congruent with their specific beliefs, worldviews, developmental levels, and current positions.

By taking care with the language we use, we can enhance the positive mpact of what may be our one and only meeting with a person who is struggling with suicide.

WORK WITH SYSTEMS

As a solution-focused therapist, my primary interest in any kind of systemic work is in *utilizing systemic resources,* rather than in uncovering systemic pathology or pathogenesis. There are many good reasons to work systemically with someone at risk for suicide. First, no one who is in such pain that suicide seems like a solution should be alone with that pain. What is needed is a network of support, a team. Certainly a therapist can be one member of such a team, but I do not and cannot constitute a team all by myself. Discovering other team members or potential members who are available both inside and outside of the therapy room is a useful way to spend some of our time with individual clients. Bringing those people or groups "into the room" is still more useful. Ideally, we can do this in person. When potential "team members" are not present or readily available to attend sessions, we can still "bring them in" by eliciting and utilizing details and stories of our clients' connections to them. Any relationship that is potentially helpful is worth exploring: with a family member, friend, co-worker, boss, teacher, service provider, neighbor, new acquaintance, pet, or celebrity hero; whether young or old; living or dead; visible or invisible; imaginary, fictional, or real.

A second benefit of systemic work is that a helping team can provide a more stable and secure "safety net" for the person at risk. A third benefit is that team members can provide a broader source of information about what may be helpful, including information on client histories of success and resiliency, and on clients' needs, wants, strengths, and resources. A fourth advantage to working systemically is that members of a helping team provide a ready-made, appreciative "audience" for change that can do much to reinforce and solidify the person's efforts (White & Epston, 1990). Fifth, organized, collaborative teamwork means that there is a more rational and workable sharing of responsibilities. More than that, however—a sixth, critical benefit—therapeutic activation and engagement of individual support networks can have direct therapeutic impact, specifically in diminishing two of the risk factors cited by Joiner (2005): the painful perception of perceived burdensomeness and the painful experience of thwarted belonging.

In utilizing systemic resources in my work with clients, one of the biggest challenges for me has been to escape the family therapy "box," to consider more of the multiple, overlapping systems in which humans live, and the resources available there. I find it helpful to remember the work of Michael Rutter (1987). Long before the current interest in protective factors and resiliency, Rutter began his Isle of Wight studies on "invulnerable" children, that is, children who do well in life despite long lists of "risk factors" in their personal and family histories. One of the outstanding findings of those decades-long follow-up studies was the powerful positive influence of *one good relationship* in a vulnerable child's life. Wondering about such relationships and their helpful impact in my clients' lives keeps me alert for these possibilities.

Systemic thinking and practice bring other challenges. One such challenge is learning to think not just in terms of diverse individual relationships, but also about how an individual's relationship with diverse *communities* may be helpful. Connections with communities of

Tips for Thinking Systems

Wonder about the following:

- Who are the *important people or communities* in this person's life?
  — Family/daily routines
  — Friends, hobbies, recreation
  — Work, school, online
  — Neighborhood, animals
  — Spiritual or religious connections/imagery
  — Heroes—fictional or real
- How are they or can they be *helpful* to this person?
- How can I *reinforce or facilitate* that helpfulness?
- *Whom should I call first?*

faith, of common background or common interest, and of mutual support or with mutual goals can make a difference.

A second challenge lies in understanding one's own systemic participation well enough to act in useful ways. A third, related challenge is developing collaborative working relationships with potential "team members" whose views of what is helpful for the client may be very different from our own.

COLLABORATE WITH CLIENTS

Opportunities for vulnerable people to "fall through the cracks" in overburdened helping systems abound. This occurs despite the well-documented finding that most people who die by suicide have met with a health professional within a few months or weeks of their deaths (Appleby et al., 1996; Luoma, Martin, & Pearson, 2002). Also, adherence to treatment has been shown to be a serious problem; that is, individuals most likely to die by suicide are also among the most likely to avoid treatment altogether, drop out, or fail to follow through with referrals or transfers (Appleby et al., 1996; Vieland et al., 1991). Building collaborative relationships from our first contacts with people at risk for death by suicide may facilitate them getting and using the help they need.

Clients with a wide range of problems and in a wide range of helping situations do better when they see themselves as engaged in a collaborative relationship with their helpers (e.g., Geller, Brown, Zaitsoff, Goodrich, & Hastings, 2003). Mutual participation in treatment decisions—an aspect of what I would call collaborative treatment—has been associated with better outcome in a variety of health and mental health conditions (e.g., Brown, 2001; Holman & Lorig, 2000).

Solution-focused therapists actively seek to understand clients' views and preferences, and to focus on possible solutions that follow directly from that understanding. These individualized solutions can become alternatives to suicide:

> By taking suicide as an attempted solution to a problem (but only one of many) you reduce blame for the client and value the difficult nature of their situation. You invite the client to wonder if this is the only valid solution. This can generate intrigue and curiosity which maximizes cooperation with the client, rather than causing them to have to explain the seriousness of the situation and the correctness of their choice. (Hawkes, Marsh, & Wilgosh, 1998, p. 103)

Such an interactive process seems more likely to be perceived by clients as mutually participatory than would be treating the client as the passive recipient of a risk assessment questionnaire, or as the object of a treatment plan designed and implemented by the therapist. There are advantages for helpers as well, in terms of sharing responsibility and workload more equally. Such sharing may be especially important in work with suicide, where the load can sometimes feel heavy.

Much has been written about issues of "countertransference," or helpers' personal reactions to working with suicidal clients (e.g., Maltsberger & Buie, 1974; Zimmerman, 1995). Such reactions can form barriers to collaboration. These barriers may occur readily between therapists and two groups of clients: (1) those who are seen either as noncooperative or "resistant," such as young people diagnosed with "conduct disorder" and often viewed as "untreatable," and (2) those who make repeated suicide attempts and are often described as "acting out," "chronically suicidal," or "borderline," and interactively as "manipulative," "attention-seeking," or "just holding the

therapist to ransom." This language seems unlikely to promote positive relationships!

Helpers can take a number of steps to encourage more collaborative relating. Briefly, these might include the following:

1. *Watching for, telling, and retelling stories about positive outcomes* in cases that might initially have been described in some
   of the ways cited previously.
2. *Taking care in our record keeping:* One useful guideline is to assume that clients are going to read whatever we write about
   them (an increasingly likely event), and to consider our language in that light. I see this approach as helpful primarily in assisting therapists to maintain a respectful and balanced view of
   clients at every level of communication, and in ensuring that
   when clients do read their treatment records, they encounter respectful and balanced documentation.
3. *Shifting our perspectives on "resistance":* for example, from a
   "thing" that lives inside some especially "difficult" clients, to a
   sign that something is awry in the interaction between two people. The second position leaves much more possibility for
   change and improvement in the relationship.
4. *Attending to the messages we give in our actions:* For example,
   David Jobes (2006) recommends that the clinician sit beside
   "the patient—who is the expert of his or her own experience"(p. 41) for assessment and treatment planning, in order to
   communicate:

   > The answers to your struggle lie within you—together we
   > will find these answers and we will work as treatment part-
   > ners to figure out how to make your life viable and thereby
   > find better alternatives to coping than suicide. (p. 41)

   Whatever seating arrangement we choose, finding concrete
   ways to convey this message can contribute to a collaborative
   relationship.
5. *Practicing mindfulness and acceptance*—the simplest, most
   powerful, and perhaps the most challenging route to a collaborative treatment relationship. I think of the acceptance implicit
   in a statement I have heard Insoo Kim Berg make many times to
   a suffering person who was doing or saying something that from

the outside might seem irrational, self-defeating, or "resistant": *"You must have a good reason."*

Collaborative Goals

I assume that if a client is talking with me, there remains some possibility that problem-solving options other than suicide can still be considered. Therefore, there is already a basis for collaborative work. A client might have goals with which I would choose *not* to collaborate, such as developing an effective plan for death, or convincing significant others (including the therapist) to agree or help with suicide plans. So part of the therapeutic conversation would be a search for goals that are important, salient, and relevant to the client and on which we *could* cooperate. These might involve getting some relief from current pain or worry, finding ways to communicate more effectively with significant others, or just help in dealing with institutional or bureaucratic barriers. A goal's immediate significance to the client is more important than its specific content. Our efforts to discover some non-self-destructive (or, at least, less self-destructive) goal that will truly make a difference are often therapeutic in and of themselves.

COLLABORATE WITH COLLEAGUES

There are obvious advantages of collaborative practice with colleagues for clients. When we (helpers) work well together, there are fewer "holes" in the safety net. Clients are more likely to get the help they need in a timely way, and to have access to a broader range of helping resources that may contribute to positive outcomes (e.g., housing support, vocational rehabilitation, life skills training). In addition, helpers working with suicidal people need to be part of a team, just as clients do: we function more effectively and are more likely to work well with clients when we have the backup that we need.

Just as in my clinical practice, in working with colleagues I can be overwhelmed by all that I know, or think I know, and miss opportunities to understand the other person's views. Collaboration with colleagues can be a challenge, especially when colleagues who could be helpful to our clients think and practice very differently from the way we do. (When will those workers at the school board/hospital/welfare

**Tips to Enhance Collaboration with Clients
and Colleagues**

- Find *common ground.*
- Establish *mutual goals.*
- Recognize and compliment *partners' expertise.*

agency realize that if they only understood *my* approach . . . ?) Mindfulness is perhaps even more of a challenge in good teamwork than it is in good therapy.

We have the skills as trained helpers to form collaborative relationships, even under difficult or stressful conditions. Indeed, we do it every day with our clients. Simply taking the time to acknowledge the difficulty of our colleagues' work, the efforts they exert, and the value of what they do can often make subsequent discussions much easier, more congenial, and thus more collaborative.

EVALUATE EFFECTIVENESS

How do we know that our therapeutic efforts are useful to our clients? Given the seriousness of suicidal behavior and the limits of our time and influence in clients' lives, we need to know that our efforts are making a difference. I am talking here about how we evaluate effectiveness in the "micro" context of our everyday clinical practice, not in the "macro" sense of large-scale outcomes research. How do I discover what in my treatment relationship and procedures is working, and what is not working, for this particular client, here, today?

Furthermore, how do we evaluate effectiveness in ways that are (1) valid, (2) timely, (3) time efficient, and, most of all, (4) helpful in maintaining positive efforts and improving the immediate quality of our helping work? Such questions are especially challenging, given that it is really what goes on *outside* the treatment context that determines usefulness. While gathering information about the impact of our interventions in the wider context of clients' family, peer, work/study, and community networks helps with answering these questions, it is rarely feasible on more than a very limited basis, and not immediately helpful in the treatment session.

The solution-focused answer to these questions lies of course in asking the client. It is a routine aspect of solution-focused practice to evaluate the usefulness of treatment from the client's perspective. Often this is accomplished with scaling questions (e.g., Franklin, Corcoran, Nowicki, & Streeter, 1997). We ask clients to evaluate their progress, the general usefulness of sessions, and the helpfulness of specific courses of action. Then and most important, we apply this ongoing feedback to improve the treatment environment, process, and results. Standardized questionnaires also can be used to solicit clients' input and to put clients' wisdom to work in their treatment. In the selection of instruments, it is helpful to keep in mind the goal of balance between life- and death-oriented, or between problem- and solution-oriented, materials. The sequencing of materials is also important; I would always suggest ending a session with a more "hope-friendly" instrument, such as a coping inventory or one of the Reasons for Living inventories.

Of course, these ideas about evaluation are not unique to solution-focused therapy. For example, in the Collaborative Assessment and Management of Suicidality (CAMS) model "the patient's perspective is treated as the assessment gold standard" (Jobes, Wong, Conrad, Drozod, & Neal-Walden, 2005, p. 484). The Outcome Questionnaire–45 (OQ-45; Lambert et al., 1996) is used to assess progress and change at every session. Jobes' patients are asked to evaluate both their reasons for living and their reasons for dying, and assessment sessions end with a question about the "one thing" that would help them to not feel suicidal (Jobes et al., 2005, p. 486). Miller and colleagues utilize both a short form of the OQ-45 and the Session Rating Scale (SRS; Johnson, Miller, & Duncan, 2000), a four-item questionnaire that asks clients to evaluate aspects of the helping relationship (Miller, Duncan, Sorrell, & Brown, 2004).

Tips for Evaluating Effectiveness

- Make evaluative questions and/or formal evaluation instruments a *regular* part of your practice.
- Collect systemic and contextual information when possible.
- *Always ask the client.*
- *Apply the feedback* that clients give.

DO WHAT YOU CAN DO

"Doing what we can do" is a simple principle, although, like many simple ideas, not necessarily straightforward or easy to apply. In suicide prevention work, both client *and therapist* can sometimes be overwhelmed by the number and seriousness of client problems. In this circumstance, it is all too easy to lose perspective, direction, and hope. A focus on doing what *can* be done—rather than on doing everything, or doing the perfect thing—allows us to move forward. Taking this realistic, instrumental position may be a useful model for clients. Doing what we can fits well with an emphasis on concrete, attainable, measurable goals, and, it specifically includes "harm reduction" approaches, for example, limiting or complicating access to an individual's chosen method for suicide.

In my own work, I often have to remind myself of this principle. For example, when I feel overwhelmed by a client's multiple, complex needs and all the things that could be done, I ask myself, "What is one telephone call that I can make?" While there is always more to do in terms of working with relevant systems than I can possibly manage, it is a very rare day when I cannot find time for a single telephone call.

I remind myself often of the groundbreaking work of Jerome Motto (Motto & Bostrom, 2001). His "postcard study" remains the only example of controlled research demonstrating a decrease in deaths by suicide as the result of an experimental intervention with people at risk (Comtois & Linehan, 2006). The intervention in this case was remarkably "doable": Motto sent simple notes to half of the patients who were discharged from a state facility after hospitalization for depressive or suicidal states and who subsequently refused or discontinued follow-up treatment. The notes, individually typed and worded differently each time, expressed concern for the patient's well-being and invited the patient to respond. "We hoped to show that our intention was simply and entirely to let the person know that we remained aware of his or her existence and maintained positive feelings for him or her" (Motto & Bostrom, 2001, p. 829). The number of people who died by suicide in the two years following hospital discharge was significantly fewer in the group who received the letters.

Tips for Doing What You Can Do

Ask yourself:

- What is one thing I can do right now that will make a difference to my client?

If you don't have an answer:

- *Ask the client.*
- *Do something.*

Following the principle of doing what we can helps us to maintain an essential balance. On one side of this balance is the understanding that suicide does happen, sometimes despite our best efforts. On the other side is the need to continue intervening with energy and optimism—both to prevent suicide when we can and to lessen its destructive impact.

Chapter 2

Putting Principles into Practice: Asking Useful Questions

> All questions are leading questions. (Hoyt & Berg, 1998, p. 209)

> The Nobel physicist Isaac Isador Rabi said, "There are questions which illuminate, and there are those that destroy. [We should] ask the first kind." Therapists who have cultivated an appreciation of the efficacy of questions understand that to question is to wield a powerful linguistic blade. It is necessary to ensure that the blade is used to reveal strength and beauty rather than to carve away these same qualities. (McGee, DelVento, & Bavelas, 2005, p. 381)

Solution-focused questions function as a "tap on the shoulder" (Berg & de Shazer, 1994) in therapeutic conversations about suicide. They draw suffering people's attention to more positive or constructive aspects of their lives and experiences. Often these aspects have been ignored—"untapped"—in preoccupation with the sources and details of pain and perturbation.

In the movie *Schindler's List* (Spielberg, 1993) is a scene in which industrialist Schindler takes leave of the group of Jews he has saved from death in the concentration camps and prepares to drive away in his big car. He begins to chastise himself for not selling the car; he could have used the money for bribes to save more people. Schindler becomes increasingly distressed and agitated until the workers reach out to him, literally tapping him on the shoulder to say, "Don't look at that. Look at us. You have saved so many" (Spielberg, 1993). A solution-focused therapist might shape this intervention as a question, inviting Schindler to reflect for himself on a very different reality than the painful one he was so fixed on: "What about what you *did* do?"

It is as if the questioner points in a particular direction and the answerer must stop, look where the questioner is pointing, take in all the background of the scene, and then use this context to formulate a response. The answerer is thus involved in a process of meaning making, using both logic and imagination, in which the questioner's perspective both penetrates the answerer's discursive world and is enveloped by it. (McGee, DelVento, & Bavelas, 2005, p. 381)

BEGINNINGS

Therapy is really just two people talking, trying to figure out what the hell one of them wants. (attributed to John Weakland, in de Shazer, Berg, & Miller, 1995).

Is suicide the only way of achieving their goal? (Hawkes, Marsh, & Wilgosh, 1998, p. 98).

Knowing what clients want is critical. As early as possible in our conversations, often well before developing specific goals, we need at least a general idea of what can make a difference. Only when we know what clients want can we provide help that will be relevant, important, and salient to them; that may shift their thoughts or their actions, their "viewing" or their "doing" of problems.

Shneidman (1993) saw suicidal people *as trying to solve a problem.* Other suicidologists have echoed his view of suicide as problem-solving behavior (e.g., Chiles & Strosahl, 2005; Michel & Valach, 2001), as have adolescents described as "previously suicidal" (Paulson & Everall, 2003, p. 309). From this perspective, suicide is a means to an end rather than the actual goal. This understanding allows the clinician to collaborate with clients who are suicidal. Even if clients' thinking is constricted and they are "stuck" in the "SOS" mindset—"Suicide [is] the Only Solution"—*there is something that they want to change.* If we can discover what that is, we can begin to look for alternatives to suicide that may give them at least some part of what they want:

> By taking suicide as an attempted solution to a problem (but only one of many) you reduce blame for the client and value the difficult nature of their situation. You invite the client to wonder if this is the only valid solution. . . . By investigating alternative solutions to the problem, and a different map for reaching their overall goal . . . you help the client feel valued and open up options. (Hawkes, Marsh, & Wilgosh, 1998, p. 103)

In focusing on what they want—in Shneidman's (1993) terms, on what they are trying to achieve using suicide as a problem-solving strategy—we also interrupt the mental "rehearsals" of suicide that may pave the way for eventual suicidal behavior. "They begin to separate suicide (the act) from what they want to be different (which may have nothing to do with death)" (Hawkes, Marsh, & Wilgosh, 1998, p. 103).

After welcoming clients for a first session, most therapists provide some orienting information and discuss legally required consent-to-treatment issues. In my practice, for example, I discuss how I work, ask permission to take notes during the conversation and explain the limits of confidentiality, always including my duty to warn in case of imminent danger of suicide. (As far as I know, this forewarning has never prevented anyone from disclosing suicidal thoughts or plans.)

I might then ask, "So, what brings you here? How can I be helpful to you today?" More often, I ask a question more explicitly shaped to elicit something about what change the person wants.

Opening Questions

- What needs to happen here today so that next week, when you look back on this meeting, you can say that it was a good idea to come here?
- What are your best hopes for this session? (Brief Therapy Practice, London—Iveson, 2003)
- Suppose that this conversation turns out to be helpful to you. How will you know?
- What are you hoping can be different for you as a result of coming here?
- What do you want to be different in your life by the time you are ready to end therapy? (Kreider, 1998, p. 346)
- What would your best friend say could be helpful to you? (de Shazer, 2004)

It is my clinical impression, after many years of opening conversations with clients in these ways, that for clients experiencing great
pain and perturbation and struggling with thoughts or plans of suicide, such questions go to the heart of the matter. *Is* there something
to hope for? *Could* something make a difference? What could possibly be helpful? Often their responses to such first questions tell me
immediately that they have been considering suicide, as well as giving glimpses of what might make a meaningful difference. Questions
about how the client will know that a session was worthwhile also
have the function of "implicitly communicating your faith in the
client's expertise" (Dolan, 2002, p. 3).

Each of the questions in Table 2.1 invites individuals to consider
the possibility of change. Even if clients respond—as in fact they often do—by relating their problem stories, they are talking about them
in the context of something that they want or hope to change. The
therapist can reinforce this possibility even in the course of listening
and empathizing, for example:

CLIENT: And then after all that the plant was sold and I got laid off. I
   couldn't even support myself; I'd have to depend on charity. So
   then I just gave up. I knew that it was hopeless.

THERAPIST: So it seemed hopeless, after all you went through, to lose
   your job too. This is so important to you—to work and support
   yourself, to feel independent.

CLIENT: Yeah.

THERAPIST: It's something that you really want.

We now know about three things that could make a difference to this
client:

   1. To work
   2. To support himself
   3. To feel independent

The therapist can now explore each of these important aspects of the
client's life and begin to look for ways that this client can achieve
some part of what he wants without surrendering to hopelessness.

TABLE 2.1. Shifting Assumptions

When clients see the problem as	Use language to suggest that it is
Permanent	Temporary
Unchanging	Fluctuating
Out of their control	Predictable, subject to client influence and choices
Unbearable	More tolerable at some times
All-powerful	*One* of the important things in their lives

BALANCING ACKNOWLEDGMENT
AND POSSIBILITY*

I shall advocate a synthesis of the extremes: the richer therapeutic narrative is the one that embraces both the positive and the negative, allowing each its due salience and proper role. . . . The aim of the intervention is thus to make room for a more complex narrative and for options that would have been banned out of existence by a more simplistic frame of mind. (Omer, 1998, pp. 414-415)

Sometimes the most effective moments of therapy occur when you as the therapist are able to model an acceptance of these competing forces. (Chiles & Strosahl, 2005, p. 99)

Clients need to tell us their stories, and to know from us that they have been heard. Reflective, empathic listening—*ting*—is the heart and soul of helping conversations.

Often I have told of a phone call I received around three o'clock in the morning. This woman had decided to end her life, and she was curious about what I had to say. I offered all the arguments against such a step and we discussed the pros and cons. We finally reached the point where she promised to postpone her plans and to come to see me at nine that same morning. She appeared on time and began: "You would be mistaken, doctor, if

---

*This phrase is based on a discussion in Butler & Powers (1996), who cite O'Hanlon (1993) as the basis of their understanding.

you thought that any of your arguments last night had the least impact on me. If anything helped me, it was this. Here I disturb a man's sleep in the middle of the night, and instead of getting angry, he listens patiently to me for half an hour and encourages me. I thought to myself: if this can happen, then it may be worthwhile to give my life another chance." (Frankl, 1997, p. 12)

One of the mistakes I made when I first began trying to incorporate solution-focused attitudes and methods in my practice was to give short shrift to clients' problem stories in my hurry to get to solutions. Fortunately, the process is resilient. My clients quickly taught me that I must listen fully, before even the most artful solution-building questions could be helpful.

For me, full listening can include asking a question such as, "Has it been so bad that you have thought about suicide?" Asked with sincere concern, such a question can help to convey the therapist's appreciation for the client's pain and distress. If the answer to the question is "no," then I can be curious about how the client has found life-affirming ways to bear such difficult problems. If clients are in fact engaged in suicidal thinking or behavior, it is important for me to know that— for ethical, professional, and legal as well as therapeutic reasons. I see a strengths-based, solution-focused approach as consistent with being clear and direct about suicide-related thoughts, plans, and actions. I suspect in fact that solution-focused practitioners may be *more* comfortable than many other clinicians engaging in conversation about suicide or other "difficult" topics because

1. they know that the conversation will also include hopeful content and solution building;
2. there is genuine sharing of accountability for change; and
3. solution-focused clinical experience leads practitioners over time to have greater confidence in client capacity to resolve even major life problems: "At this point, I'm surprised when something *isn't* better" (Korman, 2005).

Occasionally clients require significant time to tell us about their problems before they are ready to move on—on rare occasions, more than one session. More often, they are open to considering alternatives to their problem stories early in the first session. It was at first surprising to me that clients grappling with pressing issues of suicide, what Shneidman (1993) called "highly lethal [suicidal] patients" (p. 147), are no different in this regard. Receptivity, careful pacing in tune with their needs, and the various ways, including silence, that we show our appreciation of their troubles can all help the client move from problems and troubles to solutions and goals. The simple phrase "of course," spoken with conviction, can convey a great deal about the therapists' understanding and empathy:

CLIENT: I just . . .* It's just been so hard, since John died.

THERAPIST: . . . Of course it has. . . . How have you coped so far?

In any helping conversation, we walk a tightrope between accepting and validating the client's struggle and helping the client build solutions. If we become too mired in understanding and elucidating the problems, then neither we nor our clients can move forward; if we fail to acknowledge clients' suffering, they may feel isolated, rejected, misunderstood—poor platforms for collaborative work. One of our tasks, then, is to gauge how and how much to acknowledge client distress, and how and when to introduce "solution talk." There is no formula for this balance; mindful attention to the client's words and reactions is what makes it possible.

CLIENT: Everything seems so bleak and hopeless. I can't bear it.

THERAPIST: It seems unbearable.

CLIENT: Yes.

THERAPIST: When was the most recent time that you remember feeling even a tiny glimmer of hope?

CLIENT: Well . . . I guess maybe when my boss called to say that I should take as much time as I needed, that my job would still be there.

For this particular client and therapist, on this particular day, the previous exchange represented a workable balance between acknowledging (using client language) what the trouble was and beginning to look for solutions (in this case, to ask an "exception" question).

---

*Ellipses in case transcripts indicate a pause.

Language Use

Part of maintaining a workable balance between acknowledgement and possibility is using small shifts in language to offset clients' negative assumptions about themselves and their problems. For example:

CLIENT: I don't see any way out.

THERAPIST: Right now you don't see any way out.

The therapist's statement both accurately and sympathetically reflects the client's assertion and modifies its meaning from permanent and irrevocable to a temporary point of view. O'Hanlon (Bertolino & O'Hanlon, 2002) calls this *partializing* totalizing statements.

Consider a second example:

CLIENT: Nothing else seems to matter to me anymore.

THERAPIST: It seems like nothing else matters.

CLIENT: Yes.

THERAPIST: That is really troubling to you.

CLIENT: Yes, it is.

THERAPIST: You want things to matter to you.

CLIENT: . . . I guess I do.

THERAPIST: What is it that you feel should matter?

"Nothing seems to matter" is a very different statement from "nothing matters." Even "wanting to want to" (de Shazer, 2004) is a small step toward challenging the tyranny of the problem. Knowing what should or could matter is a useful first statement about goals for the future.

A third example of small but significant shifts:

CLIENT: I had to stop [my suicide attempt] when my friend Jack came in.

THERAPIST: So you decided to stop when he arrived.

The therapist reflects the client's action and introduces the idea of the client making a decision or choice.

A final example:

CLIENT: I'm still here just because I'm too lazy.
THERAPIST: So being lazy is one of the things that has kept you alive.

The therapist acknowledges the client's view of what has made a difference while shifting the context from laziness being the solitary (and probably negatively valued) exception to it being one of the things that has kept her going.

These small language shifts can begin to open up possibilities for change.

EXPANDING POSSIBILITIES FOR CHANGE

"Exceptions"

Exceptions is a troublesome term. It was originally intended to define the nonoccurrence of a problem, an "exceptional" event from the standpoint of clients who see their problems or complaints as "always happening" (de Shazer 1988a, p. 4n). Narrative therapists speak in a somewhat similar way of *unique outcomes* (White, 1991). However, "nothing always happens" (de Shazer, 1988a, p. 52). No problem, however apparently overwhelming and ubiquitous in a person's life, happens 24/7 with the same intensity, frequency, and impact. There are *always exceptions. Exceptions,* then, are not actually "exceptional" (and unique outcomes are not unique). They are, in fact, to be expected—and sought after—and used to build solutions. Often the simplest and most workable solutions are to be found in existing exceptions—whatever the person is doing when not fully engaged with the problem. Some practitioners have suggested that exceptions are "just so many different ways of perceiving and acting—mere pointers to other new perceptions and acts" (Omer, 1996, p. 330). Put differently, exceptions

> . . . signify examples of "micro-solutions" already happening within clients' experience and ways in which clients have been successful. They can be conceived of as clues that signal how progress can be made. If understood and explored they can be

amplified and repeated. (Sharry, Madden, & Darmody, 2003, pp. 45-46)

For clients who see suicide as a solution to their troubles, exceptions are "chinks in the armour of the problem" (Sharry, Madden, & Darmody, 2003, p. 45) that offer glimpses of pathways to alternative solutions.

Examples of Exception-Seeking Questions

- What was different about the time you were in an emotional crisis but did not consider suicide as an option?
- When recently have you had even a few moments of relief from the pain?
- What is different about those times when you are not thinking about suicide?
- What else?
- Tell me about the most recent time that you felt even a moment of satisfaction in your work [or closeness with your family or interest in the future] despite the pain you are suffering.
- What is one small sign that things
  — are beginning to get back on track?
  — might be getting back on track?
  — are not getting any worse?

For example, consider a sixty-seven-year-old man who lost his wife of forty-five years to heart disease one year ago. He is despondent and focused on his loss and on the daily pain of his rheumatoid arthritis. Recently he has become increasingly preoccupied with suicide as a solution to the pain of his life.

CLIENT: I spent almost every day last week in bed.

THERAPIST: Oh my. What was different about the days when you somehow managed to get up?

CLIENT: That only happened when I had to babysit my grandchildren.

That this man, who can hardly get out of bed, still somehow manages to babysit grandchildren, is a startling, heuristic, *and not uncommon or unlikely* "exception." How then might the therapist work toward amplifying and repeating it? Many possible lines of solution-building enquiry could follow from such an "exception." Consider how a conversation developing from one or two of the example questions provided here might make a difference for this client.

Examples of Follow-Up Questions for Amplifying "Babysitting My Grandchildren" Exception

- How were you able to do that?
- What did you do first?
- How did you get yourself out of bed?
- What did you tell yourself?
- What else helped you to get out of bed?
- What would your grandchildren say made a difference for you?
- How did what you did make a difference for your grandchildren? For their parents?
- Who else knows that you managed to do this?
- Who would be surprised to know that you were able to do this?
- What difference would knowing this about you make to that person?
- What would your wife have said about you caring for your grandchildren?
- On a scale from 1 to 10, if 10 stands for completely safe from suicidal thoughts, and 1 stands for completely vulnerable to suicidal thoughts, where are you on that scale right now? When you are lying in bed? When you are with your grandchildren?
- Tell me about your grandchildren [detailed questions, especially about activities and interactions with them].
- Supposing that your grandchildren were able to put this into words, what are their hopes for you?
- How are your grandchildren like you?
- What are your hopes for your grandchildren?
- What is one of your best attributes as a grandfather?
- What would your grandchildren say about that?
- When your grandchildren have children of their own some day and tell them about you, what do you think they will say? What do you want them to say?

Reasons for Living

Reasons for living may be viewed as a special kind of "exception," and they play a particular protective role in therapy with people who are struggling with suicide (Malone, 2000). In the case example given previously, it is likely that the first exception, babysitting grandchildren, will also turn out to be a reason for living. Probably the most reliable method for discovering clients' reasons for living is to listen for such possibilities and to comment on them, for example:

CLIENT: When my marriage fell apart and I couldn't even take care of my kids properly; that's when I really lost it. I can't do anything worthwhile with my life.

THERAPIST: Sounds like taking good care of your kids is really important to you.

CLIENT: Of course it is. Any father wants to do that.

THERAPIST: It obviously matters to *you*. Could you tell me a little bit about your children?

Any opportunity to expand on reasons for living, to hear details, and to bring these critical entities "into the room" (i.e., draw the client's attention to them in the present conversation) should be utilized. We can also ask questions directly about reasons for living; some examples are provided here.

Examples of Questions About Reasons for Living

- What are your reasons for living?
- What about reasons for living?
- What is your most important reason for living?
- What would your [important relationship] say is your most important reason for living?
- What keeps you going?
- What helps you fight back?
- How did you know that it was important for you to keep living?
- How have you decided to keep living, day by day?
- If there were one thing that might be worth living for right now, what would it be?
- What kept you alive when you felt this way before?
- When you look back on this time a year from now, what will you say was most important in keeping you going? What else?

Presession Change

Presession change, also known as *pretreatment* or *preintervention change,* has been operationally defined as "changes clients make between the initial telephone call and the first therapy session" (Johnson, Nelson, & Allgood, 1998, p. 159). Clinical practice and research findings suggest that presession change is a common phenomenon, that it predicts progress on therapeutic goals (i.e., positive outcomes) as well as improved treatment adherence, and that the helpful impact of presession changes may be reinforced by therapists' interest in such changes (Allgood, Parham, Salts, & Smith, 1995; Howard, Kopta, Krause, & Orlinsky, 1986; Johnson et al., 1998 Lawson, 1994; Weiner-Davis, de Shazer, & Gingerich, 1987).

Presession change can be identified by the therapist as clients tell their stories, asked about directly, or assessed via a scaling question early in the first session, for example:

> Let's say 10 means how you want your life to be when you have solved the problem that brought you here, and 0 means how bad things were when you picked up the phone to set up an appointment, where would you say the problem is at today between 0 and 10? (Berg & Miller, 1992, p. 83)

Any number different from 0 indicates that something is different already, and those differences are typically a rich source of exceptions and building blocks for further change. For the client who decides to call a therapist instead of developing or acting on plans for suicide, presession exceptions may be key reasons for living.

Coping Questions

Coping questions take this general form: "How have you managed to *x* [do or say or think something useful] in spite of *y* [difficult problems]?" They often provide useful exception information as well as helping to maintain the acknowledgement-possibility balance. Often, a coping question includes an implied compliment, for example:

THERAPIST: How have you managed to keep working day after day when you are feeling so unhappy about your life?

CLIENT: I never really thought about it as anything special. I just told myself I had to keep going. I knew that the boss counted on me.

In this exchange, the therapist has learned a great deal about the client's strengths—that she is responsible, hard-working, and loyal—and about an existing coping skill—positive self-talk. Responsibility and hard work are certainly useful factors in successful therapy; loyalty is a positive relationship factor; and her practice of motivating self-talk may become an important intervention.

With clients who are talking about suicide and may feel overwhelmed, therapists should look for "ways to phrase coping questions that respect clients' immediate perception of life's hopelessness but still invite them to think about how they are surviving" (De Jong & Berg, 2002, p. 228).

Protective Factors

I have a magpie relationship with the literature of my profession: I observe it carefully, watching for shiny things to add to my collection. In particular I collect information about what works, what helps, what balances or even outweighs risk for suffering people. I am interested in what therapists can do, but before that I am interested in client behaviors, statements, beliefs, experiences, and relationships that have protective value. I remember that it is *client factors* that account for the largest proportion of variance (40 percent) in successful therapeutic outcomes (Bohart & Tallman, 1999; Lambert, 1992, 2004). Noticing such factors in my own clients helps me to stay hopeful. Pointing them out to my clients, directly or more subtly, may contribute to their hopes as well. Sometimes I include observations about such factors in my end-of-session feedback to clients. I may also look for ways to utilize protective factors in constructing solutions with clients.

More important, however, than generic protective factors cited in the literature are the idiosyncratic positive experiences, abilities, and beliefs of individual clients: their unique exceptions, coping strategies, and reasons for living. The ways in which we as therapists notice, mark, and highlight such client strengths and resources are core aspects of solution-focused practice.

Responding to and Utilizing Exceptions

Insoo Kim Berg is a master of the wide eyes, the head tilt, the soft-voiced "Really! You did that?!" to signal to clients that something in what they have said is a good or significant thing. Such "punctuation" of the therapeutic conversation to underline the importance of client capacities, ideas, or achievements can be achieved in many ways: verbally through exclamations, grunts, or "Hmms"; nonverbally with raised eyebrows, surprised looks, writing a note. The emphasis on client strengths may also be more verbally explicit, as in the use of compliments throughout the conversation or as part of formal feedback at the end of a session.

Murphy and Duncan (1997) describe a "Five E" method for utilizing exceptions: eliciting, elaborating, expanding, evaluating, and empowering Some possible applications of their method are presented in Table 2.2.

A note about "empowering": I agree with Steve de Shazer that "[n]o therapist ever empowered anybody. People empower themselves, and the best we can do is to provide some conditions or circumstances that make that just a little bit more likely" (de Shazer, Berg, & Miller, 1995).

A BETTER FUTURE: THE MIRACLE QUESTION ("YOU ASK THEM WHAT?")

The future is both created and negotiable. (de Shazer et al., 2007, p. 3)

Future thinking and the ability to better plan and foster hope are central to helping tip the balance from a preoccupation with reasons for dying to a preoccupation with reasons for living. (Jobes, 2006, pp. 86-87)

The aim is to invite clients into conversations about alternative perspectives and to open up the possibility of a future where life is better for them, with suicide sidelined as a potential method of moving forward. (Sharry, Darmody, & Madden, 2002, p. 302)

TABLE 2.2. Applying Murphy and Duncan's (1997) Five-E Method for Utilizing Exceptions

Method	Definition	Example Questions
Eliciting	Using listening, observation, and questions to discover exceptions	You said that you hardly ever feel safe. What has been different about those rare times when you have been able to feel safe?
Elaborating	Evoking the details of the exception	When was it that you were able to feel safe with your sister there? What was it about being with your sister that helped you to feel safe? How do you make arrangements to see her? How often? What do you do together?
Expanding	Opening up possibilities for accessing exception conditions or doing more exception-related behaviors	What difference might it make for you to see your sister more often? What would need to happen for her to take the time? What do you say to yourself when your sister is around?
Evaluating	Asking qualitative and quantitative questions about differences	With regard to you being able to feel safe, would you say that you feel about the same, less safe, or more safe when you spend time with your sister? On a scale from 1 to 10, if 10 stands for feeling completely safe and 1 stands for completely unsafe, where are you when your sister is with you? When you are on your own? When you are on your own but looking at a picture of the two of you together? When you are on your own but talking to her on the telephone?
Empowering	Questions that invite clients to look at what they are doing that helps to create exceptions	How have you built a relationship with your sister that helps you to feel safe? What difference does it make to know that you have this safe relationship with her? How do you think it makes a difference for her? You said that last week just talking to her on the telephone made a difference. How were you able to use those conversations to help yourself feel safer? What did you pay attention to?

The miracle question (see Appendix A) is a core practice—perhaps *the* core practice—of SFBT. It asks clients to envision a personal future without their current problems. In doing so, they have to imagine, not just positive change, but the myriad tiny *consequences* of positive change in their daily lives.

> The miracle question makes supreme strategic sense: It works like parachuting behind the enemy's lines. It lands the therapeutic dialogue, at one stroke, in a world of pure solution.
> Change is to be experienced as all-pervasive, as a daily matter, as something with which the client is so familiar as even to fail to perceive it. (Omer, 1996, p. 330)

The miracle question requires "a dramatic shift from problem-saturated thinking to a focus on solutions" (De Jong & Berg, 2002, p. 85). Suicidologists sometimes ask me if a person trapped in the cognitive and perceptual constriction common in a suicidal state can respond to such a complex, hypothetical question. My first answer is, "I don't know until I ask." So far, every person but one* of whom I have asked the miracle question (conservatively, several thousand people) has given me a more or less useful answer. My next answer is that the miracle question is the single most powerful tool I have for interrupting or disrupting that constricted state. When clients are so trapped in a view of their problems as interminable, intolerable, and inescapable that suicide seems like the only answer, it can take the idea of a miracle to break them out. Ordinary future-oriented questions may not do it.

I don't mean by this that either client or therapist necessarily believes or expects that a miracle will happen. The miracle question, when phrased and used as intended, does not suggest to clients that a miracle is coming. It is a hypothetical question, beginning with that wonderfully useful word "Suppose . . ." It is the *idea* of a miracle that is useful because it surprises people and gets their attention, and because it frees their solutions from their problems.

---

*One client could find no answer to the miracle question. Eventually we went on to other things. An hour later she left a message on my voice mail to say that on her way home she had realized "That was a trick question! You tricked me! You wanted me to figure out that I already have everything I need to solve my problems. I don't need a miracle. Well, I figured it out. I can do this myself."

What was that last part again? *Because it frees their solutions from their problems*. The perceived need to understand and solve every aspect of the problem(s) before moving toward options for solution is a heavy and unnecessary burden. In suicide intervention work, that burden may also be dangerous, diverting precious time and energy from what could make an immediate difference. Real-life solutions frequently bear little or no relationship to the problems they assuage. Consider a medical example: Having a dog or cat as a pet protects against stress-induced high blood pressure (Allen, Shykoff, & Izzo, 2001; Jennings et al., 1998; Odendaal, 2000). Living with a small furry nonhuman creature is thus one useful and practicable facet of a solution to a life-threatening condition. However, we could spend a very long time investigating the general and particular causes of high blood pressure and amassing information about the problem without ever catching sight of this possibility. Framing solutions only as answers to particular problems limits the scope of available and usable options. Protective factors are not just the absence of risk factors. Reasons for living and reasons for dying are separate continua.

Answering the miracle question shifts clients' focus to the details of the preferred future and away from the problem perceptions that push people toward suicide. In answering, clients begin to focus instead on options for change that may be unrelated to the problems or the sources of the problems, options that enhance, reinforce and bring to the forefront their reasons for living. Answering the miracle question can create "future pull" (Bertolino & O'Hanlon, 2002, p. 140), evoking a possible future that is uniquely compelling for the client. "For things to get better, we have to see more than their present state" (Kast, 1991/1994, p. 139).

The miracle question belongs to a category of interventions that are relatively simple conceptually but far from easy in application. Timing and pacing of the question to be "in sync" with the client are critical. One general rule of thumb about when to ask the question is "as early as possible" in the first meeting with clients (de Shazer, Berg, & Miller, 1995); another is at the point when clients have identified something that they want, at least in general terms (Berg, 1989). (Clients generally identify what they *don't* want very quickly. Getting clear and concrete ideas about what they *do* want can take more time and effort on the therapist's part.) Useful suggestions for effective pacing and emphasis in asking the miracle question can be found in de Shazer and colleagues (2007) and in De Jong and Berg (2002, 2007).

Remember Snyder's (2000; Snyder, Michael, & Cheavens, 2000) findings about hope requiring pathways thinking and agency thinking? As a visual thinker, I sometimes imagine that when the "miracle picture" gets really clear and bright, the light that it casts shines back along the pathway from here to there. One of the most important parts of my job is to help clients to illuminate their pictures—and thereby their pathways. I do that by asking follow-up questions to elicit detail upon interwoven detail of the results of these hypothetical miracles in my clients' lives.

Details, Details, Details

The aim of follow-up questions to the miracle question (see Appendix A) is to elicit as complete a portrayal as possible of how the miracle will affect daily life activities. The more mundane, everyday, particular, and "trivial" the details are, the better.

> Concrete, detailed descriptions of behavior and action constitute a virtual rehearsal of what a person wants to do in his or her life. The more detailed the description, the more vivid and "real" the experience becomes for the client, thereby making it easier and more natural to carry out in real life. Furthermore, the experience of creating a richly detailed behavioral description allows the client to pre-view some of the future rewards of the contemplated changes, thereby increasing motivation. . . . if the contemplated behavior involves a much desired but initially difficult change . . . the feelings evoked . . . can be a source of much needed "courage for the journey." (de Shazer et al., 2007, p. 46)

Descriptions that include thoughts, feelings, and actions have the broadest application (de Shazer et al., 2007). Questions that bring the descriptions into context, and especially relationship context, are crucial (e.g., Who will notice this change in you? What will they see? What will they do in response?).

If you examined the questions that I use in my work, I am sure that the most frequent one would be "What else?" I keep asking as long as the clients can give more details about how their daily lives will be different after the miracle. It is useful to persist with details of the miracle picture until you think that clients can "see" the miracle; that is, there is enough diverse detail to make it live for them. At that point, we can turn to constructing a "bridge" between the miracle picture and the present.

Miracle Picture Exceptions

Sometimes miracle picture exceptions (i.e., instances of part of the miracle already occurring) come up spontaneously in the conversation. Most often I ask directly, "When was the most recent time that you experienced even a small part of your 'miracle picture'?" Eliciting and elaborating these exceptions, however trivial they may seem, is a key step in helping clients construct pathways to solution.

GOALS

Goal setting ideally follows clients' answers to the miracle question because then their goals can be derived from and connected to their pictures of a better future, instead of to their pictures of the problem. As discussed earlier, this provides the largest possible scope for useful goals. Goals become the action plan for achieving the future envisioned in the miracle picture. The "future pull" of the miracle picture helps to animate and motivate goal setting and progress. Thus, goals might be related to the problems clients have described (e.g., "to be able to calm myself down when my boyfriend threatens to leave me, instead of thinking about suicide"), or they may be apparently unconnected (e.g., "to volunteer twice a week at the food bank").

There are other advantages in building goals after a miracle picture is in place. One is that clients are more likely to focus on something that is part of the miracle picture and that can therefore be described in concrete, everyday terms rather than being vague or general. And even if clients do suggest very vague, general goals, we can ask, "Would playing soccer like you talked about in your miracle picture be an example of that? Yes? And what else?"

Much of the work of goal setting is helping clients to modify goals to be small enough and practical enough that they can quickly put them into action and see positive consequences. For clients battling helplessness and hopelessness, the challenge is helping them to find goals for change that are relevant enough to make a difference while being within their current capacity to accomplish, so that they are likely to achieve immediate, hope-engendering results. Chiles and Strohsahl (2005) recommend interventions that are "bite-sized, concrete, and 'doable'" (p. 66). According to Jobes (2006):

> I whittle away at the patient's reluctance [to act] by breaking down the behavior goal into (sometimes comical) minigoals that even the most depressed patient will ultimately admit they can do. I once had an obese patient who insisted she could not exercise; the prospect was just too overwhelming for her to even consider. I insisted that we break down the goal and work toward successive approximations of the larger goal. Again she refused. When she refused to consider a 30-minute walk each day, I nevertheless persisted. Finally with mutual laughter we negotiated an agreement where she could commit to walking for 3 minutes each morning. . . . In the coming weeks we increased the walking by 5-minute increments until she reached a point where she voluntarily felt comfortable increasing her walking regimen on her own. In 2 years she was up to walking twice a day for 45 minutes and had lost 60 pounds. (p. 86)

A solution-focused therapist would probably use questions to achieve similar results, for example, "What is the shortest possible walk you could take?" or "How far have you walked recently?" and "How soon would you be willing to try that again?" (See Appendix A for questions that are helpful in setting doable goals.)

*"MAKING NUMBERS TALK"**

Scaling questions are a powerful, effective, and efficient tool. In suicide intervention work they are in my view indispensable. Scales allow clients—even clients whose verbal facility is limited—to evaluate for themselves and communicate with others about their current emotional and cognitive states, their views and opinions, their success at coping, their goals, and especially about differences: small next steps, movement and progress toward their goals. A number of

---

*Partial title of 1993 article by Berg and de Shazer.

practitioners have commented on the utility of scaling questions in clarifying ongoing issues of risk and safety (Callcott, 2003; Fiske, 1997, 2002, 2003, 2004a; Hawkes, Marsh, & Wilgosh, 1998; McGlothin, 2006; Sharry, Darmody, & Madden, 2002; Softas-Niall & Francis, 1998a, 1998b).

Examples of Scaling Questions about Risk and Safety

On a scale from 1 to 10, if 1 stands for you are definitely going to kill yourself today and 10 stands for the day after the miracle,

- where were you before you decided to come here today?
- where are you now?
- what needs to happen so that you can maintain that number, or even move up slightly?
- where do you need to be on the scale to be safe from killing yourself?
- where do you need to be on the scale to be safe from thoughts of killing yourself?

Let's say 1 stands for the moment when you were ready to pull the trigger, before you decided to come here, and 10 stands for pulling the trigger is not an option:

- Where are you right now?
- [For any answer greater than 1] What is different now? What else?
- [If the answer is "1"] What has to change in order for you to say "2"?

If 10 stands for "I can see some light at the end of the tunnel," and 1 stands for "I see no hope at all,"

- where are you right now?
- [if 1 or more] what gives you (even) that much hope?
- what would it take for you to move up just one-half point on that scale?

"On a scale from 0* to 10,

- how much do you want to find an alternative to this situation?
- how realistic is it that you can stay safe this weekend?

(Continued)

(Continued)

- how confident are you that you can stay safe this weekend?" (Hawkes, Marsh, & Wilgosh, 1998, p. 104)

On a scale from 1 to 10, if 10 stands for "I believe that I will live a long and satisfying life and die of natural causes," and 1 stands for "I will die soon by suicide,"

- where is your belief right now (adapted from Bertolino & O'Hanlon, 2002)?
- where was it at the worst point?
- where will it be when you are able to get a night's sleep without nightmares? To tell your wife that you came here to talk with me today? When you go for a walk with her in the evening instead of going to the bar?

On a scale from 1 to 10, if 1 indicates the pain you feel is unbearable and 10 indicates that you can handle the pain, where are you?

On a scale from 1 to 10, if 10 means that you are determined to live and 1 means you don't know if you can make it, where are you?

*Some solution-focused practitioners use 1-to-10 scales, and some use 0-to-10 scales. Steve de Shazer used 0 to 10, and Insoo Kim Berg uses 1 to 10. I know of no evidence that it makes a difference.

Solution-focused scales are self-anchored rather than normed: the client, not the therapist, defines what a "3" or an "8" means on the scales.

> I remember one case fairly recently [Berg & de Shazer, 1993] where I asked a scaling question and she said she was a 2. . . . I can imagine the people behind the mirror saying, "Oh, Christ, she's only a 2." . . . I was just waiting for her to expand some on what "2" might mean, without having to ask her. Then after a pause she said, "You know, that's pretty damn good for me." I shook her hand. She thought it would be a God-damned miracle for her ever to reach 3 or 4. So, to her 2 was halfway to her goal—she knew she would never get past 4. If she maintained that 4, she would be satisfied. (de Shazer, in Hoyt, 1996, p. 71)

The client-generated, client-specific meaning of the numbers differentiates this application from therapist-defined scales used, for example, to assess clients as being at predetermined levels of lethality or perturbation. McGlothin (2006) defines the scales he uses in this way: clients are assessed as "low" risk between 1 and 3, "moderate" risk between 4 and 7, and "high" risk between 8 and 10. While this approach to numeric questioning may still be a useful tool, it lacks the flexibility and client-centered focus of solution-focused scaling questions. Also, McGlothin defines 10 as the most lethal or perturbed and 1 as the least (i.e., 10 is the negative pole and 1 the positive). In my experience, this approach to scaling does not lend itself to tracking change and progress with the same intuitive ease as a scale where positive change means increasing numbers.

Other Quantitative Questions

- How much of what you have been going through do you think is a normal response to the multiple losses you have had recently?
- What percentage of your son's problems do you think is common to adolescents? To kids with learning disabilities?
- [If the answer is, "I don't know"] How could you find out? And how could you learn about how other parents deal with that?
- How much of your company's loss is due to your management and how much to the recession? To your partner's misappropriation of funds?
- Out of 100 percent, how much of the time are you thinking about suicide?
- What are you thinking about at other times?
- What is the highest percentage of time thinking about that [i.e., something other than suicide] that you have had recently?
- How did you manage that?

COMPLIMENTS

Never lose a chance of saying a kind word. (William Makepeace Thackeray, in Eisen, 1995, p. 44)

Compliments act to highlight and reinforce clients' strengths and resources. For people who are so lost in negativity and self-denigration that suicide looks like a desirable escape, the significance of such results can be profound. Morrissette (1992) describes how the use of compliments about observed strengths is surprising—and therefore attention getting—to homeless youth, a group at high risk for suicidal behavior (Kidd, 2006; Kidd & Kral, 2002). Compliments are often a forceful and telling "tap on the shoulder," and a much-needed counter to painful feelings of being unappreciated or burdensome. Solution-focused therapeutic conversation is riddled with compliments—some explicit and direct, but most of them implicit in our questions.

For example, I ask people the kinds of detailed questions already described about what they want to change and about their preferred futures. In asking, I make implicit attributions of clients' understanding, judgment, positive intention, and agency. Both our thoughtfulness in asking such questions and our interest in the clients' responses are complimentary (and complementary!) postures. Most people appreciate being consulted seriously on their opinions and treated as partners in the therapy enterprise.

Indirect verbal compliments most often take the form of "how" questions, for example, about clients' decisions to get help, their understanding of what would and wouldn't work for them, their use of coping skills, their capacity to tolerate or overcome pain and problems: "How did you do that? How did you figure that out?" Such questions in effect invite clients to reflect on their own competence, to compliment themselves. Such tributes to their own positive qualities often surprise and intrigue clients and, especially when reinforced by therapists, can become the basis for new ways of knowing and telling their own stories.

There are still more subtle means of complimenting in therapeutic discourse. Berg and Dolan (2001) describe the many ways in which therapists' positive perceptions of clients "slip out":

> . . . raising an eyebrow, opening your eyes wide, or leaning forward to get more information all convey to the client that you admire his or her courage, fortitude, and impressive accomplishments. Since this kind of exchange of information is inevitable, why not use it deliberately, more thoughtfully, and to the benefit of the client? (p. 81)

MESSAGES: THERAPIST-TO-CLIENT FEEDBACK

I try to include a feedback component even in very brief helping conversations that may occur in relatively casual contexts, such as in the hallway, lounge, or kitchen area of a treatment facility, group home, or shelter. I usually do the same in telephone calls. (Because I sometimes travel for teaching work, I occasionally arrange brief telephone sessions with clients or supervisees when I am unavailable to meet with them.) I might say, for example, "Just let me think about all this for a minute, and see if there are any thoughts that I want to leave with you."

In my therapy office, I explain either in the first telephone call or early in the first session that I will be taking a short break and then providing feedback. There are several advantages to a routine of pausing (a five- or ten-minute break) and then giving feedback:

1. Knowing that I will have the opportunity to "have my say" at the end of the session helps me to listen more mindfully to clients and to intrude my ideas less. Typically, by the time we get to the end of the session, any "good ideas" I might have thought about have been replaced by the clients' own good ideas, which are much more fitting.
2. Clients listen very carefully to feedback when it is set up in this way. We know also that people tend to remember what they hear at the end of a conversation, the "take-home message."
3. The break gives me a chance to catch my breath and sort out my thoughts, feelings, and impressions. This may be especially needed if I am deciding how to respond to someone who is in a suicidal crisis. On occasions when I need to get information or to consult with a colleague, the break provides an opportunity to do that.
4. Feedback gives us the opportunity to focus on how clients' goals for change can be activated outside the therapy context.

Compliments

The first and most important part of a solution-focused feedback message is compliments. Beginning the feedback with compliments often surprises clients:

Most clients, struggling under the weight of their problems, are not expecting to hear a series of affirmations about what they want and what they are already doing that is useful. . . . More often, they are feeling discouraged about their past choices and prospects for the future. (De Jong & Berg, 2002, p. 118)

Thus, beginning with compliments further helps to get clients' attention.

It is important to be selective in the compliments we give, choosing those which are well grounded in what we know so far about clients, which can be delivered with sincerity, and which are likely to be seen by clients as plausibly related to their goals. For example, I might say:

I am so impressed that you have somehow kept your sense of humor through all this. I always remember my grandmother telling me that humor was a saving grace for us humans, and I believe that. I also believe what they taught me in psychology school: that a sense of humor is a sign of flexibility in a person's thinking, and a very good sign of your ability to find solutions, even to very tough problems.

Bridges to Suggestions

Practitioners learning solution-focused therapy are often puzzled by the idea of the "bridge," the second part of a solution-focused feedback message. The bridge is simply a rationale for the homework suggestion: a statement or perhaps a way of describing the suggestion that makes sense to the client. Often taking care to include the client's language in describing the suggestion is sufficient as a bridge. More explicit bridging statements often begin with such phrases as "I agree with you that . . . " or "Because x [e.g., staying calm, taking care of your children] is so important to you right now . . ."

"Homework" Suggestions

Therapy is about living life rather than a shelter from life. (Kreider, 1998, p. 349)

I refer to the third component of solution-focused feedback as suggestions, or occasionally as "experiments," rather than as homework or tasks or assignments. Our ideas for clients are not intended to be prescriptive. If clients don't do them there is no penalty; we assume that there must be a good reason and that perhaps something else would be a better fit. "The practitioner suggests; the client chooses" (Murphy & Duncan, 1997, p. 43). In general, the more closely we follow clients' ideas about what will make a difference for them, the more likely they are to follow our suggestions and to find them useful. "It is rare for an SFBT therapist to make a suggestion . . . that is not based on the client's previous solutions or exceptions" (de Shazer et al., 2007, p. 5).

Clients can also create their own suggestions or be asked, e.g., "If you were to give yourself a homework assignment this week, what would it be?" (de Shazer et al., 2007, p. 12) or "What is one thing you'd like to take from today's meeting to try out until we meet again?" (Kreider, 1998, p. 350).

Of the suggestions we make, one has been used frequently enough to be called the "solution-focused formula first session task" (de Shazer, 1985, p.137). In its generic form, the suggestion to clients is, "Between now and the next time we meet, notice the things in your life that you want to have continue." Yvonne Dolan describes how this suggestion can form "a bridge across the problem":

> Often in work with people who have had recent and severe trauma there is something about answering the question about what you would like to have continue that for many people provides an ongoing connection to hope, to something under their control. A lot of clients tell me they have written down the things they want to have continue and slept with them under their pillow so that they realize that this terrible thing that happened that is not all there is to their life! (in Malinen, Cooper, & Dolan, 2003, p. 6)

Tasks that, like this one, invite clients to notice exceptions, can be very helpful for those whose thinking has been overwhelmed and constricted by negativity.

Readiness for Change

I have struggled, both in my clinical work and in writing this book, with how (or whether) to include this concept. Earlier versions of so-

Examples of Suggestions for Clients

- Pay attention to the times when you are able to think about the future.
- Observe when the urge to harm yourself is not quite as strong and you are able to overcome it just a little more easily.
- Notice what you say to yourself when you talk yourself out of the idea of suicide as a solution. What arguments do you use?
- Make a list of every time you act on your reasons for living.
- Notice what other people do and say that shows that they value you (Thorana Nelson, personal communication, November 15, 2006).
- You and your husband were able to give me a long list of things that you have done in the past that seemed to make a difference. [Review list.] I suggest that you choose one option from this list and, before you go to sleep tonight, picture yourself doing this and the difference it makes for you, for him, and for the relationship. [Or] I suggest that you choose one option from the list, put it into action, and then discuss with him to evaluate how much difference it makes for each of you.
- I am really impressed with this idea of yours. I suggest that you take the first small step toward implementing it and notice what difference it makes for you.

lution-focused brief therapy (e.g., Berg, 1994) used the rubric of "customership": clients might be (1) *customers* for change, ready to do whatever could make a difference in their problems—so that the therapist's complementary role is as active partner, helping them investigate solutions; (2) *complainants,* wanting change but neither taking active responsibility nor believing that they have the power to initiate change—so the therapist's part is to listen respectfully and inquire what is possible *within the clients' frame of reference;* or (3) *visitors,* seeing no need for change, often puzzled about what they were doing in a treatment session at all—so that the therapist is more in the position of a host, making clients comfortable and inquiring about their needs (Thorana Nelson, personal communication, November 15, 2006).

The problem with this approach is that, although presented as an aspect of therapeutic *relationship,* the customer-complainant-visitor language lent itself to assessing and labeling the client. As such, it could limit rather than expand therapeutic possibilities. Prochaska and colleagues have developed a "stages of change" model (Prochaska, 1999; Prochaska, DiClemente, & Norcross, 1992) that has been broadly applied and is often understood as an assessment of "motivation" (Sharry, Madden, & Darmody, 2003). Sharry and colleagues see the model as linked to the customership approach, with the "precontemplation" stage equivalent to a "visitor" relationship; the "contemplation" stage equivalent to "complainant"; and the "preparation-action-maintenance-termination" stages as equivalent to "customer." Applying these stages also involves assessing and labeling the client, but at least in a stage model there is an explicit expectation of change. Indeed, much of the explication of Prochaska's model deals with therapeutic facilitation of such change.

I discuss this here because I think that the "readiness for change" construct can be useful in helping therapists to stay on track with clients. There is particular application in making homework assignments or suggestions congruent with the person's readiness for change. When dealing with suicide risk, it is important not to overwhelm clients with suggestions for steps toward change that seem to them to be more than they can handle, perhaps inadvertently confirming a belief that they are helpless. So when clients seem to be less ready for change, less arduous tasks, such as observation of exceptions, may be a better "fit." Conversely, when clients are more ready for change, it is important to seize the moment and make suggestions for more active tasks that may move them closer to alternative solutions (and away from suicide as a solution).

I find it most helpful to access readiness for change (or "motivation") primarily through a direct question to the client: "On a scale from 1 to 10, if 10 stands for 'I would do anything to solve this problem' and 1 stands for 'I wouldn't lift a finger,' where are you?"

It is important to acknowledge that the person may be too exhausted, discouraged, or afraid to take strong action. At the same time, this is another of those questions to which the answers are often a surprise: sometimes someone who is actively planning suicide and has been caught in pain and hopelessness for a long time is a "10": "What have I got to lose?" This is a moment when a crisis becomes an opportunity for change.

SAFETY PLANNING

The central theme of a solution-focused [suicide] assessment is that extensive and persistent interest is shown in the indicators of safety and constructive ways of living. (George, Iveson, & Ratner, undated training handout, cited in Callcott, 2003, p. 75)

The SFBT therapist does his or her best to use the client's ideas and vision to maintain safety. . . . Therapists need to think in terms of developing a detailed safety plan that fits the client's experience and life realities. (de Shazer et al., 2007, pp. 157-158)

When clients are treated with respect, given hope, and supported to develop their own criteria for success, they can bring safety home (either together or individually) and include it as a valued member of the family. (Johnson & Goldman, 1996, p. 194)

With disclosures of suicidal intent: Whenever possible, suspend all assumptions about the meaning of the client's words or the action to be taken until later in the session. (Hawkes, Marsh, & Wilgosh, 1998, p. 98)

I have deliberately situated this discussion of safety planning toward the end of this chapter. When suicide first comes up in a therapy session—typically in the first few minutes—I acknowledge this disclosure as an indication of how terrible things seem for the client right now and I continue to ask solution-focused questions. I do not drop the therapeutic conversation in favor of a prescribed risk assessment and management protocol. I shift to active planning for client safety only toward the end of the session, if no alternative pathways open up in the conversation, and if clients continue to indicate, through answers to questions and in other ways, that suicide remains their immediate problem-solving option of choice. (As mentioned earlier, almost always, the necessary risk assessment information will emerge in the course of a "regular" solution-focused therapy conversation. Whatever questions I still need to ask I can ask later in the session.)

In practice, it is extremely rare for me to need to move from a solution focused therapeutic position to an active rescuing stance. Even if therapist-initiated rescue were necessary, I would attempt, if possible, to engage the client's cooperation and I would try to incorporate some of the client's preferences, resources, relationships, and goals. One way of doing this is to continue to offer some choices, however limited those choices may in practice become, for example, "Shall I call the security guard to help us get to the Emergency Department, or will you agree to walk there with me?" or "Do you want to let your mother/husband/boss know that you are going to the hospital or would you prefer that I do it?"

Idiosyncratic safety plans that require clients to work on what they want to achieve using their own personal and relationship resources are always preferable to plans we devise for them. Positive ideas and plans for moving forward on personally meaningful goals are inconsistent with suicide and subvert the suicidal process.

Getting to a relevant safety plan often requires persistence with key questions. For example, Insoo Kim Berg interviewed a teenaged boy, Carl, following his suicide attempt the night before (Berg, 2004; de Shazer et al., 2007). Carl described the frustration and despair triggered by interactions with an older brother who was newly released from prison and sharing Carl's room. Having established that the brother's aggressive, taunting behavior was unlikely to improve, Insoo asked, "So what do you need to do differently so that it doesn't happen again like last night?" She asked that same question, with minor variations, four more times, each time after listening carefully to the answer he gave. It is not uncommon for clients to respond to solution-finding questions as Carl did, with problem-focused talk. Clients see obstacles to solutions. It is important that both the client and the therapist be aware of such obstacles, of how hard it is to surmount problems, both in one's perception and in the real world outside the therapy room. It is equally important that solution building not be derailed by the obstacles.

In her conversation with Carl, Insoo utilizes the information Carl gives her to augment the safety plan, inquiring in detail about concrete steps for overcoming the obstacles he has cited. For example, they developed a list of indicators (heart pounding, head hurting, the wrong words coming out of his mouth) that would tell him he needed to avoid a particular situation and viable plans for what he would do and where he would go instead of staying in a situation that could trigger dangerous reactions.

A Note on No-Suicide Contracting

No-harm or *no-suicide* contracts (e.g., Drye, Goulding, & Goulding, 1973) have become part of standard and expected practice in suicide assessment and treatment, despite lack of evidence for their efficacy and the potential limitations (Center for Suicide Prevention, 2002; Miller, 1999; Reid, 1998; Rudd, 2006; Rudd, Mandrusiak, & Joiner, 2006; Stanford, Goetz, & Bloom, 1994). I see potential value for a conversation similar to what Rudd (2006; Rudd, Mandrusiak, & Joiner, 2006) describes as a *commitment to treatment* or *commitment to living*. Such interactions have most value for the client when they serve as a structure or scaffolding for a therapeutic conversation rather than as an end in themselves ("Sign here").

EVALUATIONS: CLIENT-TO-THERAPIST FEEDBACK

If practitioners are using formal evaluation methods, such as the SRS (Johnson, Miller, & Duncan, 2000) and/or the OQ-45 (Lambert et al., 1996), then the therapist's break is a natural time for the client to complete the forms.

More informal evaluation can occur at any time but generally makes most sense near the end of the session, either before or after the feedback. My own bias is to ask such questions after the feedback, since feedback is an important part of the session.

CONTINUING: A FOCUS ON PROGRESS AND CHANGE

The EARS paradigm describes a solution-focused approach to second and subsequent treatment sessions: Elicit, Amplify, and Reinforce any indicators of change or progress—and then Start over and look for more progress. EARS has particular application when there is risk for suicide. First, asking about the details and effects of even small changes reinforces the message that change is expected. Second, any conversation about real positive change is hope inducing and can make the client more open to thinking about possibilities when the conversation shifts again to problems and struggles. Third, if there is no observable change, then the therapist and client can dis-

Examples of Evaluation Questions

On a scale from 1 to 10, where 1 stands for "I might kill myself in the next twenty-four hours," and 10 stands for "I will definitely choose to be alive twenty-four hours from now," where were you at the beginning of this session? Where are you now? [If numbers are different]

- What made a difference?
- What else?
- What could help you to move up another half point on the scale?

On a scale from 1 to 10, if 10 stands for as helpful as it could be, and 1 stands for not helpful at all, how helpful was this session? [If greater than 1]

- What tells you that it was helpful? What else?
- How could it have been more helpful?
- What was the most useful thing about this conversation for you?
- What was the least useful thing? How could that be improved?
- What do you see right now that says to you that this was a useful thing for you to do?
- What should we keep doing next time? What should we change?
- What surprised you about this session?

cuss what needs to happen differently. Where suicide is a possibility, there is no room for false security just because the person is "in therapy." It is essential that therapy produce change—change that is significant to the client.

Consolidating and Maintaining Positive Change

Sustainability is an important consideration in therapeutic change. Facilitating, observing, and celebrating change is not enough; we must take steps to see that changes achieved can persist.

Change can be consolidated in a number of ways: by compliments and "cheerleading"; through questions about difference; by facilitating an appreciative "audience" for change; and by utilizing concrete reminders of change and progress.

Examples of Consolidation Questions

- How will these changes make what you have to do now easier?
- Whom would you like to share this change with?
- How would this situation have affected you if it had happened six months ago? And now? (adapted from Kreider, 1998, p. 351)
- What are you going to do to recognize this step forward?
- What have you been doing to get yourself on the right track?

Concrete Reminders

Especially when clients are subject to states of extreme distress and perturbation, I like to write down some of my feedback for them to take away with them. Compliments are the most important aspect. People in distress may find it hard to retain verbal information and harder still to focus on anything positive, and notes or other symbols may act as useful reminders of our positive opinions.

Examples of Maintenance Questions

- How will you continue to stay safe?
- When you have a bad day, what have you figured out that will be helpful?
- How will you apply these strategies? How will you remember?
- When you notice signs like these again, how do you plan to respond differently?
- How do you know that this will be effective?

TERMINATION

The essential criterion for duration in SFBT is however many sessions are required for clients to achieve workable, satisfying solutions (in their terms)—and not one more (de Shazer, 1991a; de Shazer et al., 2007). There is no time limit, and brevity is not the goal; solution-focused therapy is usually brief as an artifact of its process. Solution-focused methods will not, however, guarantee that therapeutic change will always occur in a brief amount of time. They simply help to find a difference that makes a difference; this tends to make therapy briefer by effectively using whatever time we have with any given individual. (Kreider, 1998, p. 355)

Therapeutic habits of orienting toward goals, progress and difference shape clients' expectation of treatment as a temporary, change-focused process. In this context, termination is more likely to be seen as "a graduation rather than a rejection" (Kreider, 1998). Sometimes the decision to terminate happens quite naturally and spontaneously as clients notice their own progress on goals and feel more confident. The processes of goal consolidation and maintenance described earlier are helpful both in facilitating such client decisions and in responding to them. Questions that help clients to notice or increase their readiness for termination may also be helpful.

Examples of Readiness for Termination Questions

- "What will be a small sign that you are one step closer to being ready to come in less frequently?" (Kreider, 1998, p. 355)
- "If 1 is when the problem was at its worst and 10 is where you'll be when you feel confident handling it (at least most of the time), where are you at today?" (Kreider, 1998, p. 352)
- What signs have you seen already that you are becoming more confident in handling this? What signs will tell you that you are continuing to get more confident?
- "Since most things in life aren't perfect, how close to 10 would you have to get to feel that you have accomplished enough for this round of therapy?" (Kreider, 1998, p. 352)
- What is one thing we could do in this session today that would help you to be a half step closer [to "enough"]?
- What is one thing that you could do between now and our next session that would help you to be a half step closer?

PUTTING IT ALL TOGETHER:
THOUGHTS ON "FLOW"

Take time for all things: Great haste makes great waste. (Benjamin Franklin, in Eisen, 1995, p. 320)

An essential part of "listening with questions," which is one way to describe counseling, is that each question is somehow based on the previous answer. In solution-focused therapy, another essential part is to ask questions to which the answer is in some way affirming to the client. (Iveson, 2002 p. 70)

Because there is no universal "script" for a solution-focused interview, therapists are required to adapt and adjust constantly. This may mean that we fumble for the most useful words and questions and that we have to tinker with and sometimes correct our verbal constructions. I remember my colleague Lance Taylor saying to a client, "I asked you the wrong question! Let me try again" (Taylor, Gallagher, Campbell, Nelson, & Fiske, 2005).

Effective timing and pacing in therapeutic conversations come from practice and observation and refinement of one's practice based on interaction with individual clients in a continuing feedback loop.

EXAMPLES OF POSSIBLE QUESTION SEQUENCES

I present these "possible question sequences" very tentatively. Although based on typical questions I might use, they are artificial constructs, not scripts for a solution-focused suicide interview. They are very bad examples of solution-focused practice because they omit (except perhaps by inference) the voice of the client. I include them because I have found that students and practitioners find such examples useful. I think that one might review these questions, or the case transcripts elsewhere in this book, in the way that I sometimes browse recipe books—and then set them aside—before cooking: to inform or color or "tune up" my approach to the ingredients in my own kitchen. Those ingredients may be similar to those in the books but will also have critical differences, just as my style, talents, and interests as a cook differ from the cookbook writer's. The differences are magnified and complicated by the fact that in solution-focused cuisine we are always working with another cook—indeed, a master chef.

Possible Question Sequence: Example 1

1. What could your best friend say that would be helpful to you?
2. How would that make a difference?

3. When you are still alive, what will you be doing?
4. How can that be useful to you?
5. How will you know that it was a good idea to live?
6. What else?
7. How have you been coping so far?
8. What else has helped you to cope?
9. What else?
10. How did you figure that out?
11. Suppose that tonight, while you are sleeping, a miracle happened and these problems that have brought you here today were solved. But, because you are sleeping, you don't know that this miracle has happened. Tomorrow morning, after you wake up, what is the first thing you will notice that will tell you something has changed?
12. How will that make a difference?
13. What else? What else? What else? How will that make a difference?
14. Who in your life would be first to notice that something was different for you?
15. What will that person notice?
16. What else?
17. What difference will seeing that change in you make for that person?
18. What will you do in response to that person's reaction?
19. How will this change your relationship?
20. On a scale from 1 to 10, if 10 stands for the day after that miracle, and 1 stands for the worst things have been for you,* where are you right now?
21. Where were you before you made the decision to come talk to me?
22. What did you do to go from 2 to 3?
23. Where do you have to be on that scale to know that you are going forward on the right track for you?
24. What is the first small step you can take in that direction?
25. What will you notice to be different when you take that step?
26. How will doing this help you to stay alive?

---

*I would not always use the "worst case" as the anchor for 1 on the scale, but in this instance, where the conversation seems to be overtly about living versus dying, I might want to suggest that the person has already survived "the worst."

27. What else needs to happen between now and when we meet again to help you keep living?
28. Who in your life will want to help with this plan? How can that person make a difference? Shall I call or do you want to make the call?
29. On a scale from 1 to 10, if 10 stands for focusing on staying alive, and 1 stands for focusing on being dead, where are you right now?
30. What do we need to do to keep that number at 6? To increase it by one-half point?

Possible Question Sequence: Example 2

1. What are your best hopes for this meeting?
2. Has it been so bad that you have thought about suicide?
3. How far have you gone with those thoughts?
4. How have you kept from acting on those plans?
5. Suppose that you did still have just one or two small hopes left. What might they be?
6. When you are feeling less pain than you do now, what else will be different?
7. What else? What difference will that make for you?
8. Suppose that tonight, while you are sleeping, a miracle happened and these problems that have brought you here today were solved. But, because you are sleeping, you don't know that this miracle has happened. Tomorrow morning, after you wake up, what is the first thing you will notice that will tell you something has changed?
9. What will you be feeling instead of constant pain and fear? How will that make a difference for you? What will you be able to do that you are not doing now?
10. How will that make a difference for you?
11. How will that make a difference for your family? For the shelter staff?
12. When was the most recent time that you experienced even a small part of that "miracle picture"? What does that tell you?
13. On a scale from 1 to 10, if 1 stands for how things were when you decided to get help, and 10 stands for the miracle picture, where are you right now?

14. How is it that you are a 2 and not a 1?
15. Where do you want to be on that same scale?
16. On a different scale from 1 to 10, if 10 stands for completely confident that I can move in a better direction, and 1 stands for no hope at all, where are you?
17. What gives you that much hope?
18. Who else is hopeful for you?
19. Who might be silently hopeful, without saying a word?
20. Is your dog male or female? What is her name? Do you have a picture of her? What tells you that she is hopeful for you? What difference will it make for her if you begin to feel better? How will she show it? What else? What will you do then?
21. What is one small thing that you could do that would make it more likely for Mitzy to act in that way?

CONCLUSION: VOICE OF EXPERIENCE

Slowly I began to come up again, as one does from a dive in deep water. I gradually stopped wondering, What life do I have? and began to consider, What life can I build? Is there a way to be useful, maybe to other people in my predicament? Is there a way to be creative again? A way to get back to work? Most of all, is there a way to be a husband and father again? No answers came, but raising the questions helped. (Christopher Reeve, 1998, p. 51, on finding reasons for living as a quadriplegic)

PART II:
APPLICATIONS

Chapter 3

Three Conversations About Dying and Living

All answers are leading answers. (Dan Gallagher, in Miller, Gessner, & Korman, 2006)

TALKING WITH GEORGE

The following transcribed session was my first meeting with George. George was forty-eight years old and worked as a technical consultant, designing and managing computer systems. I heard about George when I answered an urgent telephone message from his wife Penny, who had come home unexpectedly from work in the middle of the day to find George in the basement taping a suicide message for her and their son. He had a gun and ammunition and had planned to kill himself that day. She had already asked that he surrender the gun to her and he had done so. I was calling from an airport in another city and walked Penny through the process of getting George some immediate help. In the end she offered him the option of going to the hospital emergency room immediately with her or being taken there by police, and he agreed to go with her. I contacted the hospital to let the crisis intervention team know to expect him and to ask them to let me know that he arrived.

In a subsequent telephone conversation with Penny, I learned that George had been involuntarily committed to the hospital for seventy-two hours of observation because he was found to be a threat to his own safety. Penny told me that George had no siblings or close friends and that his mother, who had been his principal confidante throughout his life, had died two years before. His father had died by suicide when George was nine. For the past six months, George had been leaving home and work and disappearing for periods of a few hours to a few days. Penny had recently discovered that he was gambling heavily and had wiped out their savings and gone into debt. In her anger and frustration she had for the first time threatened divorce.

George declined hospital follow-up after the three-day admission but agreed under pressure from his wife and family doctor to take the prescribed medication and to make an appointment with me at my private practice.

George, a massive, deep-voiced man, was very sloppily dressed, unshaven, and with lank, shoulder-length hair. He began our first meeting slouched in his chair, half turned away from me, looking at the wall.

George, Session 1

[*The excerpt begins a few minutes into the session.*]
HF: So, what brings you here today, George?
G: [*Smiles*] My wife and my doctor thought I should come.
HF: Ah. And you?
G: I'm the bad boy. I don't know anything.
HF: Nothing at all?
G: . . . I know something's gotta give.
HF: Something's gotta give?
G: [*Laughs, shakes his head*] Can't go on the way it is.
HF: How is that?
G: Didn't she tell you?
HF: You mean your wife?
G: Yeah.
HF: She told me some things. I want to hear from you how you see it.
G: Oh, she's right about everything.
HF: Like what?
G: I keep taking off.
HF: And is that a problem for you or just for her?
G: It's a problem for a lot of people.
HF: For you?

G: Not when I do it, just after.

HF: How is it a problem for you then?

G: She gets mad.

HF: And how is that a problem for you?

G: I hate it. . . . I feel like a bad person.

HF: So . . . what are you going to do about that?

G: [*Looks at HF, looks away*] Aren't you supposed to tell me?

HF: Pretty presumptuous, don't you think?

G: Yeah. I do.

HF: So what is your plan?

G: I had a plan, but she stopped me.

HF: A plan?

G: To kill myself.

HF: Ah. How did you allow her to stop you?

G: [*Shrugs*] She cried. It was easier to promise.

HF: So you promised her you wouldn't kill yourself?

G: Yeah.

HF: So, what are you going to do?

G: Stay alive, I guess. I haven't broken a promise . . . yet.

HF: Not everyone can say that they haven't broken a promise.

G: I don't make many promises.

HF: So . . . the promise meant something to you as well as to her.

G: At the time.

HF: How is a promise important to you?

G: I won't promise her not to take off.

HF: You won't.

G: Can't be sure I could keep it. And when I take off . . . anything can happen. Promises . . . [*Waves his hand*]

HF: Taking off is something that has some control over you?

G: Yeah.

HF: And you're not sure how much control you have over it?

G: Right.

HF: When have you been able to show some control over taking off?

G: [*Laughs*] Good question. . . . Only time I know was my kid's birthday.

HF: What was different about your kid's birthday?

G: I didn't take off.

HF: Even though the urge was there, somehow you fought back.

G: . . . I guess so.

HF: How did you do that?

G: . . . I'm not a good father.

HF: And that helped you?

G: No, but I wanted to do at least that much.

HF: [*Nodding*] To show up for his birthday.

G: [*Nodding*] Yeah.

HF: So . . . even though you don't think of yourself as a good father, you still want to do what you can do as a father for your son.

G: Yeah. Of course I do.

HF: Being a father to your son is important to you.

G: Yeah. Not that I'm much good to him.

H: But a father means something to a son, nonetheless.

G: I guess so. . . . [*Strongly*] *He's a good kid.*

HF: Tell me about him. What's his name?

G: Alex. [*Smiles, straightens in chair, voice softens*] He just turned eight. Not very big for his age, but fast, loves to play ball, loves to ride his bike. Likes me to come with him.

HF: Likes you to come with him!

G: [*Smiling, nodding*] Yeah. We went to the park yesterday . . .

Time Out

Reviewing one's old tapes and case transcripts is not a comfortable activity.

There are many things that I wish I had done differently in this conversation. I wish that I had started differently. (What could make coming to this session worthwhile for you?) I *really* wish that I had asked about presession change. (What is different since you decided to give the gun to your wife?) I wish that I had picked up on how he didn't want to feel like a bad person and asked about the kind of person he did want to be. I wish that I had used the language of him promising to stay alive instead of the language of him promising not to kill himself. I wish that I hadn't started a sentence with "but" because *but*-ing people can create an argumentative framework and their natural reaction is often to argue back. I wish, I wish.

If you are wondering why I included this transcript at all, one reason is that all of the people I talk about in this chapter taught me a great deal about the value of a solution-focused approach in helping someone who is grappling with suicide as a problem-solving option. Also, they are individuals on whom I can offer some follow-up information—more of the story. And because I like to see that, in spite of my ineptness, there is resiliency both in the client and in the process. George himself went beyond not killing himself and introduced the idea of staying alive. (These are different ideas, with different possibilities attached.) I did some useful things too: I managed to stick to my position of not knowing what was right for him, and to look for differences that might make a difference. And despite my "but," George went along with the idea that a father means something to a son, an idea that helped us to focus on the most important therapeutic factor in the room with us so far: Alex.

I hope that the transcript adequately reflects the noticeable change in George's demeanor and volubility when we started to talk about his son. We spent several minutes talking about the real and simple pleasure of their time in the park, and George contrasted it with the absence of joint activities and "bonding things" with his own father when he was a child, and voiced a desire to do better with Alex. To me, this clear statement about something that George wanted was a sign that it was time to ask the miracle question.

HF: George, I want to ask you this kind of strange question.

G: Stranger than the ones you've asked so far? [*Slight smile*]

HF: Maybe. You decide.

Suppose that, after we finish this conversation we're having, you leave here and carry on with the rest of your evening. Eventually you go to sleep and it happens that tonight you have a very deep, restful sleep, and while you're sleeping, a miracle happens. . . .

And the miracle is that this problem that has brought you here today . . . is solved [*snaps fingers*] just like that; it's a miracle. . . .

But, because you're sleeping, you don't know that this miracle has happened. So, tomorrow morning, when you wake up, what will be different that will tell you that this miracle has happened?

G: There's a Rolls Royce in the driveway.

HF: Great! What else?

G: . . . Maybe I don't feel so angry and on the edge.

HF: Okay, so what will you be feeling instead of that?

G: I'll be Mister Rogers.

HF: Oh dear, I never watched Mister Rogers, so can you explain to me what it would mean to be more like him?

G: You never watched Mister Rogers?

HF: No, sorry.

G: Well he was just this nice guy, to everybody. Wore sweaters. People knew they could trust him.

HF: Okay, thanks. A nice guy that people can trust.

G: They *know* they can trust him. You really never saw him?

HF: I don't think so. So, people in your life will know that they can trust you.

G: I need to regain Penny's trust.

HF: How will it be different for you when you have regained her trust?

G: . . . A lot better.

HF: In what ways?

G: I'll feel more comfortable with her, more at ease.

HF: What will you be doing when you are more comfortable, more at ease?

G: We'll be making each other laugh.

HF: Making each other laugh. That sounds good.

G: Yeah, we used to laugh a lot.

HF: Laughing together. What else?

G: We used to do things together.

HF: So, after this miracle, you'll be doing things together again?

G: Yeah.

HF: What else?

G: I'll be able to talk to her.

HF: You'll be able to talk to her.

G: Yeah. I need better "intimacy skills." [*makes quotation marks with fingers*]

HF: Okay. What difference will it make when you have better intimacy skills?

G: Penny will be happier.

HF: And that would make a difference for you, for Penny to be happier?

G: Yeah, sure. She deserves it.

HF: You think highly of her.

G: She's an amazing mother.

HF: And that's important.

G: Yeah, Alex comes first.

HF: Alex comes first—with Penny, or you, or both of you?

G: Both of us. But she's better at it. I just do my thirty percent.

HF: The two of you agree on him coming first.

G: Yeah, I guess we do.

HF: And you do your thirty percent.

G: Should be more.

HF: What percent would you want it to be for you guys?

G: I think it should be at least fifty percent. I mean, he's not a baby anymore, and lots of fathers spend a lot of time doing stuff with kids his age.

HF: So you'd like it to be more than thirty percent.

G: Yeah, should be fifty.

HF: Sounds like you've been doing some observing, noticing other fathers who spend time with their kids too.

G: Yeah. And we need more things we can do together.

HF: More things you and Alex can do together?

G: Sure, but I meant all three of us.

HF: Oh, so that's something else that you'd like to see more—more time together for the three of you.

G: I thought it would be good, but what do I know?

HF: Well, you know Penny, and you know Alex, and you know how you want things to go between you.

G: Yeah.

HF: What difference will it make when the three of you are doing more things together?

G: Penny will see that I am more responsible.

HF: How will that help, for Penny to see that you are more responsible?

G: . . . Maybe I'll really be more responsible. [*looks at HF directly*]

HF: What will that look like?

G: Maybe I'll be able to conquer my wild side.

HF: Conquer your wild side.

G: Get some control anyway.

HF: That's something you want, more control than now.

G: Yeah.

We went on to talk about what more control would entail (he said focusing more on his family), and about what Alex would see to be different after the miracle. I asked about the most recent time when he experienced some part of the miracle picture, and he went back to the previous day in the park with Alex.

HF: On a scale from one to ten, if ten stands for the day after that miracle, all the things we talked about on that day, and one stands for the day when you thought death was the only option you had, where are you right now?

G: Two point five.

HF: And where do you want to be on that scale, to say, things are definitely on that miracle-day track, on the right track?

G: Seven.

HF: How is it that you are up to two point five?

G: I don't know. We took a nice drive on Sunday

H: The three of you?

G: Yeah. Want to do that again.

HF: Great. That's a very good plan. What else?

G: Well, Penny was willing to come to the hospital with me and everything. It helped.

H: That made a difference, her willingness.

G: Yeah.

HF: What did that tell you? That she was willing to do that?

G: We're not divorced yet.

HF: You're still together, so things could go in a better direction.

G: Maybe. Yeah.

HF: What would it take to get you up to a three? Just a three, from two point five to three?

G: A good day at the office.

HF: What's a good day?

G: Start something, finish something. Job pride.

HF: I see. Start something, finish something, that would feel good, sense of pride in the job.

G: Sure. If I could go a week without disappearing I'd get up to a four.

HF: Wow! Conquer the wild side for that long.

G: Yeah. Lately I only last four to five days max.

HF: How do you control it for that long?

G: One day at a time.

We spoke a little more about what made for a better day, and then I took a break and gave him feedback. I complimented him on how clearly and openly he spoke with me, and how this boded well for his goal of being able to talk more with Penny; on his courage to do something different; on his love for and commitment to Penny and Alex, which was the foundation for any meaningful intimacy skills; and on the usefulness of his practical ideas for improving his life. I suggested that George begin by following through with specific family activities and plans he had already mentioned. I also suggested that, since he had already been making useful observations, he continue this by noticing what Penny and Alex did or said when he spent time with them that told him how being with him was valuable for each of them; and we booked another appointment.

I did not make a "no suicide" contract with George, in part because I felt that his promise to Penny was far more important than any agreement he could make with me. I knew that problem gambling was a risk factor for suicidal behavior (Pfuhlmann & Schmidtke, 2002), although the basis for the relationship may be a common association with mental illness (Newman & Thompson, 2003). I also knew that Alex was a big, bright, shining reason for living for George, and I saw my task as reinforcing and supporting that priority. I saw George as actively engaged in a positive safety plan of his own that involved working on goals of spending more time with his family and developing better skills for being with them. I was struck by how relevant progress on these goals would be helpful both for strengthening his reasons for living and also for his goal of conquering his "wild side."

George: More of the Story

I saw George eight times. He told me in our second session that he thought it would probably make sense for Penny to come with him to see me sometime, but that he wasn't ready for that and that he would let me know when he was. (He hasn't yet.) He discussed his gambling only in oblique terms ("running away" or "the wild side"). I gave him some information about available help for problem gambling; he thanked me and said he wasn't ready to talk about that yet (or still). He did provide me with a 1-to-10 scale rating and a brief scorecard report on running away at the beginning of each session, e.g., in the second session, "I'm a four, no running away this week." He did run away once more, between our second and third meetings, and returned home a few hours later, having driven to the casino but not gone inside. Moreover, he understood this event as the victory it was, both in controlling his "wild side" for his own good reasons and in his ability to tell Penny about it when he got home. He told me in our third session that suicide was not an option for him anymore because he had made a commitment to himself as well as to Penny: "If it's really for me too, then I'm in control."

Week by week his parental contribution increased: 32, 33, 33.5, 38 percent! He also spent time regularly with both Alex and Penny, and the three of them started a weekly dinner-and-a-movie ritual, an idea George had heard about from a co-worker. George decided that one of the things that he needed in his life was hobbies or, as he put it, "ways to run away without leaving." He had no idea what would appeal to him, so he began a methodical process of testing out various possibilities. He ended up "keeping" reading, photography, and tae kwon do. He explained to me that these were all activities that had a start and a finish, and in which you could feel pride.

George's family doctor works in the clinic where I have my private practice. I saw George in the waiting room there about two years ago (ten years after our last meeting), with a big handsome young man in a university sweatshirt. George smiled and introduced me to Alex.

TALKING WITH LAURA

Laura was seventeen and had been living with her thirty-five-year-old boyfriend since leaving home and dropping out of school the year before. Laura had been sexually abused and had been previously diagnosed with multiple personality disorder (aka dissociative identity disorder). She had also lived through a major depression from age thirteen to age fourteen, and during that time, she had made two suicide attempts, the second of very high lethality. Her relationship with her previous therapist, a colleague of mine, had been positive. Laura had actually tried to contact Dr. Smith and, when told that Dr. Smith had left the clinic, remembered being given my name as a backup, and then asked for me.

When we met, Laura was struggling with two major current stressors: (1) an impending court case against one of her abusers and (2) her increasing dissatisfaction with her relationship. Her desire to leave her boyfriend was complicated by the realities that she lived with him and worked in his business. Her family home was not a safe place for her to go.

Laura, Session 1

HF: How can I be helpful?

L: I'm getting depressed. I went through it before two years ago, and it was awful. It lasted almost two years. I know the signs; it's getting worse.

HF: What have you noticed?

L: [*Sighs*] Can't sleep, when I do I wake up really early in the morning and feel awful. Don't want to eat, don't want to do anything, feel like crying when I feel anything. *Everything looks like shit to me.*

HF: Hmmm. Has it been so bad that you have thought about suicide?

L: Yes. Not so that I would do anything—not yet—but I've been thinking about it, and I *like* the idea. I never wanted to feel like that again.

HF: You really don't like thinking that way.

L: No. It means the depression is getting even worse, and I just can't live through that again. Anything would be better than that. Dying would be better than that.

HF: It's that bad—that dying looks like a better option?

L: Not all the time—not yet. But I know how this goes. Drugs don't work for me and I *can't* go through another two years like that.

HF: So, how did you overcome it last time?

L: I don't know. . . . Dr. Smith was nice and she cared about me—that was good—but I don't know if therapy can really make a difference.

HF: What have you learned from that past experience of living through depression that could help you overcome it this time?

L: I don't know.

HF: [*Waits*]

L: That's a hard question.

HF: Yes, it is. Take your time.

L: . . . All I did for the worst part of it was to lie on the couch and sleep and read horror novels.

HF: How did that help?

L: I don't know.

HF: [*Waits*]

L: Well [*long pause*] the only time I was ever really safe was when I was reading. [*Head down*] I could never go ahead and kill myself before I knew how the story ended.

HF: That makes sense to me. How can that help you now?

L: [*Small smile, shrug*] I don't know. Stephen King hasn't written that many books, and I'm a fast reader.

HF: Right. So, how *can* this knowledge help?

L: [*Looks at HF, shakes head, shrugs, waits*]

H: [*Waits*]

L: Well, I think maybe what I need to do is to *write* a horror novel. I've often thought about it.

HF: Oh! Write one of your own. How will that help?

L: I won't be able to kill myself before I see how the story turns out. It should take longer to write one than to read one—and I guess it would keep me busy in the meantime until something else changes. . . . I have ideas already.

HF: Already! Wow. . . . How does coming up with this plan make a difference for you?

Reflecting on My First Conversation with Laura

Laura presented with many risk factors: her history of past attempts, childhood sexual abuse, lack of family support, relative social isolation except for the boyfriend, court involvement, diagnoses of depression and multiple personality disorder and current suicidal ideation. However, the picture at this point was one of serious (and increasing) risk rather than of imminent danger (see Appendix C).

There was also ample evidence of Laura's resources and reasons for living. She was intelligent, verbal, candid with me, and highly motivated: after all, she had sought help on her own and persisted even when she found that her previous trusted therapist was gone. Such determination is unusual for anyone, much less a seventeen-year-old functioning on her own. Laura had learned from her past negative experience and was proactive in her attempts to prevent a recurrence. At seventeen, she already had a history of making a comeback. Despite her overt pessimism about therapy, she remembered that Dr. Smith had cared about her. And in spite of considerable distress and pressure, she had not dissociated, even though dissociation had at one time been her primary method of coping with life. She used both reading and writing as coping strategies, and there was considerable flexibility in her thinking. Wanting to see how the story turned out was for her an important reason for living—one that had already helped her to survive a very dark time in her life.

(Many years later, I was reminded of Laura when I listened to Marsha Linehan's acceptance speech on receiving the Dublin Award from the American Association of Suicidology [Linehan, 1999a]. As she described her own struggles with suicidal thinking in adolescence, Linehan said with evident emotion that the only thing that kept her alive was wanting to see how *her* story would turn out.)

Imagine if you will, the reaction among my professional colleagues or the hospital administrators if I suggested that a good suicide prevention plan for a depressed seventeen-year-old girl with a history of abuse would be for her to write a horror novel. (Horrors!) And yet, for Laura, at that moment in her life, that solution was more uniquely suited than anything that I could possibly have offered. I have told Laura's story many times (e.g., Fiske, 1995, 1998a) because she taught me in such a memorable way to trust that the client truly knows what he or she needs, a lesson confirmed for me over and over since then. Of course, Laura's write-a-horror-novel solution makes an unusually good story, unlike many of the more apparently mundane solutions that clients find. Also, while those moments of waiting for her to answer my questions seemed very long to me at the time, she was actually able to focus on a workable solution with remarkable speed. However, my conversation with Laura was in certain ways absolutely typical of solution-focused work: when I maintained a not-knowing position, focused on what had worked for her before, and continued to ask what she could do now, she came up with something—something that was relevant, salient, and important in her own terms.

Laura's Story: Further Chapters

At our next session, Laura told me that she had already written two chapters(!), and that she was stuck. Something terrible was about to happen to her young female protagonist, and Laura could not write about it until she had sorted out some things in her own life. So we began sorting. We sorted how she could go to court without being debilitated by flashbacks, and we sorted plans for her to get a new job and a new place to live, and soon after she sorted plans to go back to school as well. I saw Laura once a month for a year (her frequency of choice), and in that time she went through a great deal, with her characteristic focus and resourcefulness, and without ever taking the irrevocable slide into depression that she had feared.

I have a little more to tell about Laura because she experienced anxiety and sleep disruption during her first pregnancy eight years later and came back to see me. She had already researched her symptoms, knew what treatments were available, and wanted to try a desensitization approach. My assigned role was to teach her relaxation strategies. So I did that, and she came back a month later, doing much better, and said that she hadn't liked my strategies and so had developed one of her own, a self-guided-imagery exercise based on a long-standing wish. She had always imagined herself as one day living in her own "dream home," and her relaxation strategy involved picturing her arrival at this home, and then a slow, appreciative progression through the rooms, deciding on paint colors and furnishings. Her only complaint was that it worked so well she barely made it to the front door anymore without falling asleep: "The basement is never going to get finished!"

My last meeting with Laura was a few years later. Laura was thirty, busy raising two young children, finishing her bachelor's degree, and still writing—and beginning to publish—her stories. I was called to testify in the last of the long series of criminal and civil court cases against the people who had hurt her when she was a child. I dislike going to court (all that tension!) and I couldn't find a place to park, and I finally came flapping into the building worried about being late and not knowing where exactly I was supposed to go. Laura came up to me as I dithered in front of the elevator, took my arm, and said soothingly, "It's okay, Heather, we have half an hour. Take a deep breath, let it out sloooowly—and let's get a nice cup of tea."

TALKING WITH MARCO

Marco and I met when he was twenty-five and about to leave the city to take a teaching degree. Although as a student he was covered by his parents' extended health insurance, he paid me in cash for the session so that no one in his family would know that we had spoken. Marco had been struggling for years with profound feelings of despair. He had known since his early teens that he was gay and had achieved a level of self-acceptance despite having a minimum of external support and understanding. However, he had not been able to resolve his love and pride for his large, close immigrant family and their vibrant community with his belief that their religious and cultural convictions would never allow them to accept his orientation. Sadly, his beliefs were well-founded: two young men in the community had been rejected by both their own families and Marco's when they came out, and they had been ostracized ever since. Marco's fears had prevented him from connecting with a new, more accepting community, and from developing strong relationships outside his family. Several months before he came to see me, Marco had found a package in his room, with no note, containing pamphlets about "conversion therapy" (i.e., "therapy" with the goal of changing a person's sexual orientation).

Marco had always wanted to be a policeman (an ambition that was unusual in his community and perhaps a disappointment to his parents, who hoped that Marco, with his intelligence and academic achievements, would become a professional). To mollify his family, Marco had completed a bachelor of science degree, but instead of applying to medical school, he had followed his own dream and entered police college. It took only four months there to convince him that being a gay cop, in or out of the closet, was not a path he could take. He left.

When he decided to apply for a teacher's program in another city, it seemed like a chance to develop a life for himself away from his family (and, in my view, a remarkable display of resilience), but now he was overwhelmed at the idea of being alone in a strange place. Being away would also mean leaving behind the three people in his life who knew that he was gay: a woman friend from university, a former teacher, and his family doctor (I was the fourth). The idea of coming out to new people seemed overwhelming. Marco had thought about suicide "off and on" for years and recently had become preoccupied with plans for shooting himself (he had access to a gun owned by an uncle), although "I'm not there yet." I noticed, however, that he was continuing to prepare for university and that he talked about teaching as more than just a consolation-prize career—as a way of life with real satisfactions for him. His miracle picture was very active and detailed and included going for a bike ride, playing with his neighbor's dog, packing for university, finishing a book he had been trying to read in preparation for one of his courses, helping his elderly neighbor with his garden, and talking to his friend on the telephone. When I asked him about how these things would make a difference, he said that it was important for him to do "good life" things, not just sit and think. According to Marco, his thinking tended to become more and more negative, and he was very good at using logic to convince himself that there was no hope. Good-life things shook him out of this, providing immediate, in-his-face evidence that some things were still worthwhile, "even with everything," that he *could* take action.

We talked about how he could plan to make good-life actions part of his life at university, beginning right away in order to ease the transition, and how he could get further help in his new city. Marco left with a list of possibilities and a commitment to do something on his list each day. He left the conversion therapy pamphlets behind. (Because of his logical mind, I also recommended *Choosing to Live,* a cognitive therapy self-help book by Tom Ellis and Cory Newman [1996]. Among other things, the book helps readers understand that negativity can masquerade as "logic" and apply evidence-based logic to finding reasons and plans for living.)

I exchanged e-mail messages with Marco soon after he arrived at university. He had some very difficult days but followed through with the plans we had discussed, and they did seem to help. Two months later, Marco e-mailed to ask if we could arrange a long-distance telephone consultation, as he had a "critical life decision" to make and wanted my input. When we spoke, he told me that he still had emotional ups and downs, although it seemed to be getting a little bit easier, and that he had a dilemma. As part of his commitment to regular good-life actions, he volunteered at the local animal shelter once a week. One of the dogs that he walked was a timid, lab-sized mixed-breed with a traumatic history, Pippa. Pippa had fallen in love with him, and he with Pippa. The shelter staff were thrilled and wanted him to take the dog, and his apartment building was animal-friendly. So what was the dilemma?

M: I love dogs.

HF: Yes, I can tell that you do. And this dog in particular.

M: A dog is not just a . . . a . . . a *possession*. A dog deserves respect.

HF: Yes.

M: And good care.

HF: Okay. Yeah, you have a very responsible attitude—

M: [*Interrupts, sounding a little exasperated*] It's a *commitment,* having a dog.

HF: Right.

M: Especially this dog.

HF: That's right; she's going to need some extra care.

M: *I'd have to be here.*

HF: Ahhhh. *You'd have to be here.* [*I'm finally getting it.*]

M: Yes. Suicide would be impossible. No matter how bad it was. And I just can't decide. I've thought, and thought, and looked at the pros and cons, and I'm stuck, right on the fence. I've gone over it and over it. I haven't slept in two nights. So, please, just tell me what you think.

HF: Okay, let me get this straight. You're giving *me* the tiebreaker vote?

M: . . . I guess. Yes.

HF: Committing to the dog would be a real commitment; you couldn't go back on it.

M: Yes. I don't want to bring her home and then change my mind. That's not fair to her. If she comes, it's for good.

HF: And if she comes, suicide just isn't a possibility for you anymore. No going back. Every time you look at this dog, you will be reminded that you are committed to life.

M: Right.

HF: And I'm a therapist, and you know me a little, and you've chosen *me* to make the final decision.

M: [*Long pause*] You think I'm loading the dice?

HF: Well, I'm honored that you would include me in this. And, yeah, I think you're making your own decision.

M: . . . You're right. I was loading it. [*Sighs, begins to laugh*]
[*Both laugh.*]

M: [*Still laughing*] Say it anyway.

HF: Marco, *Go get the dog. Get the dog right now.*

Marco sent me an e-mail with a picture of him and Pippa and, three years later, another message to say that he had a teaching job on the West Coast and that he and Pippa were well. I would love to know more of their story—but I don't need to.

Chapter 4

Solution-Focused Approaches to Crisis

There is a luxury in being quiet in the heart of chaos. (Virginia Woolf, in Eisen, 1995, p. 260)

Many problem-focused practitioners tend to view a crisis as a disruption of the person's equilibrium and crisis intervention as a restoration of that balance. We have found it useful, however, to view traumatic change as an opportunity that calls for an incredible marshaling of strengths. (De Jong & Berg, 2002, p. 219)

Let's learn a lesson from tea. It shows its real worth when it gets into hot water. (Anonymous)

CRISIS INTERVENTION AT FIRST CONTACT

Renée: Getting the Client's Help to Help the Client

In 1994 I was in Iqaluit, in what is now Nunavut (Canada's eastern Arctic territory) for a national suicide prevention conference. The conference planners, experienced in suicide prevention efforts in general and in the northern context in particular, knew that for many conference attendees, discussion of suicide, even in prevention terms, could stir up painful memories. This was always true at such meetings, and most salient in the north, where so many families and whole communities have been devastated by suicide losses (Katt, Kinch, Boone, & Minore, 1998; Leenaars, 2006b; Royal Commission on Aboriginal Peoples, 1995; Sakinofsky, 1998). Nunavut suicide prevention trainer and advocate Caroline Anawak once determined that in a twenty-year period, this sparsely populated region had lost the equivalent of ten classrooms of children and teenagers to death by suicide (Anawak, personal communication, June 12, 2001). Part of the conference planning was to make "quiet rooms" available to participants at all times, with supportive counseling available in several languages from qualified volunteers. Attendees with relevant credentials were asked to indicate on the conference application form their willingness to serve shifts as volunteer counselors. I checked off the volunteer box, was informed of my three-hour shift, and didn't think much about it until I had been in Iqaluit for a few days and the conference was under way.

By then I was slowly learning how little I really knew about life in the North or life as a First Nations person anywhere, and realizing anew that language is the least of the translations required among cultural groups with very different assumptions, experiences, and worldviews (Ross, 1992, 1996). I approached my shift in the quiet room with some anxiety. All went well until the moment when both of the Inuktitut-speaking counselors were busy with clients, and I heard a terrible keening noise in the hall. The noise grew louder, and a woman entered. She was shaking and sobbing and making the terrible sound. When I approached and asked how I could help, she keened more loudly and then tried to answer me, gasping, in a language that I didn't even recognize. I offered her a chair and a glass of water, with gestures and English. She replied in broken but clear French (which I could understand but which I speak poorly), and a few words of English. We sat together.

I learned that her name was Renée. One of the sessions had triggered the memory of her son's death by suicide in a very powerful and immediate way. She kept saying that she couldn't do it, couldn't do it. She had many other losses in her life, and she felt overwhelmed by her efforts to help other people with similar problems. I said, *"Vous aidez les autres, aussi?"* (Roughly—very roughly—"You help others too?") She told me she was a nurse in one of the small communities in northern Quebec (Inuvik), that no one else was around to help the people there, and that she couldn't do it all herself. She sobbed, and rocked, and keened a little more. We sat together.

I said, "You are a nurse! It must have been hard to get there." She nodded. I said that because I didn't know her it would help to know something about that part of her life also. I spoke in English and bits of high school French, and I don't know how much she understood. Apparently it was enough, because she began to tell me how she had overcome poverty and childhood abuse and a bad early marriage and alcoholism and being a single parent and the strain of living for a time in the South, all in order to learn to help her community. She had raised three children of her own and two nieces whose mother died by suicide. She hadn't had a drink in fourteen years and she had a good marriage now.

As Renée talked and I struggled to understand both her words and her story—to see how such remarkable endurance and resourcefulness were possible—other things happened. Renée gradually stopped rocking and sobbing and keening, she drank the water and asked for more, her voice became stronger and her English better. After a few minutes, she took a deep breath and sighed it out and asked me my name, apologizing that she didn't remember. Then after a time she said, "Most days now, I have peace about my son." She talked about her son and his life and death and about the beliefs and the people who have helped her to cope with his loss—one of them a younger sister who was also at the conference. She cried some more, but quietly, and she took the hand I offered her and held it, for comfort. Comfort, I would say, for us both. Renée said that although she is still sometimes overwhelmed with pain, she will not kill herself because she knows that her children and other people in her life look to her as a model, as an elder, and that her husband would miss her scolding him. And we laughed, and made tea, and her sister came looking for her.

Helping in Crisis

It has been our experience that a thorough exploration of [clients' personal] resources can often reduce the level of risk. Choices other than suicide are identified by the caller and his or her self-esteem is bolstered by time spent exploring their strengths and resiliency. (Wright & Patenaude, 1998, p. 332)

In our experience, most clients in crisis situations stabilize and make progress as they participate in the solution-building process. Like any other clients, clients in crisis improve by focusing on what they want to see different and drawing on their past successes and strengths. (DeJong & Berg, 2002, p. 218)

A Focus on Strength, Resource, and Coping

I'm glad you made it here. I wonder how you did that? (DeJong & Berg, 2002, p. 309)

When I talked with Renée, I was floundering in my own ignorance: about her, her language, her background and culture. My most viable option was simply to learn from her. Although the specifics were different, this is the position of most crisis counselors on distress lines and in walk-in crisis centers: they have minimal information, they can't make any assumptions, and they have to listen to the client and try to speak the client's language.

My assumption as I spoke with Renée was that this terrible pain and grief could not be her whole story. There must be something more, something that had helped her survive. I didn't know then about the work of Snyder and colleagues (Snyder, Cheavens, & Michael, 1999; Snyder, Michael, & Cheavens, 2000) showing that the review of past achievements and the self-perception of competency engender hope, but I could perceive the shift in Renée as we talked about her history of overcoming obstacles to accomplish her goals. Other practitioners have suggested the value of exploring clients' strengths and resources as a key aspect of crisis intervention (e.g., De Jong & Berg, 2002; Greene, Lee, & Trask, 1996; Greene, Lee, Trask, & Rheinscheld, 2000; Hoff, 2001; Hopson & Kim, 2005; Kids' Help Phone, 1994; Korhonen, 2006; Roberts, 2000; Roberts & Ottens, 2005; Wright & Patenaude, 1998; Yeager, 2002; Yeager & Gregoire, 2000). Looking for information about past and current success and competence uncovers useful content, that is, information about internal and external resources that can be utilized to help the client; but I think that it does more than that.

My perception is that, as Snyder might predict, the experience of explaining one's success and competence also creates an immediate change. The outcome is a noticeable calming of the physiological and emotional activation (Shneidman's "perturbation") that impels people toward desperate action, and a perceptible shift toward a more positive emotional state. We know that positive emotional states are characterized by greater openness to alternative viewpoints and new learning (Frederickson, 2000, 2001; Frederickson & Joiner, 2002), and by more positive cognitions (Isen, 2002; Wingate et al., 2006), in contrast to the cognitive constriction and extreme negativity typical of suicidal ideation. I look forward to research that further investigates such cognitive, emotional, and physiological concomitants of solution-focused conversational processes.

De Jong and Berg (2002) emphasize the value of "coping dialogue" in crisis situations, because coping questions are "tailored to make sense to clients who are feeling overwhelmed" (p. 224). They suggest further that dialogues built around such questions are especially useful in situations in which both therapist and client are at risk of giving in to hopelessness (one of the sometime pitfalls of accurate and successful empathy). Coping exploration promotes a "process of mutual discovery" (De Jong and Berg, 2002, p. 227) in which both parties to the conversation become more and more aware of the unique personal strategies the client has developed and implemented. "We have come to think that this awareness, more than anything else, builds hope and motivation in clients to continue to work in the toughest of circumstances" (De Jong and Berg, 2002, p. 227). The work of Alan Wade (1997, 2006a, 2006b) also suggests that conversations about how people resist, stand up to, and cope with their pain and trauma may change both their immediate experience/state and their longer-term probability of continuing or increased symptomatology.

SFBT in a Comprehensive Crisis Intervention Model

Roberts (2000, 2002; Roberts & Ottens, 2005) recommends the use of solution-focused interviewing in Stage 5 of his seven-stage crisis intervention model.

Roberts' Crisis Intervention Model

Stage 1: Crisis assessment, including measures of lethality (suicide risk)
Stage 2: Rapid establishment of rapport/working relationship
Stage 3: Problem identification
Stage 4: Dealing with feelings and emotions
Stage 5: Generating alternatives
Stage 6: Development of a specific action plan
Stage 7: Establishing a jointly agreed-on plan for follow-up

He cites both the view of clients as resourceful and resilient and some specific solution-focused techniques—including the miracle question, exception, coping and scaling questions—as useful in tapping into memories of past successful coping strategies as well as possibilities for new, as-yet untried solutions. Further commonality exists in Roberts' explicit recognition that helpers must work with clients in crisis where the clients are, both literally and metaphorically. Roberts recognizes that clients are more likely to "own" solutions that are generated collaboratively, and that solution-focused questioning facilitates collaborative helping. His model has been applied successfully in a variety of contexts (e.g., Yeager & Gregoire, 2000).

I see room in Roberts' model for greater incorporation of solution-focused thinking and practice. For example, including reasons for living and signs of safety can improve the accuracy of lethality assessment (Stage 1). Scaling questions about attraction to or connection to life may also be helpful in Stage 1 as well as in follow-up assessments (Stage 7). Discussion of clients' reasons for living may contribute both to the relationship (Stage 2) and to the easing of negative or painful emotions (Stage 4), as well as providing useful groundwork for generating alternative solutions (Stage 5).

Solution-focused care in the wording of some questions may change the client's experience of the problem identification process (Stage 3). For example, asking, "How did you decide that it was time to get help?" is different in subtle but important ways from asking, "What happened today that got you in here?" Both questions seek information about proximal crisis precipitants (triggers), but the first one also implies that the client is an active agent who is engaged in a decision-making process, and invites the client to respond from that position. Repeated implicit acknowledgment of the client's agency creates an environment of respect (Stage 2) and may contribute to a more positive emotional state (Stage 4) and therefore to greater openness to alternatives (Stages 5 and 6).

In these and other ways, solution-focused practice can enhance Roberts' vision of a model whose "components . . . take into consideration what the persons in crisis bring with themselves to every crisis-counseling encounter—their inner strengths and resiliency" (Roberts & Ottens, 2005, p. 338).

Means Restriction

Blocking the exit is a powerful intervention. This means taking any possible steps to prevent, limit, or delay a vulnerable person's access to preferred methods of suicide. Means restriction is one of the few prevention/intervention activities that has been shown to have significant impact on death by suicide, an impact that persists across countries and methods (Ajdacic-Gross et al., 2006; Appleby, 2000; Beautrais, 2004, 2006; Cantor, 2000; Daigle, 2005; Killias, van Kesteren, & Rindlisbacher, 2001; Mann et al., 2005).

Studies have followed victims of nearly lethal attempts and found that ten to 20 years later, 90 percent or more had not gone on to commit suicide . . .
Not all suicide victims had a sustained desire to die. For some, their impulse is short-lived, and what weapon they reach for during that impulse determines whether they live or die . . .
The best form of suicide prevention may be as simple as putting time or distance between the impulse to die and the weapon at hand. (Barber, 2005, p. 26)

Reducing access to firearms is especially important, given their leading role in North American suicide deaths, the increased risk conferred simply by living in a home with firearms present, and the reduced likelihood of survival with use of guns compared to most other readily available means (Bridges, 2004; Lester, 2000). "The differentiating factor between attempters and completers may be access to a lethal method rather than a cognitive, developmental, or psychological factor" (Goldman & Beardslee, 1999, p. 428). Active collaboration with family members often helps to facilitate protective action.

(—But, is means restriction a solution-focused method?
—You bet it is. We like to do what works.)

Grandmother Strategies

Provide safety, sustenance, and comfort. People in crisis may be in shock; they may have primary needs for safety, food, warmth or cooling, water, sleep, or medical attention. These are priorities. Even when people are physically safe and unharmed, fed and rested, their *sense* of safety may be an issue. They may be emotionally shocked or numbed and need reassurance, quiet, simple kindness, and steady, undemanding care and attention. Soothing tones of voice and taking care not to startle or confuse them further are important. Connections to familiar people, places, and routines are often calming, as are simple tasks. Information can be orienting, but providing too much or too complex information can overwhelm. Sometimes people are unable to respond verbally for periods of time; in general it is better not to push. Keeping our own verbalizations simple and direct and repeating important messages makes it more likely that the person in shock will be able to take them in. Physical connection (as available and appropriate) with pets, small children, family members, friends, stuffed toys or blankets may provide solace and grounding. Music can be helpful, and of course there is always the ultimate comfort (from my own personal and cultural viewpoint): a good pot of tea.

These "strategies" of basic human kindness are also state-changing interventions that can offer relief, calming, and connectedness: anodynes for suicidal despair, perturbation, and loneliness.

Quinnett (2000) utilizes the HALT steps of Alcoholics Anonymous: "The depressed, suicidal person is more likely to pass through the threshold to a suicidal act if he or she is hungry, angry, lonely or tired" (p.124). He recommends teaching clients four actions:

- If you are hungry, eat a meal.
- If angry, count to 10, walk around the block, or find a way to forgive and forget.
- If lonely, call or visit a friend or family member, or get to an Alcoholics Anonymous or Narcotics Anonymous meeting
- If tired, take a nap.

These protective factors can also be evoked and reinforced through questions such as:

- "Suppose you got some sleep, how would that be helpful to you?" (DeJong & Berg, 2002, p. 221).
- How long has it been since you last ate?
  —How has that been helpful to you?
  —How did you get yourself to eat? (DeJong & Berg, 2002, p. 311)

The Core of Solution-Focused Crisis Intervention: Questions

Examples of Useful Questions in Crisis Situations

A. General

What do I need to know about you in order to be helpful to you?

What can you tell me about your strengths and your capacity for survival so far in your life?

What can give you some immediate relief?

"What have you found helpful so far?" (De Jong & Berg, 2002, p. 225)

What would [an important person in your life] say that you have done to cope?

What do you want to be different in the next twenty-four hours so that you can feel even a little bit better?

What will be one small sign that you are heading toward feeling a little bit more in control of your life?

Which of the skills or strengths that you have used in the past can help you hold on until our next meeting/until the paramedics arrive/until you feel calmer?

What needs to happen first?

Who (else) in your life has been helpful in the past when things were bad? Who would be most likely to be helpful now? Who else?

(in first therapy session following a crisis) What would you prefer to figure out today, something on your recent trouble or on the goal you stated for therapy? (adapted from Kreider, 1998)

B. Questions about a suicidal crisis that "suggest the event could be a turning point" (Callcott, 2003, p. 77), such as:

Do you think that after this you will be more or less likely to hurt yourself again?

(If less likely) What is different that makes it less likely?

What are you more likely to do instead?

What are you thinking now that didn't occur to you when you made the suicide attempt?

How might some good come out of this?

How would [an important person in your life] say that this could be make a positive difference?

Suppose that in six months, you look back and see this as something that turned out to be for the best. What will allow you to look at it that way? What will be different as a result?

Case Example: A Distress Line Call

Unlike most of the others in this book, the script that follows is not taken from my practice (although most of the therapist's questions and responses are virtually identical to ones I have used in real conversations with people in crisis). I wrote it in response to a request to present to a conference of crisis line workers (Fiske, 2003, 2004a). Since I do not do telephone counseling on a regular basis, I had no case material available that was directly applicable to the work that the participants were doing.

The young man in this script has just learned of the unexpected death of his beloved new wife. Rushing to her, he is confronted by the sight of her dead body and, overwhelmed with grief, decides to take his own life. This is neither his first recent loss nor his first resort to violence: just days before, he himself had killed a cousin of his wife's. The cousin had killed one of the young man's closest friends. These deaths had intensified long-standing conflicts between the young man's family and his wife's, conflicts so intense that the couple were forced to marry in secret with the help of her nurse and a Franciscan brother.

This story may have begun to sound familiar: it is of course Shakespeare's tragic drama, *Romeo and Juliet* (1599/1954). However, in our version of the tale, Balthasar, Romeo's servant, returns to Juliet's tomb as Romeo prepares to stab himself, intervenes, and insists that Romeo talk to a distress line counselor on Balthasar's cell phone. (*Pace* to all those who might reasonably feel that in adapting this story I debase a classic).

As you read the transcript, and based only on what is said in this fragment of conversation, note any or all of the following:

- Romeo's views and beliefs: what is important, salient, and relevant to him, and the particular words or idiosyncratic "potent phrases" (Chevalier, 1996, p. 24) that he uses to express these
- Romeo's current, past, or potential reasons for living
- What Romeo wants, including what he thinks his death would achieve (how suicide is a "solution" in his eyes at this time).
- Romeo's strengths and resources

Romeo Calls the Crisis Line

VOLUNTEER: Distress line. How can I be helpful?

ROMEO: I don't know.

V: Mmhmm. . . . .

R: You can't help; no one can help.

V: And you made the call because. . . . ?

R: Balthasar wanted me to, and he was so upset.

V: Balthasar?

R: He works for me, but he's my friend—he came in and saw what I was going to do. He freaked.

V: So, he's a friend—is he there with you?

R: Yes.

V: I'm glad you have a friend with you. You said you were going to do something that got him very upset. What was it?

R: I'm going to end my life, I have poison. Look, you don't understand! *Juliet is dead!* She's dead; nothing else matters.

V: Juliet is terribly important to you.

R: The sun and the moon. She was my life.

V: Tell me about her.

R: We were just married. . . My perfect, beautiful little wife, full of laughter. Such a gentle soul. She would not harm a living thing. I would have done anything to keep her with me, safe and happy. Why did this have to happen?

V: It's incredibly difficult—to lose her, when you were just married, when you would have done anything to keep her with you.

R: Yes. Friar Laurence would say it was the will of God, but how could such a thing be the will of God? She was so good, and so young, and so happy. No one really knows how good she was, how brave.

V: You knew her, you saw this goodness and bravery in her, even if others did not.

R: Yes. Our love for each other showed us things others could not see.

V: So—because of that love, and what it showed you, no one else will be able to remember her as you will.

R: No one.

V: And that knowledge of her, as she truly was, that is important.

R: . . .Yes.

V: So—how *will* she be remembered? If no one else truly knows her?

R: I . . .what do you mean?

V: What memories of Juliet will remain in the world?

R: . . .You want me to say that without me, no one will ever know her. You want me to live to keep those memories alive.

V: I want you to live, yes, *and* I think that only you can decide what is truly important to you. How important is Juliet's memory?

R: Without her, it is . . . it may be the only thing that is important. But you don't understand. I can't do anything, everything has fallen apart. I have done terrible things. Everyone will be against me.

V: Everyone? . . . *Every*one?

R: Yes! . . . well . . . maybe not Balthasar, I guess . . . and Friar Laurence.

V: Balthasar is your friend, the one who was so distressed that you . . .

R: That I was going to kill myself.

V: Yes, and you care enough for your friend that even in that most desperate moment you were able to stop yourself when you saw his pain.

R: I . . . yes.

V: And Friar Laurence?

R: My confessor, and priest.

V: And he is not against you? How do you know that?

R: He helped us to elope, Juliet and I. And. . . . he has never been against me. He is truly a man of God.

V: So, he helped you, and he has always been for you. And what you know about him convinces you that he really is a man of God.

R: Yes.

V: You have known him for a long time?

R: All my life. I have spent more time in his company than I have in my father's.

V: Mmmm . . . so, knowing Friar Laurence as you do, if he were here right now, what would he say to you?

R: . . .he would say, that Juliet is with God, and that . . .

V: [*Waits*]

R: . . . that if I want to see her again I must live out my life as a good man.

V: Live out your life as a good man. How have you already begun to do that?

R: I haven't! I ran away, I failed Juliet, I tried to take poison . . .

V: And you didn't.

R: But only because I just couldn't stand to see Balthasar that way.

V: And to stop, out of love for your friend, was that the act of a good man?

R: . . . Perhaps.

V: Who else in your life, if they had come in when Balthasar did, might have reacted in a similar way?

R: Not . . . well, my father . . . not out of love perhaps, or not only out of love, but for the family honor.

V: The family honor? How would that be important?

R: [*A little indignant*] My father is the head of the whole Montague family. He must always think of the family's good name, and to him my death would be shameful.

V: Family honor is a responsibility.

R: Yes, a very important responsibility.

V: Just to your father? Or to you also?

R: Of course to me also! I have always tried in my own way to protect the honor of my family, to uphold our good name.

Reflecting on the Conversation with Romeo*

Romeo's Views. Romeo is a talker, and he very quickly lets the volunteer know that he is experiencing the loss of his beloved, idealized Juliet as unendurable. In terms of salience, relevance, and importance, this loss is absolutely central. Her importance to him is reflected in his language: "the sun and the moon." His thinking is considerably constricted at the moment: "nothing else matters." Yet, he was aware of the distress of his friend, and it mattered enough to him that he stayed his hand and engaged in this conversation. (In this he is like every other person on the brink of suicide who talks with a crisis

---

* I am indebted for much of this section to the many fruitful conversations I have had about the "case" of Romeo with colleagues, literary friends, and workshop participants.

worker: *something* causes the person to delay or interrupt self-destructive action.) He believes that his life is unworkable because of the "terrible things" that he has done. When asked, he predicts the reactions of both Friar Laurence and his father, and the reasons for each. In the course of the conversation, his respect for and attachment to Friar Laurence, and his intense sense of responsibility for the family honor, also emerge.

Reasons for Living. Even in the immediate aftermath of his loss, Romeo's reasons for living become evident, among them:

- His love for Juliet
- Maintaining her memory
- His friendship, loyalty, and perhaps sense of responsibility to Balthasar
- His religious faith and beliefs
- His connection to Friar Laurence
- His connection to his father
- The family honor

What Romeo Wants. Initially Romeo talks about wanting to die, but his actions at the time, talking to the distress line counselor, are in fact aimed at calming Balthasar's distress. As he talks with the counselor, it appears that he has other things he might want:

- To cherish and protect Juliet's memory
- To understand her death
- To respect Friar Laurence's (and his own?) beliefs
- To defend his family's honor

Romeo's Strengths and Resources. Romeo is articulate, polite, respectful, and honest, even in this extreme circumstance. He has a strong facility for verbal expression, including emotional expression, and a readiness to engage with people—even with a stranger/counselor. He has a friend with him, a friend who he cares for and who has already acted to protect him. He has other strong attachments, including those to Friar Laurence and his father. With Balthasar, that is three important people who *he knows* want him to live and who would be negatively affected by his death, and Romeo has a strong sense of responsibility to and for other people. He is courageous (enough to face the fear and pain of death) and we might hope that his courage could help him to live without Juliet and bear his grief. He has a lifelong history of religious belief and practice, a critical factor in providing some answers to his "whys" and potentially in helping him to live a meaningful life again.

Moving on with Romeo. In spite of his devastation and the intensity of his intent to die, Romeo was an active participant in the conversation with the distress-line volunteer. One could say that he tapped *himself* on the shoulder; it was the answers, not just the questions, that redirected his attention toward reasons for living, or, perhaps, some process that went on between the two.

How might you, as Romeo's crisis counselor, further enhance the presence and impact of his reasons for living? More generally, where would you go from here? Before you go on to read the questions below, make a list of questions you might ask him at this point, either to pick up on any of the possible threads already present or to develop others. Then look at the ones in the table and consider how they would fit (or not fit) for you.

Possible Further Questions for Romeo

So, how *can* I be helpful to you?
What would Father Lawurence say could help you now?
What would your father want you to do?
What would family honor say?
What other responsibilities are important to you?
You knew Juliet so well, and loved her so deeply.
(wait for agreement)
She loved you also?
(wait for agreement).
What would she say to you now?*
On a scale from 1 to 10, if 10 stands for, "I know that I will live out my life and try to be a good man," and 1 stands for, "I know that I will kill myself today," where are you?
(if 1) What can happen to move you to 1.5? To 2?
(if greater than 1) How is that you are (e.g.) a 3 and not a 2 or 1? How does that make a difference? What else?
What did you think of in realizing that you have moved from a 1 to (e.g.) a 5? How did that make a difference? What else?

(Continued)

(Continued)

Suppose a miracle happens and you no longer think of suicide as the
    solution to your problems. What will you be thinking of instead?
What can I or anyone in your life right now do for you?
Who would you want to come and be with you right now?
(if Romeo is unable to respond) Can I call Friar Laurence for you?
If I ask you, will you turn the poison over to Balthasar?

*This is a powerful question sequence, and probably not one to be asked if you
have any inkling that there is or may have been a suicide pact. However, even
if (unlikely as it seems) Romeo said that Juliet would want him to join her in
death, he has already provided a basis for questioning this statement, asking
again about her love for him, her kindness, her "gentle soul," etc.

The preceding questions for Romeo are all designed to follow and
build on the previous conversation with Romeo. Obviously, timing
and pacing, which are not represented in the table, are crucial in making any of these lines of questioning helpful to him.

CRISIS INTERVENTION IN THE CONTEXT
OF ONGOING RELATIONSHIP

Mrs. Boomer and Daisy

My first on-the-job encounter with what I now think of as Ericksonian utilization came in 1972, soon after I was hired for my first
full-time job in the helping field, as a counselor in a juvenile correctional facility in Nova Scotia (despite my complete lack of any skills
or experience that would qualify me for such work). One of our in-
mates attempted suicide in my first week by jumping from a poorly
secured second-story window in a new building. She survived with
minor injuries, and the institution survived a string of suicide attempts in the ensuing weeks and months. For me the most terrifying
of these deeply disruptive events occurred on a Saturday morning,
when a senior girl came screaming for me to come to the laundry, that
Daisy was trying to kill herself. Daisy was fifteen, physically a big,
strong woman but intellectually much younger (my memory is that
she had been assessed as having a mental age of about eight, and her
verbal skills were quite limited). Our school could not provide an appropriate program for her, and so she spent much of her time work-

ing—apparently happily—in the kitchen. She had also made herself chief caretaker to the cats that lived on the property, and staff turned a blind eye to the kittens in her dormitory space.

In the laundry I found Daisy huddled in the corner flourishing a sharp knife and sobbing that she wanted to die. There was already blood on her neck and chest. When I tried to approach, speaking to her as calmly as I could, she began to saw at her neck, which bled more. The other girls in the room screamed louder, and one, and then another began to laugh hysterically. I was terrified that Daisy would hit an artery, and was virtually paralyzed. Into this bedlam arrived Mrs. Boomer, our head housekeeper, who was not usually at work on Saturdays: she had come to drop off a load of magazines for the girls. She strolled in, took in the scene, and in her sternest voice, said "Daisy! How can you ever be a good mother if you behave this way!" Daisy stopped sawing. She stopped crying. She stood perfectly still, and her eyes got big. She began to hiccup. Mrs. Boomer walked up to her and took the knife, which she passed to me. Then she took Daisy by the hand and led her off for bandaging and a good strong pot of tea.

Mrs. Boomer was not doing magic (although it certainly seemed that way to me at the time). She was being wise, that is, making good use of something she knew: that Daisy dreamed of being a mother, that caring for the small and helpless was what she most loved, that doing this well was of utmost importance to her. The dream of motherhood was Daisy's African violet, and Mrs. Boomer used it to get her attention, to tap her on the shoulder, to remind her of something that was radically different from whatever pain-filled thoughts and feelings had overwhelmed her in that dark moment.

Daisy was apparently calm and happy for the remaining months of her stay with us, and then she went home. I eventually went back to school. I have been blessed since then with some fine teachers, both in and (mostly) out of school—but only a few as effective as Mrs. Boomer and Daisy.

A Solution-Focused Approach to the Crisis of Relapse

> The path was worn and slippery. My foot slipped out from under me, knocking the other out of the way, but I recovered and said to myself "It's a slip and not a fall." (Abraham Lincoln)

The idea of "relapse" in connection with any life problem—substance or other addiction, relationship problems, depression, self-harm behaviors—can be dangerous (Gallagher & Korman, 2006). In its wake all too often come assumptions of inability, helplessness, and hopelessness. *Relapse prevention* approaches (e.g., Marlatt & Gordon, 1989) typically focus on predicting relapse via identification of triggers and then finding ways to avoid, prevent, or defuse the triggers. Solution-focused practitioners take a different tack, based on evidence about recovery: "Relapse is a normal learning experience. *Relapse means that there was a success*" (Berg & Reuss, 1998, p. 58, emphasis added). They suggest that rather than a back-to-square-one approach, "most clients simply need a reminder of what they already know how to do" (Berg & Reuss, 1998, p. 59). Therefore:

> When a client who has relapsed returns to treatment, it is more important to discover what caused him to *stop* drinking again and how he is *regaining* his recovery than to impute his motivation or go on a safari for relapse triggers. (Berg & Reuss, 1998, p. 58, emphasis added)

Practitioners can focus on what went right instead of what went wrong. This focus can be conveyed through language: for example, calling the event a "setback" instead of the more laden term "relapse." An attitude that is matter-of-fact, caring, respectful, and (still) hopeful will help. Questions that ask for "news of a difference" often have an immediate impact, for example: "How did you manage to get back on track after only five days (instead of three years like before)?" Berg and Reuss (1998) suggest eliciting "rich [i.e., highly detailed] descriptions" of the "'getting ready to stop again' solution-moment" (p. 58). And the "setback" experience can be utilized in a practical, hope-friendly coping conversation: "What have you learned from this that will help you to stay on track in the future?"

Concrete Reminders, Cues, and Symbols

There are good reasons why we are trained for emergency response with simple mnemonics: "the ABCs of crisis response," "the 4 steps for clearing an airway," etc. In high-stress situations it is easier to respond by rote or to read instructions from a handy wallet card than to think things through or remember details. When clients in crisis are able to agree with us on plans of action, it is useful to provide, or ask them to create, concrete reminders.

This is also the case when the primary outcome of a crisis-counseling conversation is that people access or develop more helpful ways of viewing either a situation or themselves. I often write such ideas or realizations on the back of a business card for clients to take with them. List-making is another easy and practical way of concretizing parts of a helpful conversation (Dolan, 1994; Esposito-Smythers, McClung, & Fairlie, 2006; Freedman & Combs, 1997). For example, I often begin a list of reasons for living as clients talk, make them a copy to take away, and invite them—and perhaps their family or friends—to add to it. (See Chapter 7, "Annie," and Chapter 9, "Tom Session 3," for other examples of therapeutic list-making.)

Symbols or reminders of positive connections to people, places, or activities can serve as lifelines. "Do you have pictures of your children with you? Yes? Can you keep them in front of you?" If we have supportive relationships—even brand new ones—with clients in distress, then we can sometimes contribute a strand to such lifelines. A note on the back of a business card is simple to do and provides a tangible reminder. When I worked in the same office every day, I had a number of small mementoes on the shelves—pretty rocks, small carvings, etc. This gave me the option of inviting clients to take something from the office to remind them that I was available as a resource to them. (I once made such an invitation to a young woman who was in considerable distress immediately before going into hospital for emergency cancer surgery. She thought for some minutes, and then decided to take my Persian rug. She kept it with her in her hospital room and during her difficult recovery and subsequent chemotherapy treatment, bringing it back eighteen months later. I am very glad that it made a difference for her—but I have learned to say "something small.")

Case Example: Utilization with a Client in Distress

On a Wednesday evening at about ten o'clock, I was in my home office, struggling to finish a report. The phone rang, and at first I could not understand what the person was saying or even who was on the line. My client, Kay, was sobbing so hard that it took several seconds before she realized that she was speaking to me directly and not to my voice mail. Then she made frenzied apologies for "bothering" me and sobbed harder. I spoke to her softly and told her we had time, to talk when she was ready, I was there. Eventually she was able to tell me that she had just heard from her lawyer about the final judgment in a civil suit she had brought against a family member who had abused her physically, emotionally, and sexually for years. Although he had previously been found guilty in criminal court and had served time in prison, the civil judgment was that she was not entitled to any damages. She said over and over that "he had won again," "they always win," "there's nothing I can do." Then she began to repeat "I should be dead, I should be dead, I should be dead." This was very concerning in and of itself, because it was something that she told me the abuser had said to her on many occasions, and because I knew that Kay had made two previous suicide attempts, each time with that statement running through her head.

The file drawer with Kay's file in it was open beside me. I grabbed the file, with its record of our therapy sessions together, and flipped quickly to my notes from a session two weeks before. (Most of what I write in my case notes is direct quotes from clients.) I worked to keep my voice quiet and my tone level. The pace of the conversation was slow, with long pauses.

HF: Kay, I want to read to you what you said to me two weeks ago about this possibility.

K: Oh! . . .What I said?

HF: That's right. Here it is: You said, "I do have good reasons for doing this. I don't want Nicky [stepdaughter] to think that I didn't stand up for myself. How can I tell her to be an assertive woman if I run away from this?"

K: . . . Nicky. . . That's right. That's what I thought.

HF: And then you said, "And it's for me too. I want to stand up and say my say. Even if I don't win the case and don't get any money, that's not what it's about."

K: I said that?

HF: I wrote it down. You know how I'm always writing down things you say? [*Hoping to remind her of the scene in my office, to shift her attention to that context*]

K: [*Slowly*] Yeah. You do.

HF: And that's what you said. You said that it was for Nicky, and for yourself. You said, "Even if I don't win the case and don't get any money, that's not what it's about. It's about not letting him win. If I do nothing, he wins again. *If I stand up,* then win or lose, *he's history."*

K: . . . If I . . . if I didn't go to court, then he would win.

HF: That's what you said.

K: Yeah.

HF: And you did go.

K: Yeah.

HF: For your own good reasons, win or lose.

K: [*Voice strengthening*] That's right.

HF: You didn't let anything stop you. You went, you stood up, you said your say.

K: I did, didn't I?

HF: You did. So that means . . .

K: . . . *He's history.*

HF: That's what you said. Shall I read it again?

K: Yes, read it again.

HF: Shall I go slow so you can write it down?

Without the File?

I was fortunate that the file I needed was immediately available. I could have attempted to remember what Kay had told me two weeks before, and it might have helped, especially if I could recall some of her actual words. I think though that it might have been hard to avoid a position of "arguing her into" another perspective, which was unlikely to be helpful. What else might I have done? The two possibilities that occur to me are both strategies that I learned from Yvonne Dolan (1994, 2002).

An Older, Wiser Self

Adapting Dolan's question about an older, wiser self might have gone something like this (HFP = HF pretend; KP = K pretend):

HFP: Kay, I want to ask you something a little bit strange. Is that okay? [*I would want her attention*]

KP: Okay.

HFP: Imagine yourself as an old, wise person. Somehow, we don't know how yet, you have got through this terrible time. . .And you have gone on to a really good and satisfying life. . .Looking back to where you are now . . . what would you tell yourself?

Similar to the miracle question, this question allows the client to move to the idea of a better future without denying the problems of the present or first needing to figure out solutions. And, similar to the miracle question, it has an inductive, compelling quality: it gets the person's attention. Also, it utilizes the client's self-knowledge, tapping into understanding about coping and flexible problem solving that may not be readily available for someone in an emotional state whose thinking may be constricted. Henden (2005) points out that the question contains a presupposition that the client will grow both older and wiser: in answering, the client implicitly accepts this presuppositional framework. Finally, it is difficult even for clients caught in very negative mind-sets to deny the authority of their own future selves to give useful advice.

I might not ask a question such as this if the client seemed too "shocky," or too dissociated, to deal with the cognitive complexity of a future/conditional question. In that event, or if I tried this question without a helpful result, I might use the four-step process for dealing with flashbacks.

Dolan's Four-Step Process for Dealing with Flashbacks

This process is a useful tool to provide to clients who are troubled by flashbacks, which can be very debilitating. I use the process most often as a strategy for clients to learn and practice when they are feeling calm and safe, so that when they do encounter a flashback the response is well-rehearsed. Whether Kay's experience qualified as a flashback is less important than whether the tool could still do the job. (I have also used the process with clients experiencing panic attacks.)

With Kay, who was already familiar with the process and had practiced it with positive results, I might simply have suggested that we "try the four steps for dealing with flashbacks." Given her familiarity

Four Steps for Dealing with Flashbacks

1. *Describe* the experience.
2. What is *similar* to a past experience?
3. *What is different?*
4. What do I want to *do now* to feel better? (Dolan, 1994)

with the method, this would probably have been enough to get her started. If she had difficulty, I could have initiated the process with the first question and "talked her through" (an approach I have also used with people in extreme distress who have never heard of the four steps). In addition to the general reorienting, structuring, and calming effects of the method, for Kay this approach would have the advantage of positive associations with occasions when she had achieved control over what had previously been overwhelming images, thoughts, and emotions. And any method would help if it could interrupt the negative loop in which she seemed to be trapped.

CONCLUSION

In my home office I have a lovely small painting that is one of my most treasured possessions. Kay painted it and gave it to me a few months after our telephone conversation. It shows a stormy sea and sky, with dangerous-looking gray rocks. Across one corner is written a quotation from Louisa May Alcott:

I will not fear the storm,
For I am learning to sail my ship.

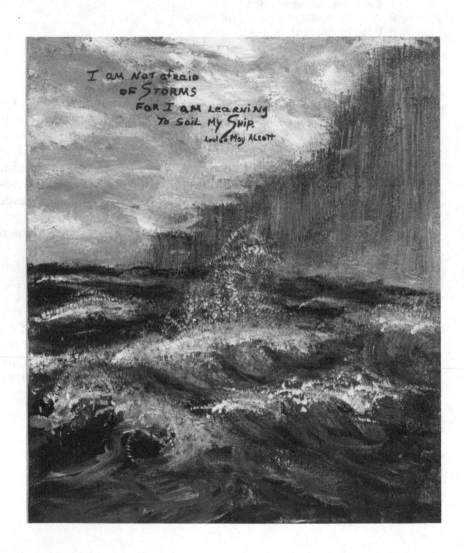

Chapter 5

Befriending the Black Dog:
Solutions for Depression

> In the midst of winter I finally learned that within me there lay an invincible summer. (Camus, 1955/1983, p. 202)

> Most of the work that is done every day in this country is done by people who don't feel very well. (attributed to Henry Ford)

Down and out. High and low. Depression and suicide.

Some words just seem to go together. In both the research literature and the public mind, death by suicide is linked to depression. Suicidal thinking is in fact one of the defining clinical symptoms of depression (American Psychiatric Association, 1994; World Health Organization, 1993). The lifetime suicide risk associated with major depression is at least 15 percent (Angst, Angst, Gerber-Werder & Gamma, 2005; Lönnqvist, 2000) and probably higher (Clark & Goebel-Fabbri, 1999), and this risk increases exponentially when depression is accompanied—as it often is—by other diagnoses, especially substance abuse disorder (Keeley, Corcoran, & Bille-Brahe, 2004; Murphy, 2000). Nonfatal suicidal behavior is also strongly linked to depression (Kerkhof, 2000; Lönnqvist, 2000). Many suicidologists view identification and treatment of depression as the most powerful secondary prevention strategy available (e.g., Goldney, 2005; Jenkins & Singh, 2000), and some point to suggestive correlations between increased rates of antidepressant medication and decreased rates of suicide (Gibbons, Hur, Bhaumik, & Mann, 2005; Isaacson, 2000; Olfson et al., 1998; Olfson, Shaffer, Marcus, & Greenberg, 2003). However, the explanations for rate changes are unclear, and conclusions based on these findings are probably premature (Beautrais,

2006; Bertolote, Fleischmann, DeLeo, & Wasserman, 2004; Bostwick, 2006). Among other things, there is the niggling question of whether differences in toxicity between newer and older anti-depressants, rather than fewer overdose attempts, may account for part of the observed change.

Recently the predominance of the mental illness paradigm for understanding and preventing suicide has been questioned (Bertolote et al., 2004; Chiles & Strosahl, 2005;). It is also important to note that most depressed people do *not* die by suicide: "Suicide and depression are not synonymous" (Shneidman, 2005, p. 119). Major depression is not only the most common, but also the most *treatable* of mental illnesses: most people get better (Depression Information Resource and Education Center, 1997). Still, there is no doubt that from a public health point of view, prevention of suicide at any level is linked to easing the very real burdens of depression. And given the ubiquity of the constellation of physical, cognitive, emotional, and behavioral experiences known as major or clinical depression (aka "the common cold of psychiatry," see Table 5.1), effective strategies for working with individuals suffering in these ways belong in the toolbox of every helper.

The ongoing Helsinki Psychotherapy Study is a prospective investigation comparing the effectiveness of four forms of psychotherapy, including SFBT, in a randomized sample of 367 patients diagnosed with depression and/or anxiety (Knekt and Lindfors, 2004). In reporting outcomes for SFBT and short-term dynamic psychotherapy based on follow-up assessments up to one year post-treatment, the authors concluded that "both types of therapy are effective in the treatment of depressive and anxiety disorders in clinical practice" (Knekt and Lindfors, 2004, p. 72). Smaller nonrandomized studies have also shown positive results (Lambert, Okiishi, Finch, & Johnson, 1998; Lee, Greene, Mentzer, Pinnell, & Niles, 2001; Reimer & Chatwin, 2006), as have studies of mixed-diagnosis psychiatric populations (MacDonald, 1995, 1997; Vaughn, Young, Webster, & Thomas, 1996). A number of practitioners have considered how solution-focused practice can be applied with clients diagnosed as depressed (e.g., Clark, Donovan, & Painter, 2003; Johnson & Miller 1994; Pichot, 2007).

TABLE 5.1. What We Mean by "Depression": "Signs and Symptoms"

Physical	Sleep disturbance Change in appetite, eating Lack of energy, fatigue Loss of sexual desire Digestive problems Pain
Emotional	Sadness Shame, worthlessness Irrational guilt Irritability, resentment Anhedonia (absence of pleasure/interest) Helplessness/hopelessness Pain
Cognitive (often shown as school or work problems)	Concentration difficulties Memory problems Indecisiveness Suicidal ideation Lack of interest Pessimism, negativity
Behavioral	Withdrawal Crying speels or "flat" response Slowing or restlessness Neglect of responsibilities Neglect of personal care Reduced coping Complaints Substance abuse

So, what can solution-focused therapy contribute?

HELPFUL APPROACHES

The Core: Solution-Focused Questions

Examples of Useful Questions with "Depression"

- What are you doing to limit the effects of depression on your life?
- What have you learned from your difficult experience?
- How are you taking care of yourself in spite of your illness?
- What are you able to do in spite of your sadness/lack of energy?

(Continued)

(Continued)

- How did you manage to make this call/get out of bed/go to school or work or the shelter?
- What else are you able to do in spite of feeling so lousy? What does this tell you about yourself?
- Who is on your side in the battle against inertia/death/the black dog?
- What are their hopes for you?
- Who knows you best? How would that person say that you manage to beat depression sometimes, even very briefly? What would that person say could make a difference for you?
- How are you staying connected with people in your life?
- What will be different for you when pain is no longer running your life? What else?
- On a scale from 1 to 10, where 1 is the worst you have ever felt and 10 is the best, where are you right now? What would you need to do to move up half a point?
- Has it been so bad that you have thought about suicide? How have you kept going?
- What do you know about recovery and change from your life experience?
- How can this information be helpful to you now?
- When you are feeling better, what do you know that depression keeps you from knowing now?
- What do you think when your mind is clear?
- What is a useful argument for you to use against negative thoughts? When will be a good time to use this argument? How will you remember? What can help you to remember?
- What was the most recent time that you were able to overcome depression, even briefly? What was different? What did you do differently? . . .think differently? . . . say differently? How did this help? How did you figure this out? How can you do more of that?
- On a scale from 1 (no help at all) to 10 (really helpful) how helpful has this conversation been? What could we do next time so that it is one point more helpful?
- What else?

Respect and Curiosity

The therapeutic stance of respect and curiosity that is fundamental to SFBT work probably contributes to positive common therapeutic factors. This stance applies to *everything,* including the possible value or usefulness of aspects of "depression" for the individual. For example:

THERAPIST: This may seem like an odd question. You've told me about how having no energy has made it so difficult for you to carry on both at home and at work . . . I'm wondering about ways that this lack of energy may also have been somehow useful to you.

CLIENT: *Useful?* It's been awful!

THERAPIST: Mmhmm [*Nods, waits*]

CLIENT: . . . Well, I suppose that I know now I'm not invulnerable. My wife would say that it's good for me to slow down. She's been telling me for years that I have to take better care of myself.

THERAPIST: And what do you think about that?

CLIENT: Well, yeah, I suppose you could look at it like a kind of wake-up call.

THERAPIST: A wake-up call. . . . a *wake*-up call. That makes sense, doesn't it?

CLIENT: Yeah, I guess . . . [*Small laugh*] Yeah, I guess it does.

THERAPIST: So, having heard this personal wake-up call—what difference is that going to make for you?

I have been repeatedly surprised by the diverse ways in which clients find validating personal meaning in their difficult experiences. Often the value they perceive in "depressive" phenomena creates a useful shift in their viewing of the problem. In the case example excerpted, the client's own idea of a "wake-up call" telling him to slow down and attend to self-care seemed to change his understanding of what he was going through in several critical ways:

1. from something "crazy" and "out of the blue" to something that was logical to him;
2. from something that "just happened" to him to something in which his own behavior and habits played an important role;
3. from something new and unknown in his experience to something at least partly in the realm of the familiar and predictable; and
4. from something that he was helpless to understand or change to something that could be within his control.

With or without an awareness of how helplessness and hopelessness are linked to suicidal behavior, I think that this new understanding offers a much more flexible and practical platform on which to build individual solutions.

Consider how this sequence might have gone quite differently. The therapist might have simply accepted that the experience was awful rather than useful in any way, and moved on to other questions, with the assumption that no value existed in the client's difficult experience. Or, the therapist could have *suggested to him* that his current problems were a "wake-up call" telling him that he needed to change. In the first situation, the possibility would simply have been lost. First rule of brief therapy: *Go slow.* Wait. Wonder. In the second situation, let's assume that the therapist was extraordinarily gifted and somehow came up with exactly the most fitting reframe at exactly the apt moment. I am sure that some therapists can do this, maybe even more than once—but I wouldn't want to risk my clients' health and well-being on the chances of doing so routinely. Even assuming that the therapist managed to do so on this occasion, the impact and "buy-in" for a useful idea are not as powerful as when the therapist buys in to the *client's* ideas. And, of course, when useful ideas all begin with the therapist, therapists have to work much harder, be much smarter, and be comfortable with being wrong more of the time than if they just get useful answers from their clients.

Finding and Building on Exceptions

> A man who feels depressed only knows he feels this if he had other times when he was happier. (Sharry, Madden, & Darmody, 2003, p. 45)

Helping clients to notice and emphasize exceptions to "depression" is critical: "it is the therapist's role to notice them [exceptions] and to gently challenge the client to exchange his or her ["depressed"] worldview for a more well-rounded one, one in which both positive and negative events are noticed" (Pichot, 2007, p. 125). Pichot suggests that it may be most useful to discover exceptions in relation to scaling questions ("So what makes the difference between three and four?"). Metcalf (1998) suggests asking clients to rate their level of control over symptoms on a "depression intensity checklist" and then asking solution-focused questions about how they are able to be more in control and what difference that makes. Another option for discovering and utilizing exceptions is use of a solution-focused rating scale for recovery from depression (Table 5.2).

TABLE 5.2. Solution-Focused Rating Scale for Recovery from Depression

	Never Sometimes Always
1. Have the energy I need	1 2 3 4 5 6 7 8 9 10
2. Able to see the humor in things	1 2 3 4 5 6 7 8 9 10
3. Able to smile	1 2 3 4 5 6 7 8 9 10
4. Able to laugh	1 2 3 4 5 6 7 8 9 10
5. Able to confide in someone else	1 2 3 4 5 6 7 8 9 10
6. Able to listen to others	1 2 3 4 5 6 7 8 9 10
7. Able to watch TV	1 2 3 4 5 6 7 8 9 10
8. Able to read a magazine or newspaper	1 2 3 4 5 6 7 8 9 10
9. Able to read a book.	1 2 3 4 5 6 7 8 9 10
10. Able to distract myself	1 2 3 4 5 6 7 8 9 10
11. Able to concentrate for short periods	1 2 3 4 5 6 7 8 9 10
12. Able to concentrate for longer periods	1 2 3 4 5 6 7 8 9 10
13. Able to seek help	1 2 3 4 5 6 7 8 9 10
14. Able to get to sleep	1 2 3 4 5 6 7 8 9 10
15. Able to sleep deeply	1 2 3 4 5 6 7 8 9 10
16. Able to wake refreshed	1 2 3 4 5 6 7 8 9 10
17. Able to eat regularly	1 2 3 4 5 6 7 8 9 10
18. Able to eat healthy choices	1 2 3 4 5 6 7 8 9 10
19. Able to go to work/school	1 2 3 4 5 6 7 8 9 10
20. Able to enjoy something	1 2 3 4 5 6 7 8 9 10
21. Able to feel love	1 2 3 4 5 6 7 8 9 10
22. Able to take responsibility	1 2 3 4 5 6 7 8 9 10
23. Able to accept a compliment	1 2 3 4 5 6 7 8 9 10
24. Able to enjoy favorite activities _____(specify)	1 2 3 4 5 6 7 8 9 10
25. Able to receive comfort	1 2 3 4 5 6 7 8 9 10
26. Able to enjoy music	1 2 3 4 5 6 7 8 9 10
27. Able to feel self-respect	1 2 3 4 5 6 7 8 9 10
28. Able to look forward to something	1 2 3 4 5 6 7 8 9 10
29. Able to get some exercise	1 2 3 4 5 6 7 8 9 10

TABLE 5.2 *(Continued)*

	Never			Sometimes				Always	
30. Able to care . . .										
a) About a person	1	2	3	4	5	6	7	8	9	10
b) About a pet	1	2	3	4	5	6	7	8	9	10
c) About school/work/volunteer job	1	2	3	4	5	6	7	8	9	10
d) About _____ (specify)	1	2	3	4	5	6	7	8	9	10
31. Able to hope for the future	1	2	3	4	5	6	7	8	9	10
32. Able to see something positive	1	2	3	4	5	6	7	8	9	10
33. Able to enjoy loving touch	1	2	3	4	5	6	7	8	9	10
34. Other _____ (specify)	1	2	3	4	5	6	7	8	9	10
35. Other _____ (specify)	1	2	3	4	5	6	7	8	9	10
36. Other _____ (specify)	1	2	3	4	5	6	7	8	9	10
37. Other _____ (specify)	1	2	3	4	5	6	7	8	9	10

The scale is structured similarly to other solution-focused scales such as the Solution-Focused Recovery Scale for Sexual Abuse (Dolan 1991) or the Substance User's Recovery Checklist (Berg & Reuss, 1998). All of the items focus on what the client is *able* to do even while feeling (or thinking or doing) "depressed." It might more accurately be called Scale for Resistance to Depression, or simply Ability Scale. Client and therapist can use the scale to notice exceptions that can be further utilized, and to monitor how clients maintain some abilities and make positive changes in others from session to session. The items have been constructed so that anyone who responds will most probably be able to do at least some of the things on the scale. The last four (unspecified) items are the most important: they allow for tracking idiosyncratic abilities, personal exceptions that are meaningful to the client, or for adding new, previously unnoticed abilities. In fact, one could (should?) scrap this scale entirely and develop an individual set of ability parameters for every client. Imagine how the co-construction of an item list delineating one thing after another that the client can do might make for a useful therapeutic intervention.

Mindfulness

Mindfulness, a long-standing component of SFBT, has been receiving considerable attention in terms of its utility in the treatment of depression (e.g., Segal, Williams, & Teasdale, 2002). The recent focus has been on providing formal training in mindfulness practice for clients. While I happen to believe that mindfulness practice can be beneficial for almost anyone, I would not suggest it (or anything) unless it seems to be a "fit" for the client.

For example, when clients describe racing thoughts that keep them awake at night, or repetitive negative thoughts that interfere with concentration and with their ability to enjoy life, I might ask, "When do you have a quiet mind?" Sometimes they describe very specific ("exceptional") circumstances that allow them to experience a quiet mind and that can perhaps be utilized. Even if the quiet-mind exception is connected to very specific times, places, or circumstances ("when I ride my horse on Saturday and Sunday mornings"), it may be possible to develop associational (reminder) cues that will help the individual to connect with that special time as needed (Dolan, 1991, 1995) or, with practice, to bring that same "quiet mind" receptivity to other times and places.

I recently worked with Julio, a soldier who had been on leave because of depression in the aftermath of traumatic loss. During his leave he found working on his uncle's woodlot to be a profoundly healing "quiet mind" experience: "I don't think about anything else, it's just me and the trees. I calm down inside just thinking about going there." He developed a self-guided meditation that involved imagining the sights, smells, sounds, and sensations he experienced entering the woodlot, walking through the trees, selecting one for culling, beginning to saw . . .

When Julio was getting ready to return to work he was very concerned about his re-adjustment to a tough work environment, made tougher by a superior who was hostile to anyone with mental health issues. I asked Julio what he could take with him into that environment that would remind him of the peace of mind he had been finding. He thought for a while, then brightened and said, "I could keep a pencil in my pocket!"

I said, blankly, "You could keep a pencil . . . ?"

"Sure! It's a perfectly normal thing! No one would think anything of it!" I was still confused. Julio explained: "A pencil is made from a tree. Anytime I put my hand in my pocket and feel the pencil, I'll remember working in the trees. I'll just breathe in that wood smell for a minute, and then get on with what's in front of me."

Because so many clients (and students, and colleagues, and friends) answer "when do you have a quiet mind?" with "never!" and "I wish," I also have a stash of simple exercises that can be taught as part of feedback to clients. The basic breathing exercise that follows is an example. It is a good beginning exercise because it includes words to replace whatever unfriendly ("depressogenic") loop the client would like to interrupt. It is readily grasped and applied; I have used it with young children. I like that individuals decide what they want to breathe in and breathe out rather than the therapist prescribing this for them. This means that clients have to "check in" with themselves to decide what they want and what they don't want—a useful exercise in itself. I usually demonstrate and then ask the client to do it with me in the session before trying it at home, describing it as an "experiment" because "there are many ways of achieving a quiet mind and you may have to try out a few to find some that are a good fit for you."

Basic Breathing Exercise

Client says to self (silently)

While breathing in:
"Breathing in _____ [something I need today, e.g., peace, courage, warmth, confidence]"

While breathing out:

"Breathing out _____ [something I need to get rid of today, e.g., fear, fatigue, pain, tension]"

Some clients may decide to pursue formal mindfulness training, for example, meditation; some will find more active, physical routes to a quiet mind more appealing. Any method that involves concentration and breath control (including yoga, tai chi, some of the martial arts, and some musical or dance practice) can offer similar benefits.

"Homework" Suggestions

The most common, effective, and parsimonious feedback suggestions utilize something that is already working for the client.

**Examples of Solution-Focused Homework Tasks
for "Depression"**

- Test this breathing exercise to see how well it works for you.
- Make a list of all the things that you manage to do in spite of being depressed. Or, keep an exception diary.
- Notice what is working for you in spite of everything, what you want to keep.
- Collect ideas and/or statements about yourself that are different from the ones depression gives you.
- Rehearse the Pretend Plan (adapted from Webb, 1999):
  — Don't do anything yet. Just *imagine* yourself doing the solution.
  — Pretend your solution at least three times per day. Think about what you will do first.
  — Each night before you go to sleep, play your "solution movie"
  — Practice your solution plan in your mind every time you see an opportunity where you might use it. For example, whenever you want to just stay in bed for the day, imagine yourself working in the garden
  — Rehearse your solution movie whenever the problem comes into your mind this week

---

My experience is that suggestions for clients dealing with "depression" issues are especially useful when they focus and reinforce attention to small changes in the direction of their goals, or what Gergen calls participation in a "progressive narrative" (de Shazer, 1991b). Evidence of such participation is an important, salient, and relevant contrast to previous narratives of being stuck, regressed, or "chronically ill."

FREQUENTLY ASKED QUESTIONS (FAQs)

Sometimes clients are already diagnosed—whether formally, by a doctor, or by taking an online quiz—as depressed. How does a solution-focused therapist work with that?

I have to respond to this question with what my husband calls the psychologist's standard answer: "it depends." It depends on how helpful it is to clients to have been diagnosed or self-diagnosed as depressed. If their previous explanations for their problems were negative, for example, "I'm crazy/weak/lazy/cursed/stupid/senile . . ., " then the news that they have a diagnosable, treatable illness may be very helpful to them. If a diagnosis is necessary in order for them to get something that they need, such as insurance coverage for treatment or flexible work hours from their employer, then I will make appropriate diagnoses myself. The very real treatment needs of people whose most evident "symptom" of depression is anger and irritability are often neglected, and (speaking the DSM language for a moment) an appropriate diagnosis of depression often helps them in a variety of ways: they may get help that they need and can benefit from, the attitudes of helpers and family may be more understanding, and, if the conversation is handled well, they may begin to see more hope for change.

On the other hand,

> . . . the label "depression" can become an all-encompassing description leading one to attend primarily to evidence that one is depressed—periods of tiredness, moments of discouragement, relationship faux pas, nettling irritation at small slights are granted foreground status while hopeful thoughts about the future, small accomplishments, satisfying interactions, and moments of contentment are either ignored completely or dismissed as naïve or untrustworthy because they do not corroborate the description of depression. (de Shazer et al., 2007, p. 221)

Clients may get stuck in such limiting mind-sets about "depression." They may view the diagnosis as an indication of weakness or unacceptable vulnerability, or believe that depression is a life sentence from which the only escape is death. In such cases it is more helpful to implicitly or explicitly challenge or deconstruct the diagnosis, to identify clients' "troubles" or "complaints" as a natural outcome of loss, of extreme stress, of physical illness, or to talk about them in more specific, everyday terms, as the sadness, fatigue, or irritability that the person wants to change. "For the solution-focused practitioner, the more crucial issue is how the client uniquely experiences depression and whether he or she can give an operationalized description of it" (O'Connell, 2001, p. 8). In a solution-focused context, clear, detailed descriptions of "depressive" experience constitute information about what the person wants to change.

Attention to alternative, more constructive stories and descriptions of depression and recovery from depression may be helpful in circumstances in which being diagnosed as depressed has increased the person's depression. Many smart, productive, attractive, famous, and otherwise admirable people have suffered with depression—and recovered (e.g., Kronkite, 1994; Solomon, 2001; Styron, 1992). It is easy to pay attention to these stories and, when useful, to mention them to clients. For example, I might refer to articles from *Moods* magazine, which regularly features first-person stories by well-known people who have struggled with depression and found personal solutions. Or, I might ask questions or give feedback suggestions that invite clients to notice or actively research stories of people who have been through this dark passage and gone on to a brighter place. These interventions are variations on Michael White's use of celebrity comebacks (White, 1996). Solution "banks," or other applications of tapes, writings, or consultations provided by former clients who are now doing well (Sparks, 1997; Sparks & Duncan, 2001), can also be used with considerable impact both for the client who is struggling at the moment and for former clients who know that their difficult learning can make a difference for someone else.

Careful attention to exception can mitigate the sometimes demoralizing impact of diagnosis. Metcalf (1997) describes using the DSM diagnostic criteria as a "map" for noticing gaps, contradictions, changes, and variations in symptoms. Clients with family histories of mood disorders usually also have family histories (often overlooked or unacknowledged) of coping, surviving, resisting, and even overcoming these disorders. When clients have a fatalistic view based on family history ("It's in my genes. There's really nothing I can do"), a solution-focused genogram (family tree) exercise (Kuehl, Barnard, & Nelson, 1998) may be useful in highlighting positive counter-histories.

What about antidepressant medication (ADM)?

Questions, concerns, fears, and frustrations about antidepressant medications arise so commonly that one of the pitfalls awaiting me as a therapist is the temptation to launch immediately into a prepared recitation of my own opinions and knowledge: how the drugs work, the pros and cons, the "best practices." Or, I could just provide an informational handout.

However, as in the earlier example of the man with no energy who came to see his situation as a "wake-up call," I am better to wait and inquire carefully as to what the client's views are, and work with those. One of the challenges is finding ways to maintain a collaborative stance when clients attribute any positive changes to the medication, effectively disempowering themselves. This attribution issue is inherent in ADM use:

> Prescribing medication throws an unavoidable emphasis on help coming from with*out* rather than from with*in*. This focus invites clients to perceive themselves as less rather than more competent—often the first step on the slippery slope to relapse and interminable therapy. (Trautman, 2000, p. 100)

On the other hand, any helpful tool—and antidepressant medication can be a helpful tool for many suffering people—is worth utilizing. Trautman (2000) suggests a "both/and" approach to deal with the problem of potential helpfulness versus potential harmfulness with ADMs. Acknowledging that much of the impact of medication is placebo (i.e., hope and expectancy) factors, he proposes that we maximize the usefulness of both the placebo effect and the active drug effect. Questions that recognize the useful effects of medication while taking care to highlight clients' agency and their contributions to their own recovery are both/and. Another useful frame for therapeutic conversation might be to "talk of medication not as a treatment for a disease but as a means of getting to certain goals" (Caron, SFT e-mail list, 1998, in Milner and O'Byrne, 2002, p. 150).

Examples of Useful Questions When Clients Are Using Antidepressant Medication

- How have you been using the medication to help you with your goals?
- How have you been taking advantage of getting more sleep/feeling more energy/thinking more clearly/[whatever improvement is attributed to ADM]?
- "What percentage of this change do you attribute to the medication, and what percentage do you think is your own doing?" (Bertolino and O'Hanlon, 2002, p. 208)
- How have you and the medication been working as a team?
- How are you and your doctor working together on this?
- The medication might help you sleep better and feel more energy—but it can't get you out of bed and dress you up and get you to work. How did you do that?

Of course, neither the previous example questions nor the answers are ends in themselves: they are the seeds for a conversation about the small, potent, everyday details of the person's efforts toward their goals.

What about those handouts? Do you provide information about depression?

"Psychoeducation" has a role in solution-focused practice, but a smaller and more focused role than in many approaches. In general, I wait to see what the client is already doing and feeling and thinking that is working, so that both of us can understand that the client is responsible for those things and gets the credit for them. I provide information, if I have it, more in response to specific client requests or concerns.

And of course everything has exceptions to everything. I do sometimes give unsolicited information, sometimes in the form of handouts, to buttress positive positions already taken by the client; to reinforce safety measures, for example, regarding how to safely stop or adjust ADM; to answer direct, specific questions; or for clients to use in educating their significant others about how to be helpful. Some clients have already done research at the library or on the Internet, and then I am interested in what they found to be useful and how they are applying what they have learned (i.e., presession change). When clients ask for recommendations, I give suggestions for them to check out so that they can decide what applies for them, what might apply, and what definitely does not. I also refer clients who think that they would find such programs useful to community education sessions. I do have some favorite written resources. They present consumer or first-voice accounts of depression *and recovery*: for example, *Moods* magazine, or a self-illustrated book called *Conquering the Beast Within*, by Cait Irwin (1998), or Kaye Redfield Jamison's (1995) extraordinary account of bipolar illness from both personal and professional perspectives, *An Unquiet Mind*.

What about when an already depressed person encounters a major stressor or even just a really, really bad day—the sort of thing that could push a vulnerable person toward suicide?

Life happens. We (therapists) are not usually waiting in the wings when things fall apart for our clients. How do we help clients use what is helpful to them from the therapy context when they are in crisis? Most of the answers to this question are proactive ones, that is, the care we take in helping clients to consolidate and maintain positive changes and to keep useful tools close at hand. Concrete reminders of resource and possibility, in the form of symbols, cues, "rainy day letters," scrapbooks, lists, crisis cards (Chiles & Strosahl, 2005), or "emotional emergency kits" (Dolan, 2002) may help clients get through a bad patch. "Quiet mind" practice can reduce dangerous perturbation. The work that we do to help clients get or stay connected with other people or communities or to their own religious or spiritual lives may pay off when clients reach out to those relationships. Most important perhaps is a commitment to working so that every encounter we have with clients leaves them with something that may be of use to them outside the therapy office, such as an idea or plan or connection or a bit of hope or relief.

Do you always assess for suicidal ideation or plans with a depressed individual?

I hope that as a solution-focused practitioner I can safely say that I don't *always* do anything—at least not when it comes to introducing my own content agenda. My job is to find out what people want, collaborate with them in constructing workable goals, and support them as they work on those goals. Conversations about "depression" in a person's life often include talk about suicide, and I would inquire about such statements, whether they were direct or indirect. In empathizing with people's pain and distress, I may ask if it has been so bad that they have thought about suicide, and if so, how far those thoughts have gone—to plans, or actions? However, my conversations more often get to this information in the course of asking solution-focused questions. My questions would typically be about the opposite of suicidal thinking and behavior: safety and reasons for living.

How do you compliment someone who is negative about everything?

Pichot (2007; Pichot and Dolan, 2003) suggests a two-step process for complimenting that may be a better fit for a client looking at life from a depressive point of view than a more direct statement of approbation:

1. Therapist expresses surprise in response to client's accomplishment, a salient exception to the problem
2. Therapist asks client how the client achieved this

An example of such an exchange might go as follows:

1. "Really! You managed to finish the assignment even though you were so exhausted?"
2. "How did you do it?"

I watched you work with a client and it looked to me like you were doing cognitive-behavioral therapy (CBT). What's up with that?

CBT methods have established effectiveness for reducing depressive signs and symptoms, including suicidal behavior (Brown, et al.,

2005). I do work that "looks like" CBT fairly often. Here's how that might happen with a client who had identified "dark thoughts" as a problem for her:

ME: So, what's been helpful for you in dealing with these dark thoughts?

CLIENT: Well, sometimes I just tell myself over and over that this will pass and tomorrow is another day.

ME: And how does that make a difference for you?

CLIENT: Sometimes it's just like a momentary little distraction from the bad thoughts. Sometimes I actually convince myself, at least for a little while, and even feel a little bit better. It's hard though.

ME: Of course it is. Still, it makes a difference: it distracts you from the dark thoughts—at least for a short while—and sometimes you convince yourself and even feel a bit better. That's pretty remarkable, when these thoughts are so powerful.

CLIENT: I guess so. I never thought about it like that.

Look at what this client is *already doing* to help herself:

1. Identifying "dark thoughts"
2. Catching these thoughts as they happen
3. Challenging them—
4. —Using positive self-talk

Similar to other determined and resourceful people I have met in my office, this woman had discovered or created some of the essential practices of CBT for herself. Given that she is already utilizing this effective methodology, I want to piggyback on her existing approach, encouraging her to use it further and helping her refine and focus it in useful ways. After inquiring further about the difference this makes for her and other things she is doing that are helpful (i.e., other "exceptions" to the problem), I might give her feedback that would sound something like this:

> You know, I am struck by how you have figured out some useful ways of challenging your dark thoughts. The strategies that you have developed—identifying how the thoughts are a problem for you, catching the thoughts as they happen, and then chal-

lenging them with positive statements that make sense to you—these are very impressive. There is a whole field of therapy called cognitive therapy that uses those very strategies. Therapists and researchers have worked for years, written all kinds of articles and books, just to figure out what you figured out for yourself. You are on a good track there. And maybe we can use some of their ideas as well, if you think they fit and would be worth a try for you. For example. . . .

What about alternative therapies?

Many paths to recovery exist. Talk therapies, medication, dietary changes, Omega 3 oil supplements, light therapy, mindfulness meditation, exercise, placebo, cortical stimulation, and even (for some) doing nothing have all been shown to work, both alone and in combination, and (except for doing nothing) to make future episodes less likely (Carson, 2002; Cooper, 2006; Dobbs, 2006; Lam & Tam, 2000; Lawlor & Hopker, 2001; Parker, Gibson, Brotchie, Heruc, Rus, & Hadsi-Pavlovic, 2006; Thayer, 2003; Tkachuk & Martin, 1999: Wernecke, Turner, & Priebe, 2006).

One important caution: a drug is a drug, and many powerful drugs come from natural sources. "Supplements" from the health food store are often unregulated drugs, and combining them with prescribed antidepressants can be dangerous. For example, St. John's Wort shows promise as an effective antidepressant (Wernecke, Turner, & Priebe, 2006), and is recognized and controlled as such in many countries. In North America, however, it is categorized as an herbal or nutritional supplement and so is not subject to the controls required for substances classified as pharmaceutical. One result of this is that products may contain anywhere from zero percent to several hundred percent the stated quantity of their so-called active ingredients. An individual taking such medications may be under- or overdosed, or take inconsistent amounts over time. Anyone combining St. John's Wort with prescribed ADMs that have a similar mechanism of action may overdose on both the therapeutic effects and the side effects. In addition, combining the two can obscure what is really helping.

As a psychologist and talk therapist, when working with individuals who are taking, or wish to take, antidepressant medications—whether prescribed, over-the-counter, or "alternative"—I prefer that they consult with a registered (licensed) health professional who is expert in the safe and effective use of such substances, such as a psychiatrist or naturopath.

Isn't this whole approach just positive thinking?

Hmmm. "Just" positive thinking? Positive thinking is a powerful force, as demonstrated by Martin Seligman's (1991) work on optimism and pessimism and Macleod's research on reduced positive future thinking in depression (MacLeod & Moore, 2000; MacLeod & Salaminiou, 2001). Aspects of solution-focused therapy certainly partake of positive thinking—and go well beyond. SFBT provides a methodology for accessing, shaping, and using positive thinking, for putting positive thinking into positive action.

Both Seligman's work on optimism and the field of positive psychology inspired by it have particular application here: first, because of an accumulation of evidence that a more optimistic and less pessimistic stance is protective against many of life's ills, including depression (Abramson et al., 2000; Chang & Sanna, 2001; Hawkins & Miller, 2003), and recent findings showing that optimism can modulate the relationship between depression and suicidality (Hirsch & Conner, 2006). Second, Seligman clearly presents optimism as a *choice:* a life discipline that can be learned. Taking an optimistic point of view, then, can be a decision that a person makes and follows through on, a new habit deliberately cultivated. In my view, the conversational process of SFBT may be an effective way to acquire, practice, and refine such habits of positive thinking.

CONCLUSION

Like all human pains, depression can also bring gifts. Andrew Solomon (2001) speaks eloquently of one such gift in *The Noonday Demon: An Atlas of Depression*:

> People who have been through depression and are stabilized often have a heightened awareness of the joyfulness of everyday existence. They have a capacity for a kind of ready ecstasy and for an intense appreciation of all that is good in their life. [There is a] . . . meta-joy, the joy in being able to give or experience joy,

that enriches the lives of those who have been through major depression. (p. 435)

Out of despair, joy. (Milton, 1990, p. 401)

Chapter 6

Chronic Attempts at Solution: Working with People Who Have Made Repeated Suicide Attempts

All therapists have had the experience of that sinking feeling in the pit of the stomach when certain names appear in their appointment books. (Duncan, Hubble, & Miller, 1997, p. ix)

We would gladly trade all we know for all we do not know about patients with suicidal lifestyles. (Chiles & Strosahl, 2005, p. 133)

Success can occur with impossible cases when therapy is accommodated to the client's frame of reference and the client's theory of change is honored. (Duncan, Hubble, & Miller, 1997, p. x, emphasis in original)

There are cracks, cracks in everything.
That's how the light gets in. (Cohen, 1992)

THE TEACHER

Ashley was seventeen when I first met her, and had already survived four suicide attempts by overdose, the first when she was only twelve. (If you prefer to read partial transcript of our first meeting before knowing more of her story, skip the rest of this paragraph.) She also had a history of nonsuicidal self-mutilation, both cutting herself with a knife and burning herself with lit cigarettes. Ashley had been sexually abused by an older cousin when she was between ages eleven and thirteen, and although she disclosed the abuse to her aunt and mother at the time, they did not believe her. The abuse ended when she told her cousin that she would kill herself if he bothered her again. Ashley had also sustained a serious head injury in a motor vehicle accident at age nine, with frontal lobe damage. Sequelae of this event included irritability, chronic fatigue, visual-spatial learning problems, and difficulties with concentration, short-term memory, and decision making. The last two issues negatively affected her school performance despite her superior intelligence and strong verbal skills. At the time of our first session, she lived with her mother, a successful executive who relied on Ashley to collect her from local bars when the mother was incapacitated by drink, and to see that her mother got to bed safely. Ashley routinely checked each night to ensure that her mother was lying on her stomach so that she would not aspirate her own vomit. Ashley had limited contact with her father, a career military officer. Her older brother lived nearby but rarely visited. A beautifully dressed and groomed young woman with considerable presence, Ashley was very dramatic in voice and gesture. In previous treatment relationships she had been diagnosed, despite her youth, with borderline personality disorder.

Ashley, First Session

HF: So, Ashley, I understand Dr. Brown suggested you meet with me after he saw you in the emergency room last week.

A: [*Sighs*] Yes. [*Sarcastic*] He seemed to think I needed some help.

HF: And you? Do you think you need some help?

A: If someone who tries *over* and *over* to kill herself and has been *cursed by God* to have an awful life needs help, then yes, I need help.

HF: Ah. So, how can I be helpful to you?

A: I don't know. I'm sure you're a nice person but lots of nice people have tried to help me, and I'm still cursed.

HF: Cursed?

A: Nothing ever works out for me. I can't depend on anyone to be there for me, and I keep failing at everything I try. The "experts" all tell me that I have so much "potential," but it never amounts to anything.

HF: Wow! Sounds like things have been really grim for you—and for a long time.

A: That's right.

HF: But still some experts see you as having a lot of potential. I'm curious about what they see.

A: It's what they *don't* see that matters. They *don't* see the pain I'm in, they *don't* see that all being smart has ever done for me is make me a social misfit.

HF: . . . So, despite the potential, your experience is really one of pain, of not getting support—-even being really smart has backfired because you feel like a social misfit.

A: [*Quieter*] That's right, that's what they all miss.

HF: What else?

A: How much time do you have?

HF: Today, another [*looks at watch*] almost forty minutes. Sounds like there's a lot to tell.

A: Oh yes.

HF: What do I need to understand first?

A: . . . That you can't possibly understand how bad it is for me.

HF: And when I understand that? How will that help?

A: *Help?* It can't *help.* I'm beyond *help.* No one can *help* me.

HF: I see. So, it's not that for me to understand how bad it is for you would *help*—that's not it. . . .

A: That's not it.

HF: But that is the first thing I would have to understand.

A: Yes.

HF: And so, for someone like me to understand that. . . .

A: Is impossible.

HF: Ah! So I can never really understand it.

A: That's right.

HF: You're right, of course. I could never really understand how bad it is for you, and I really need to know I can't. Your experience is unique.

A: I guess. Everyone I meet seems to have a much easier life.

HF: So that makes it hard for people to relate to your experience.

A: Yeah.

HF: And . . . is that something you would like to have different? . . . for people to be able to understand that your life is so hard?

A: Not really. They would have to have been through what I have, and be as messed up as I am. And I can't really wish that on anyone else.

HF: I see. You've really thought about this, haven't you?

A: What else can I do?

HF: Good question. What do you think?

A: *You're* the expert.

HF: Mmmmm . . . sounds to me like maybe you've run into a lot of experts with easy solutions for you.

A: Maybe.

HF: . . . solutions that didn't help.

A: . . . that didn't help. [*Agreeing*]

HF: And sounds like at this point, based on your experience—and very reasonably—you're even suspicious of the whole idea that something *could* help.

A: Well, du—uh.

HF: Right. It's kinda obvious. So—given that your experience has been so negative in general, and with expert helpers in particular, I'm really curious about how you decided to give it another try.

A: [*Sighs*] I don't know why I keep trying.

HF: Sounds like it's taken a lot for you to keep trying when things are so hard for you.

A: Yeah. I don't even like to think about trying, really.

HF: The whole idea is hard?

A: Yeah. Lots of ideas are hard—*hope, future, love*—all those big meaningless words. I'm allergic to all of them.

HF: Thanks for the heads-up. I appreciate that. So, how *did* you decide to come here today after so much disappointing experience?

A: Nothing to lose. And at least it might take my mind off my life.

HF: Ah. And so even if your experience didn't change, it might not feel quite as bad if your mind was on something else?

A: Yeah. I know it's just distraction, just a defense mechanism and not a very sophisticated one, but my pain is so bad that a distraction is welcome.

HF: I can see how that could be true. So distraction, you said, is, like a defense mechanism.

A: Yeah.

HF: Something that helps you cope with the pain?

A: I guess. I don't feel like I'm coping, though.

HF: I see. . . . I guess I'm just thinking about how you have managed to carry on, just to be here at all. And it sounds like distraction is one coping mechanism that maybe makes a small difference sometimes.

A: I guess so.

HF: What other defense mechanisms do you use to help with the pain?

A: Sometimes I carry a knife in my purse.

HF: And how does that help you cope?

A: Well, I know that I can cut myself—sometimes feeling physical pain helps me to deal with the emotional pain. And knowing I can kill myself and finally escape helps me go on.

HF: I see. So having larger and smaller ways to escape is important.

A: Essential.

HF: Are there other things that provide even small escapes?

A: Drinking, sometimes. But I've cut back. Don't want to end up a lush like my mother.

HF: That makes sense. How does drinking sometimes help?

A: Clouds my thoughts, so I don't just go round and round in the same old awful track about how awful everything is.

HF: So drinking interrupts that painful thought process. What else makes a difference?

A: Well, being with friends, if I had any.

HF: Yeah, tough one. I'd like to talk more about that later. What else?

A: Well, writing.

HF: How does writing make a difference?

A: Putting things on paper interrupts the bad thought process, too. Things seem to open up. And I suppose it's cathartic.

HF: Cathartic?

A: Yeah, you know, gets stuff out. Like writing poetry about death.

HF: That helps get it out?

A: Yes.

HF: What else is it about writing?

A: . . . Well, there's a . . . I don't know, a . . . almost a, a satisfaction kind of thing if you do it well.

HF: I see. Yes, that makes sense.

A: The sound of the words, and seeing them on the page, sometimes it's like, I don't know, like being a kid.

HF: Being a kid?

A: Yeah, like before everything gets ugly.

HF: So—yourself, someone who can write, but also like a kid, with that kid kind of fresh, um, is *vision* the word?

A: More like *feel.*

HF: *Feel.* [*Writes*]

(We continued to talk for some minutes about how and what she writes and various ways in which writing is a useful process in her life.)

HF: So, writing is a rather powerful survival tool for you—distraction, release, artistic expression—

A: I don't know about "artistic."

HF: Okay.

A: I could show you some poems if you're interested.

HF: I am interested. How would we set that up?

A: I could come in tomorrow evening. Or else drop them off to you and you can look at them on your own.

HF: I'm not here tomorrow evening. Can't do that, but I can book the same time again next week. I would like to be able to read them with you, if possible.

A: I guess. The day after would be better, though. And an evening.

HF: Can't do an evening, I'm afraid. *Can* do the day after, same time—deal?

A: Deal.

Ashley, Third Session: The Miracle Question

Tomorrow is our permanent address.

—Marshall McLuhan

I hesitated to ask Ashley the miracle question at our first two meetings, because I didn't think that I had been able to get a very clear idea about what she wanted from treatment, and because I thought that she would hate the question. In retrospect, I wish that I had asked anyway. She couldn't have disliked it any more than some of my other questions—and when I finally asked, Ashley, like many other people, seemed to find the question compelling. The miracle question is often the best route to finding out what people really want. Earlier is usually better with this question, and (since the proof is in the pudding) when I did ask, in our third session, her response turned out to be extremely useful.

HF: I want to ask you this very strange question. It takes some imagination, but I think that you have an excellent imagination. Is that right?

A: I suppose.

HF: Suppose that, after we finish this conversation we're having, you leave here and carry on with the rest of your day. Eventually you go to sleep for the night, and it happens that tonight you have a very deep, restful sleep.

A: That would be a miracle right there.

HF: . . . And while you're sleeping, a miracle happens. And the miracle is, that these problems that brought you to see me, they're solved [*snaps fingers*] just like that, it's a miracle. *But*—there's always a "but," isn't there—because you're sleeping, you don't know that this miracle has happened. Tomorrow morning, after you wake up, what's the first thing you will notice that will tell you that something has changed?

A: I . . . that's . . . [*Sarcastic*] You think that I believe in magic?

HF: I don't know.

A: Well, I don't know either. So how can I answer some magic question?

HF: Pretend.

A: Pretend to answer?

HF: Pretend you believe.

A: . . . First of all, I won't be at home.

HF: Where will you be?

A: At my Aunt Jimmy's.

HF: How will waking up at your Aunt Jimmy's make a difference for you?

A: I *love* it at Aunt Jimmy's. She's nutty as a fruitcake—no surprise in *my* family—but she has a great house. I used to go there all the time and she always said I can just move in if I want. I would do it too, but then who would stay with my hopeless mother?

HF: What else would be better about being at your Aunt Jimmy's?

A: I would *finally feel* as if I had a real life! Not this pathetic imitation.

HF: Wow! So, when you have left the pathetic imitation behind and are living at your Aunt Jimmy's and finally feel like you have a real life—how will your day go?

We continued to develop the details of Ashley's miracle (or, as she insisted on calling it, "magic") picture. Even in the short excerpt, I have already learned about an important new resource: Aunt Jimmy (and/or Aunt Jimmy's house), and have gained more information about how Ashley feels trapped (she has to take care of her "hopeless" mother—a determination for which she deserves credit). I have also heard the energy with which she expresses her wish for a "real life," and as we spoke it seemed that the parameters of such a life for Ashley were not un-doable: she wanted a job, her own place—a quiet place like Aunt Jimmy's, nice clothes, a friend or two who thought she mattered, books, a swing set in the backyard. Another surprise resource: one of the things that Ashley sometimes did when she felt overwhelmed was to go to the school yard near her home and spend an hour swinging gently. This was an effective self-soothing activity for her. It turned out that Aunt Jimmy, despite being—well, eccentric—had also been a haven for Ashley in many ways. Her home had provided a safe escape, and Aunt Jimmy was also a potential role model: she had done well in her chosen career and lived a comfortable, independent life. She was not a lush.

The "magic question" became a leitmotif in my conversations with Ashley. She referred to it often, generally in mocking terms ("*You* probably want to know how *magic* would solve this"). She would then go on to say how things would be different if magic worked. Her answers often provided useful ideas about what would make a difference in her nonmagic life, and often made us both laugh, which was also helpful.

RESPECTING WHAT WORKS I: WATCHING MY LANGUAGE

Talking

Many years ago, I attended my first week of training at the Brief Family Therapy Center in Milwaukee, Wisconsin, with my colleague Brenda Zalter. We came away exhilarated by what we had seen and learned, and more than a little starstruck by Insoo Kim Berg's inimitable style of finding and celebrating client strengths and resources. On our first day back at work, Brenda and I had a session with an ongoing therapy group of ten young women who had been referred for treatment of trauma sequelae. (Although it was not a criterion for this group, each of them had made repeated suicide attempts.) The group members came back after their break and said that they needed to speak with us. Then they told us, gently but firmly, that while they knew we had been to a workshop and they could see that we were excited, if either of us said "Wow!" just once more, they would put us out in the hall and continue group on their own.

Similar to those group members, Ashley was an excellent communication teacher: throughout our conversation, she was shaping my style and word choice to be more congruent with what she could tolerate. Similar to them, she was unusual in her capacity to be aware and explicit regarding the impact of my language use on her own reactions: " . . . *hope, future, love*—all those big meaningless words. I'm allergic to all of them." The reaction she describes is one that I have frequently encountered among individuals who subscribe to a worldview that can be summarized as "Life stinks and love sucks—or vice versa" (L. Champion, personal communication, October 4, 1989). Many individuals who make repeated attempts have significant histories of multiple negative life events (Arensman & Kerkhof,

2004), consistent with such worldviews. Adapting one's language to this relatively negative stance presents challenges for solution-focused therapists, whose orientation is to strengths, resources, the future, positive goals, progress, and whose preferred tools include questions about miracle futures or about improvement on numeric scales, and, of course, compliments. "Speaking the client's language" in this context means finding ways to "damp down" or shift positive word choices. The alternative to such adaptation may be a verbal power struggle, with the client responding to every attempt at solution talk with a "yes, but."

Consider the following example from my first conversation with Ashley:

> " . . . *sounds like* distraction is *one* coping mechanism that *maybe* makes a *small* difference *sometimes*" [emphasis added].

It would have been hard to insert any more qualifiers into this single short sentence. I can't know for sure that Ashley would have rejected my comment if I had simply said: "So distraction is a coping mechanism that makes a difference for you." However, at this point in our conversation I was learning from her not to be too strong or definite in my positive observations. One way to make a positive statement more palatable for her was to be tentative, to qualify (maybe, sometimes). Another way is to be uncertain: "I wonder if distraction is kind of a coping mechanism for you? What do you think?" At times I found myself using awkward constructions in order to avoid positive terminology that could shut down the conversation: "When were things a little less bad?" (rather than "better").

Ashley taught me early in our relationship that if I wanted to ask her scaling questions, a scale where 10 was the worst-case scenario and 1 was the best (reverse scaling) worked better for her. In fact, she said she simply couldn't respond to my usual scaling questions with 10 as the positive pole. Although I never tried it, a scale from minus 10 to 1 might also have worked for her, as it sometimes has for other clients; certainly it would have fit with her belief that she had a long way to go to even be on the same playing field with other people and their problems. Defining the positive pole as a more modest step forward is another framework that more easily accommodates progress and change without being "unrealistic" if clients' view of change is more pessimistic or tentative. So the positive pole might stand for "you get through the day without harming yourself," rather than "you are living your miracle day" or "you don't need to come here any more" (which might be perceived as a rejection).

"Partializing" language use can also be helpful, for example:

CLIENT: I feel this way all the time.

THERAPIST: These feelings are with you so much . . . when are they at their worst?

C: Mornings. In the mornings I hate the whole world. My head hurts, my body hurts, and I never want to get up.

T: Sounds like mornings are terrible, so much hurting. How *do* you ever get up?

C: Well, most days I don't. I wait until afternoon.

T: Somehow you hold on through the worst of it, the mornings, and get up in the afternoons.

C: The afternoons aren't much better.

T: Are they really any different at all?

C: Well, at least I get up.

T: How do you do that?

C: Well, I don't want to miss my appointments.

T: Oh, so wanting to keep your appointments is one thing that helps you get up?

Most clients caught in the grip of painful feelings will readily answer questions about when they feel worst. If they have had extremely bad moments or days or weeks, then they must also have had moments or days or weeks that were not quite as bad—not "good," perhaps, not "better"—but not quite as bad. These differences can be critical exceptions.

Use of Compliments

One of the standard solution-focused ways of highlighting and reinforcing what works is through compliments. A mistrust of compliments or an inability to take them in and allow them to make a difference is neither unique to nor universal among people who make repeated suicide attempts. However, similar to the general aversion to positive language described previously—and perhaps as a particular case of that aversion—it seems to arise commonly enough to merit special mention here.

The two-step process described in Chapter 5, as well as other more indirect ways of complimenting through questions, may work better if direct compliments are not well-received. When giving feedback to Ashley after our first session, I told her very truthfully that I was interested in how she managed to cope with such difficult and long-standing problems, and mentioned some of the coping (or "defense") mechanisms she had described. Situating these compliments in the context of difficult problems, and using her own words to describe her resources (excuse me, *defenses*) seemed like my best chance to compliment Ashley in ways that she might be able to accept.

Caveat

One important note about the kinds of language shifts that I have been describing is that I would not *begin* a conversation with a client in this way. Even if I know that a new client has a very negative outlook, or has made repeated attempts, or is diagnosed with borderline personality disorder, I begin in my usual way, being direct and explicit in my solution talk ("How can this conversation be helpful to you?" "When have things been a little bit better?"). With Ashley, I tried something different only when she showed me and eventually told me directly that positive language was difficult for her to tolerate. I try to avoid making assumptions about what will work or not work, since assumptions are based on generalities (what worked with someone else) and/or on the past (what worked with her at some other time) rather than on current interaction with the individual (what works with her today). I have found that modifications in practice based on assumptions tend to complicate, protract, and limit the work. When I manage to ignore my own "knowledgeable" predictions about what is possible, I often find that people are able to respond in ways that I could not have imagined.

Diagnosis

Because it is client-centered, SFBT is necessarily a flexible, "one size fits one" approach. There are clear assumptions and associated methods, but no universal script: solution-focused work is not rule-bound. Injunctions that do exist tend to be dos rather than don'ts. However, there are always exceptions, and this rule is one of mine:

Never refer to another individual as "a borderline."

No diagnosis fully describes an individual, and no individual fits perfectly into a diagnostic category. Instead, we can say "person diagnosed with borderline personality disorder," or better yet, "Ashley" or "Pierre," or "Captain Sanderson."

Borderline personality disorder (BPD) is the most common diagnosis attached to people who make multiple suicide attempts (Linehan, Rizvi, Welch, & Page, 2000). This is a partial tautology, in that a pattern of self-destructive behavior is among the diagnostic criteria. As with any other diagnosis, BPD is among other things a language convention, a way of communicating information. Unfortunately, much of the information connoted by this diagnosis may be pejorative. For decades, BPD has been one of the heaviest labels for clients to bear. The traits and behaviors listed in the *Diagnostic and Statistical Manual of Mental Disorders* (DSM) criteria for the diagnosis (American Psychiatric Association, 1994) portray a painful, limited, and chaotic existence. Yvonne Dolan (1991) described a client who became suicidal after she read up on the borderline diagnosis assigned to her by a previous therapist. The label itself has become "a stereotype of trouble: predictable unpredictability, impulsiveness, dangerousness, unreasonableness, neediness, unmodulated emotional lability, dismal prognosis, and more" (Duncan, Hubble and Miller, 1997, p. 5). Understandably it is likely to promote negative reactions in helpers. Many professionals view people with BPD as extraordinarily demanding of time and energy; resistant" to or "sabotaging" of treatment efforts; "manipulative" in interpersonal relations; likely to engender conflict in helping teams or networks; and "untreatable," that is, unlikely to ever improve.

In this respect, helping professionals are like the fictional woman who "got a bad story inside her," a story that then colored everything else that she experienced in its own morbid light:

> A bad story like that gets inside of you and there's only one thing to do: Prove it. Tell it over and over again, the way you tongue an aching tooth . . . It is easier to tongue a bad tooth than

> to face the pain of extraction. It is easier to keep a rotten tale
> than to find a new one. (O'Leary, 1997, p. 143)

It is not just in fiction that a bad story can prevent us from "shifting
sets," even in the face of evidence contrary to our negative expectations.

> Once set in motion, the set or expectancy of hard going or poor
> outcome can be surprisingly resilient. . . . If left unchecked, the
> expectation becomes the person. In effect, the person is ren-
> dered "deindividuated," made equivalent to the characterization
> or label. . . . observers (nonprofessionals and clinicians alike)
> will unwittingly distort information to conform with their ex-
> pectations. (Duncan, Hubble and Miller, 1997, p. 4)

Retelling the "Chronic," "Borderline" Story

Therapists as well as clients need to know with confidence that
change is possible. In working with individuals who (like Ashley)
carry this label, one useful resource for helpers is access to some
hopeful stories about BPD. Although this may sound unlikely given
the abundance of unhopeful stories about the diagnosis, more hopeful
ones are increasingly available. First and foremost, I think that it is
helpful to hear, tell and retell human stories about people who have
received this diagnosis, have been able to make positive changes and
are living good and satisfying lives. If we have not personally encountered such stories (or have been constrained from noticing them
by the pervasive influence of a bad story), then we can seek them out,
for example in consumer action groups or in therapeutic case studies
(e.g., Duncan, Hubble & Miller, 1997).

Insoo Kim Berg (personal communication, June 7, 2002) has suggested that therapists use the list of DSM criteria for BPD (American
Psychiatric Association, 1994) as a basis for constructing more hopeful stories. This task provides beneficial exercise in flexible thinking
and in the impact of freeing oneself from the limitations of negative
expectation. More than that, it is practice in one aspect of effective
solution-focused work: utilizing the very same "facts" that have been
applied in the construction of a negative, hopeless story to co-con-
struct a different, more optimistic one (Brief Family Therapy Center,
n.d.; Miller,1997).

Better stories are also available in our professional literature. I think in particular of the contributions of Marsha Linehan (e.g., 1993a, 1993b, 1999b), whose conceptualization of BPD is based on findings showing that people with this diagnosis have missed out on learning certain basic coping skills. Individuals lacking such skills can end up going into crisis mode in response to stressors that often appear relatively minor to others. The hopeful points about Linehan's model are (1) that she makes sense of "crazy" patterns of behavior, and (2) that emotional regulation skills can be taught and learned. Outcome research on Linehan's Dialectical Behavior Therapy (DBT) has demonstrated that acquisition of such skills is in fact associated with less frequent suicidal behavior (Comtois & Linehan, 2006).

Judith Herman's (1992) research on recovery from trauma also has relevance here: she showed that a childhood history of sexual abuse, which is strongly linked to suicide and suicidal behavior in adulthood (Renberg, Lindgren, & Osterberg, 2004; Santa Minna & Gallop, 1998), is also a precursor for the constellation of behaviors and characteristics we call BPD. How does this constitute a more hopeful story? Similar to Linehan's model, Herman's findings make sense of behavior that can seem illogical, self-defeating, and frustrating (to both client and therapist). Her model also suggests possible pathways toward change: experiences (including treatment) that reduce the current impact of early traumatic events can also help to free people from the behavioral patterns sometimes labeled BPD and from increased risk of suicide.

One way of expressing something that is common to Linehan's and Herman's views is to say that individuals who function in the way that we call BPD have been trained by their life experiences to adopt suicidality as a primary coping strategy—sometimes as *the* primary coping strategy. Suicidal behavior can become "a conditioned reaction to life crises" (Chopin, Kerkhof, & Arensman, 2004, p. 56). One of our roles as helpers can be to help people in this situation develop *longer lists* of coping strategies, including more life-affirming alternatives.

In keeping more hopeful stories in view, it may also be helpful to remember that in terms of long-term outcomes, many documented exceptions to prevailing pessimistic generalizations exist. Treatment does make a difference for many people diagnosed with personality disorders, and the positive effects are significant and lasting

(Leichensring & Leibing, 2003; Perry, Banon, & Ianni, 1999). A six-year prospective study by Zanarini, Frankenburg, Hennen, & Silk (2003) found that 34.5 percent of individuals diagnosed as borderline met criteria for remission in two years, 49.4 percent in four years, and 68.6 percent at six years. Fewer than 10 percent of those in remission experienced a recurrence.

Remember: "Your patients are not broken; they are just trapped in an unworkable change agenda" (Chiles and Strosahl, 2005, p. 151).

RESPECTING WHAT WORKS II: CLIENT VIEWS AND RESOURCES

Among the many things that I gained from my work with Ashley was a renewed appreciation for utilization of client resources—*all* client resources—and a recognition that it is the client, not the therapist, who decides what constitutes a "resource." Among the group of people who make repeated attempts, many regard as primary resources behaviors and viewpoints that most therapists may see as liabilities rather than assets. In order to work most effectively with Ashley, I had to make the effort to see how such behaviors and viewpoints could be helpful to her.

In our first conversation, Ashley described a series of self-destructive coping strategies: cutting, thinking about suicide, drinking. I suspect that if I had challenged her or attempted to argue her out of any of these, we would never have got to a more constructive and workable option (writing). Accepting her views and validating her need to do *something* to change an intolerable state opened the conversation to consideration of a broader range of options.

Nietzsche (1886/1997) wrote, "The thought of suicide is a great consolation: by means of it one gets successfully through many bad nights" (p. 52). Ashley said that one of the things that helped her to cope was to keep a knife in her purse. My initial reaction to both of these statements was 100 percent negative. I wished that Nietzsche had kept his idea to himself, and I made efforts to have Ashley surrender her knife. She was willing to part with it if I required her to do so, but made it plain that she would just get another one. She also patiently reiterated that what was most helpful to her was not using the knife, but knowing that it was in her purse, that she had this "out" if she needed it. Like many others, Ashley saw suicide as a solution to her problems. Having a concrete reminder that she was not trapped forever, that she could escape via death, made it just a little easier for her to carry on.

> At some point it becomes more comforting to think of death as a way out of the pain, confusion, chaos, whatever is so unbearable. Somewhere on some level it's a stress reliever—dying and not having to deal with everything. The pain and agony of whatever the situation is, the only time there's any relief is at the thought of being dead. (DeQuincy Levine, in Bright Mind, 2006, p. 14)

Was this a dangerous coping strategy? Absolutely. (That was clear even before I encountered Joiner's formulation of how people develop their capacity to die by suicide through mental and physical rehearsal over time.) Was it helpful to her at times? Yes, and I needed to respect that. Furthermore, I try not to take away a coping mechanism until a person has something better to replace it with. Could asking her to give me the knife divert the focus of therapy from improving her life to managing her suicide risk? Yes, it could. Did I still ask her to give me her knife? Yes, I did—more than once.

On the one hand, I wanted to show my respect for Ashley's solutions and her very real need for any help she could find to get through her days. I also wanted to stay focused on therapeutic goals and progress as opposed to using up our time together in a power dance about surrendering the weapon. On the other hand, I had to balance all this with other factors: my ethical and professional responsibilities, my understanding of the protective value of even temporary delays or interruptions in the suicidal process, and my own legitimate need to get a good night's sleep on a regular basis. I kept on collecting knives from Ashley until she stopped "bothering" to replace them.

Coping

Coping questions are founded in a co-constructed appreciation of how difficult life is for clients. By their very nature, they acknowledge the existence of problems and obstacles to change. The sequence in which Ashley and I discussed her various strategies for dealing with the pain in her life is an example of a conversation about coping. Her use of the term *defense mechanisms* makes explicit the link between these actions and her efforts to deal with her problems. In general, coping questions are perhaps my most essential tool with clients who spend considerable time and energy focusing on problem stories. When Ashley told me about a particularly bad moment or day or week, I was both sympathetic and also curious about how she got through it, how she kept from totally falling apart, how one horrible day didn't necessarily lead to another just as bad. ("How is it that things aren't worse?") Acknowledging the depth and difficulty of her pain and struggle made the steps she had taken to cope more salient, important, and relevant. (Questions that focused on the difference between bad and terrible were of course more palatable for her than questions that highlighted a difference between bad and better.)

Eliciting responses to coping questions in as much detail as possible can contribute to constructive, evidence-based shifts in meaning and self-labeling for the *client:* for example, from "victim" or "cursed" to "someone dealing with really tough stuff," "a coper," "a survivor," "someone holding the line," "doing what she can," "a fighter." The importance of such shifts in helping clients develop a sense of self-efficacy cannot be underestimated. Brown (2006) reviews evidence to suggest that "the hopeless thinking of ["chronically"] suicidal individuals may be based on their expected inability to tolerate future negative events rather than on expecting a high likelihood of negative events" (p. 96). The skills-training aspect of Dialectical Behavior Therapy is one route to enhancing clients' evaluations of their own tolerance. I see solution-focused coping conversations as another (and compatible) route. Repetition of such conversations over time can help clients with very negative views to consolidate and maintain positive shifts in self-evaluation. Therapeutic tasks that invite clients to notice, repeat, and expand their existing coping repertoires further reinforce and entrench a more hopeful view of their own capacity.

RESPECTING WHAT WORKS III: THERAPIST CONTRIBUTIONS

Balancing Problem Acknowledgement with Solution Talk

Sympathizing with suicidal impulses is ... designed to validate emotional pain while reframing what are often experienced as

uncontrollable impulses . . . Acknowledging a universal connection between feeling frustrated and blocked and considering
suicide is a way of slipping the problem-solving notion in the
back door.... suicidal behavior is moved off center when you
empathize with emotional pain and frustration while linking
repetitious suicidal behavior and unsolved problems. (Chiles &
Strosahl, 2005, p. 153)

Research shows that people who repeatedly attempt suicide are
more likely than control subjects to have had "problematic events and
experiences," including high rates of sexual abuse early in life
(Kerkhof & Arensman, 2004, p. 115). Such experience can understandably color a person's worldview and interactions with others
(Janoff-Bulman, 1992, 1999), especially since most victims of violence also experience negative and harmful social responses (Wade,
2004).

As we continued to work together, I realized that Ashley often reacted with either disapproval or outright refusal to respond not just to
positive idiom but also to what I think of as more general "solution
talk," i.e., conversation about goals, progress, possibility, and change.
It was helpful for me to appreciate that her reactions made sense in
the context of her life experience. Given her remarkable self-aware-
ness, we were even able to talk about this. We sometimes, for example, negotiated how much "solution talk" she could handle on a particular day. She might say "two minutes, tops." On two occasions, she
told me to "go for it" and we had an ordinary (solution-focused)
conversation about her progress and plans.

Future-oriented methods such as the miracle question that invite
people to consider the possibility of a better future may be difficult
for clients who present what Dolan (1991) calls "learned cynicism"
(pp. 22-23). Dolan (1994) describes a useful response to individuals
who "don't believe in miracles" or who are reluctant to look to the future. When she has received a negative or doubtful response, she
sometimes says something like this:

You know, I think that your ability to look ahead to a brighter future is something that has been stolen from you by your negative
experience. I would like for you to get this back. So, could you
just give this question [or exercise, or questionnaire] a try?

I have adopted this frame often with good results. Its usefulness lies in the extent to which it mirrors the individual's own view of life, that is, that something has indeed been stolen, something that other people seem to have. When the "fit" is good, this formulation often allows people to step outside the limits imposed by their fears and do something different that may be of value. The approach is based on an assumption that

> the chronically suicidal patient is a disillusioned optimist—the patient really wants to believe that things can change for the better but has had so many disconfirming experiences that *a fear emerges about being hopeful.* (Chiles & Strosahl, 2005, p.152, emphasis in original)

Deal-Making

I once heard a physician who specializes in addictions tell a story about a "borderline" patient. He said that this client had become increasingly strident and unreasonable in her demands on his time and attention. Although he tried to set appropriate limits, she virtually stalked him: showing up at his office without an appointment, accosting him on the street, sitting outside his home in her car, sending him elaborate gifts, calling him wherever he was at all hours of day and night. (He had an on-call rotation and couldn't just turn off his phones.) He said that even after he was forced to go to court and obtain a restraining order, and after changing his office procedures, his telephone numbers, and the locks on his home and office doors, she would still track him down. She was clearly a very resourceful woman, particularly adept at getting his new telephone numbers, usually within hours of the change. It was a therapist's nightmare. Finally, in desperation, when the telephone woke him at 2:00 a.m., he told her that he really needed to get some sleep, and if she was going to call, could she please call before 10:00 p.m. or after 7:00 a.m.? There was a silence, and then she said, "Okay."

When she called him the next evening, he told her that he would talk to her for ten minutes as long as he didn't have another commitment. They had ten-minute telephone calls twice a week for months. She never called between 10:00 and 7:00, and she respected the ten-minute rule and his occasional lack of availability. Eventually she accepted a referral to one of the doctor's colleagues, and the calls gradually tapered off. The doctor didn't present this story as a paradigm for working with personality disorder; his comment was simply that the difference that mattered to him (and apparently to her) happened when he stopped responding to her as "a borderline" who needed to be vigorously "boundaried" and spoke to her person-to-person.

Much of what I was taught about how to work with clients who share some characteristics with Ashley involved establishing clear therapeutic contracts, and in particular the setting of boundaries or limits in the therapeutic relationship. In fact, almost everything within the "contract" category involved expectations for the client, a rather curious phenomenon given that a contract usually implies a more mutual set of agreements between parties. The "contractual" arrangements often meant denying clients aspects of the relationship that they felt were important or potentially helpful (such as having access to a therapist outside of scheduled appointment times). I have no difficulty with the idea of boundary setting as a necessary part of what therapists do. I also believe that therapists have a responsibility to practice (and model) self-care, which includes setting those limits on our time and accessibility that work for us. *And* I think that we can save ourselves and our clients many difficult interactions by focusing at least as much on what is within those boundaries as on what is outside them. I am especially concerned with the impact of conducting "boundary-setting" conversations with people I am supposed to be helping in which my part consists entirely of telling them "no" over and over again. Chiles and Strosahl (2005) provide useful, concrete examples of alternative, more balanced approaches to therapeutic contracting and limit-setting.

Tips for Setting Limits and Boundaries in Treatment

- Generally: Be flexible and client-centered rather than rule-bound*
- Specifically: Every time you tell clients about something that you won't do, also tell them about something that you will do.
- Seek practical individualized alternatives to meet client needs, for example, a "time out" or safe-house setting rather than hospitalization.

*within professional and ethical constraints

Differences

> There is a vital difference between "intolerable" and "just
> barely tolerable after all." (Shneidman, 2005, p. 120)

Finding differences that make a difference when working with clients like Ashley can mean taking a microchange (very small differences) focus. The therapist's ability to notice, reinforce, and celebrate even very small changes is helpful for clients in supporting their understanding that they are engaged in a process of change (the "progressive narrative," de Shazer, 1991b)—and also for keeping therapists hopeful about their clients and the value of the work that they are doing together.

Therapists also need to be alert to important changes signaled by negative reinforcement—less of a bad thing, or by the lesser of two evils—a less bad thing. Such changes may be elicited or highlighted by questions such as:

- What did you do differently so that
  —you stayed out of the emergency room that time?
  —you cut yourself only twice this week instead of every day?
- How did you decide that it was better
  —to get stoned instead of hurting yourself?
  —to endure being lonely instead of going home with an abusive
    drunk?

WHEN SUICIDAL CRISES OCCUR IN THE COURSE
OF TREATMENT

> The clinician who insists that patients refrain from suicidal behavior in order to continue therapy is doing a disservice. Learn to harness your disappointment regarding a suicidal crisis. A good place to start may be to remember that although your ability to influence is great, your power to control is quite limited. (Chiles & Strosahl, 2005, p. 189)

> Do you sit perched on the edge of the seat when the patient is talking about suicide and sit back when problem solving is the focus? . . .The general rule is that at least 85 percent of the ses-

sion should be spent in the former pursuit and no more than 15 percent spent focusing directly on suicidal behavior. (Chiles & Strosahl, 2005, p. 191)

Our responses to suicidal crises during treatment are critical, because for the client and for other people in the client's life, these events may confirm (again) that nothing has changed or can change. The solution-focused response to relapse (Berg & Reuss, 1998) is again relevant. Key to this approach is a focus not only on what triggered the setback, but on *what the client did that was different* from previous occasions or from a prevailing negative behavior pattern. In particular, we should emphasize and reinforce anything that clients are doing that is consistent with their desired future, their goals for therapy, and solution-building steps they have already been taking. For clients who believe that their strong feelings are an irresistible force, evidence that they are in fact taking deliberate, constructive action even in the face of such feelings is a powerful platform for change. Utilization or even partial utilization of crisis plans or cards is one kind of evidence for such client action.

Proactive Telephone Calls

As both prevention for and response to suicidal crises, Chiles and Strosahl (1995, 2005; Strosahl, 1999) recommend occasional brief (two to three minute), unscheduled telephone calls by the therapist,

> [a] strategy designed to remove the association between escalating suicidal behavior and your attention. . . . the message is: "I care about how you're doing. I hope the behavioral homework is going well. I really look forward to seeing you next week. Take care." . . . Do not perform therapy on the phone, but support your patient in whatever activities are occurring. (Chiles & Strosahl, 2005, p. 187)

Calls do not have to be frequent: Chiles and Strosahl suggest once a month at random intervals. They emphasize that the calls should not be tied to how the client is functioning, although

> in a crisis, you can bend the rules and add an additional call or two to reinforce the problem-solving strategies that your patient

is currently using. *Even though your patient is in crisis, the message is essentially the same, and the duration of the call is short*." (Chiles & Strosahl, 2005, p. 187, emphasis added)

I have used this strategy (slightly adapted) and found it very useful. My impression is that it modulates "crisis-to-crisis" functioning and makes dealing with crises that do occur more like an aspect of ongoing goal work rather than an interruption of that work. (I wonder if occasional brief e-mail messages might have a similar impact.) Most important, "the issue of mattering to someone and being understood can be so central to your suicidal patient's view of the world that a simple 2-minute call may be a major event" (Chiles & Strosahl, 2005, p. 188).

Crisis Response Plans/Cards

Many practitioners develop before-the-fact plans for suicidal crisis with clients so that both therapist and client understand what resources are available, what each is responsible for, and what the step-by-step process should be. Crisis cards, based on Beck's "coping cards" (Beck, Rush, Shaw, & Emery, 1979), have been used effectively in several models for suicide intervention during treatment (Chiles & Strosahl, 1995, 2005; Jobes, 2006; Joiner, 2005; Rudd, Joiner, & Rajab, 2001). Use of such cards has been conceptualized as self-regulation training (Rudd, Joiner, & Rajab, 2001) and could also be understood as a specialized form of pattern interruption (Dolan, 1995; Bertolino & O'Hanlon, 2002), or more generally as a proactive, experiential approach to doing something different. Triggering well-rehearsed crisis plans offers a possible antidote for the impulsiveness that is one of the riskiest aspects of emotional ups and downs for people who use suicide as a coping strategy (Bornovalova, Lejuez, Daughters, Rosenthal, & Lynch, 2005; Links & Rourke, 2000). The card itself may act as a concrete reminder to activate the plan, and concrete reminders—useful for anyone in moments of crisis—are especially important for those who may be predisposed to dissociation (Dolan, 1994).

In developing the card, clinician and client create a list of both internal (personal) and external (relationship or community) resources that the client believes can be helpful in a perceived crisis situation. This resource explication process is itself likely to be highly therapeutic, and can be facilitated by coping and exception questions. A crisis card typically displays two lists: first, a selected list of personally available resources, and second, a short list of emergency contacts, usually including the therapist, which the client will attempt to reach if utilization of resources on the first list does not defuse the crisis.

Sample Crisis Card

- Do not drink or use, or if I am drinking or using, stop now.
- Walk quickly to the YMCA. Go in, and if the pool is open, swim ten laps. If I still feel agitated, swim ten more. If pool is not open, run laps on indoor track.
- Read the following statement to myself ten times:
- I have survived everything they have thrown at me. I am still standing.
- Call my girlfriend. (home, 232-2323; cell, 233-2332). If I get voice mail, leave a short message. If I get her, talk to her for five minutes about a plan to get together.
- Write in my notebook what happened and what helped, to talk about at my next therapy session
- Contact: Distress Line, 332-3232
  Hospital emergency room: 332 Main St.
  Dr. X (therapist): 432-4321

(adapted in part from Chiles & Strosahl, 2005, and Joiner, 2005)

Crisis cards are used in the context of a plan developed between client and therapist as to how and when they will be employed. An explicit understanding about the therapist's availability and what can be expected if the client calls is part of this context (See Chiles & Strosahl, 2005, or Jobes, 2006 for useful discussion of crisis planning).

In my own practice, I suggest developing crisis plans and/or cards when clients indicate that they want to be able to deal with life crises differently. This happens fairly often with clients who have made repeated suicide attempts, so it could look as if this is a routine aspect of my practice with such clients. However, I use this (or any) proactive strategy reactively, in response to clients' expressed preferences.

NOTES ON THE R-WORD

I remember learning when I was first studying systemic therapy approaches that "resistance" was *between* people, a difficult but useful concept—and then going to work, and hearing a family that disagreed with their therapist labeled as "help-rejecting complainers." When clients "fail to comply" with our treatments (what tell-tale use of language!), the idea of resistance allows us to place the blame on them, or rather *in* them—in their personalities, histories, neuroses, etc. This gets therapists off the hook—*and* effectively stymies any further helping process. Steve de Shazer (1984) once declared that resistance (at least in the sense I have been describing) was dead. A plaque on the wall of the Brief Family Therapy Center commemorated its demise. De Shazer's view of "resistance" was that *if* it existed at all, it resided in therapists. Now there is a useful notion: if I have the resistance, maybe I can do something about it. He suggested that the perception of "resistance" signaled the therapist's failure to understand the client's unique way of cooperating: the therapist's intervention or style of intervention was not a good fit for the client.

I have to admit that I still occasionally have moments when I think that I perceive "resistance" in the person sitting across from me. I have learned to receive such perceptions as signals that I am off track. There are several steps I can use to get back on track: most often, I can just listen better. Breathing helps. Sometimes I can adjust my questions according to what the person is showing me about level of customership or readiness for change. Sometimes I can say to the client: "I don't think that was the right question to ask. What would be a better question for you right now?" (I usually get a two-part response: a funny look, and a suggestion for a much better question). Sometimes, the thought is a sign that I need a cup of tea, or some fresh air, or a chat with a colleague, or a vacation. Sometimes I find it helpful to ask myself the following question, inspired by Parry & Doan (1994): Suppose that, instead of being "resistant," I saw this person as trying to tell me something that I am just not getting. What might it be?

NOTES ON DEALING WITH SELF-MUTILATION

If you find yourself in a tug of war, let go of the rope. (Anonymous, probably somebody's grandmother)

"Look for the pearl in the oyster." (Lamarre, 2003)

Understanding

The *most* useful option for understanding self-mutilating behaviors is listening carefully to how individual clients describe their experiences. Ashley said: "Sometimes feeling physical pain helps me to deal with the emotional pain." Other more and less useful ways for therapists to think about nonsuicidal self-harming or self-mutilating behavior are available. The more useful options include regarding such actions as a "purposeful, if morbid, act of self-help" (Favazza, 1989); as a form of coping behavior—maladaptive perhaps, but still, coping; and as a problem-solving activity—pathological perhaps, but still, problem solving. Considerable evidence suggests the immediate utility of self-mutilation for those who engage in it: research shows that it can trigger a release of endorphins, neurochemicals that relieve pain and are associated with pleasant states of relaxation and pleasure (Van der Kolk, Greenberg, Orr, & Pittman, 1989). It is this endorphin-based tension-reduction mechanism that has most often been used to explain the easing of unpleasant emotional states:

> For those who are currently engaging in the behavior, self-mutilation is immediately psychophysiologically and psychologically reinforcing . . . Significant reductions in anxiety, fear and sadness were noted following self-mutilation. In addition, frequent self-mutilation participants reported feeling significantly more relieved on commission of the act. (Brain, Haines, & Williams, 2002, pp. 207-208)

> The tension-reduction properties of self-mutilating behavior do not extend to injuries incurred in other ways. (Brain, Haines, & Williams, 2002, pp. 207-208)

A great deal of time has been spent in research and theorizing about the differences between suicidal behavior and self-mutilation (e.g., Muehlenkamp, 2003; Walsh, 2002, 2005; Walsh & Rosen, 1988), since from the outside they may "look" much the same. One useful differentiation is that " . . . a person who truly attempts suicide seeks to end all feelings, whereas a person who self-mutilates seeks to feel better" (Favazza, 1996, p. 262). However, while these discrim-

inations may contribute to shaping clinical understanding and intervention, they should not make us comfortable in assuming that we are
dealing with separate realms. Rather than one behavior excluding the
other, they overlap in many ways. For example: more than half of
people who self-mutilate also take drug overdoses, one-quarter overdose repeatedly, and one-third expect to be dead within five years
(Zlotnick, Mattia, & Zimmerman, 1999). Self-mutilation is predictive of suicide attempts: the more kinds of self-mutilation a person
engages in, the more likely they are to also make a suicide attempt
(Zlotnick et al, 1999).

Guidelines for Helping

Be calm and matter-of-fact about the behaviors. If this is not immediately possible for you, *act* calm and matter-of-fact until you can
manage the real thing. Breathing helps.
Acknowledge and validate (regularly, often) how tough the problems
are, how much pain the person is in.
Take any indications of suicidal thinking or planning seriously. Evaluate and respond separately from the pattern of non-suicidal self-
harm.
Work to understand the logic of the self-harm behavior: "You must
have a good reason for doing this."
Once you understand what it is the person is getting, or trying to get,
from self-harm, you can begin to look for alternative, less destructive ways for them to get what they need.
Recognize self-injury as the person's *attempt to cope, solve a problem, or get relief from pain.* Use their language to describe the
function of the behavior.
Understand that they may not have learned other, more positive coping skills.
Talk with people who self-harm from this (re-) frame, for example:

- How does doing this work for you? How does it help?
- "What problems did you run into that looked so unsolvable that
  cutting yourself looked like a solution?" (Strosahl, 1999)
- How is this approach working for you? Short-term? Long-term?
  What are the consequences? How are they helpful?—or

- "Sounds like it's working now. Will it work later?" (Strosahl, 1999)

Notice, reinforce, and build on any *exceptions* to the problem, for example, times when the person wanted or intended to self-mutilate, but did something else instead:

- How did you stop yourself?
- How did you think of painting the bathroom instead?
- How could you do something like that again?

Use the language of choice and possibility: for example, ask about options and make or assign lists.

Help people to build "longer lists" of coping behaviors. For example, learning and/or practicing ways to soothe or calm themselves may help.

Help people find ways to *interrupt the self-harming pattern,* including planning to do something else first (make a telephone call, write in a journal, go for a walk) when the impulse occurs.

Encourage and reinforce *positive self-talk.*

Go beyond talking about solutions; find ways for the person to observe and (better) experience new behavior and skills, for example, rehearse, role play, *practice*—with you, friends, or family

Provide *concrete, readily available reminders* of alternative coping possibilities and resources in the person's immediate environment—especially important because self-mutilation is typically an impulsive act (Nock & Prinstein, 2005) and because the person may be in a dissociated state (Dolan, 1991) in which it is especially difficult to connect with helpful ideas and habits.

Provide an appreciative *audience* for the development and use of new coping skills. Enlist other members of the person's helping team in this effort.

Remain mindful.

Summary Thoughts

If you have noticed that these guidelines for dealing with self-mutilation seem to involve applying exactly the same solution-focused postures and methods as in dealing with other issues—you're getting it.

THE TEACHER REVISITED

I saw Ashley for sixteen months, with varying frequency, until she went to another city for university. During that time we "danced," especially for the first six months, around her knife. Gradually that coping option became less salient or perhaps less necessary: she was beginning to notice that she had a longer list of constructive coping strategies than she had once believed, and to use them at least some of the time in preference to self-destructive behaviors. When she left for school, she wanted me to continue as her therapist. We struck a(nother) deal: she would see someone at the university counseling center, and she and I would stay in touch via occasional letters. I would also meet with her when she was home for breaks (two or three times a year). Although the university/independent living experience was a major challenge, she made no further suicide attempts and for the most part was able to utilize her positive coping tools. After two years, Ashley returned to finish her degree at a campus closer to home, and we met for a few more times. Shortly after she took a "break" from treatment with me that has continued to this day.

I heard from Ashley occasionally in the next few years. She found a part-time job doing promotion and sales for a cosmetics firm. Although she sometimes mocked the frivolousness of her job ("we're not exactly world-changers"), she liked it and seemed to be good at it, and her limited energy made part time a good fit. She was living again with her mother, who had stopped drinking because of serious health problems. Ashley volunteered one afternoon a week at a local facility for disabled children, which she insisted was something she did for herself: "I want it to be how it *should* be for a kid." Some of the poems she continued to write were for these children. Her social life, which included both continuing friends and occasional boyfriends, seemed to be rather . . . eventful. She still went to Aunt Jimmy's sometimes for weekends. Her life, in short, was not perfect, but it was a real life, with real satisfactions.

The last time I heard from her, Ashley left me a note to say that she had decided she needed another creative outlet and had started a painting class. She had just completed her first painting and wanted me to have it. It is a vivid watercolor of a magician raising a wand, which now hangs in an honored place in my home office. On the back is written:

Merlin the Magician.
For Heather Fiske, from Ashley.
Do you believe in magic?

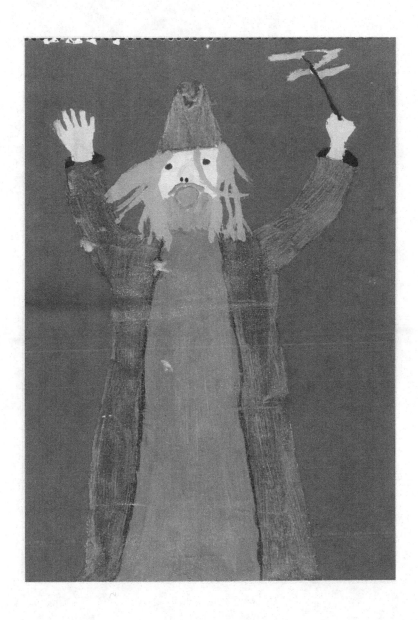

Chapter 7

Even the Children: Preventing Suicide Among Young People

> Resilience does not come from rare and special qualities, but from the everyday magic of ordinary, normative human resources in the minds, brains, and bodies of children, in their families and relationships, and in their communities. (Masten, 2001, p. 235)

I would very much like to believe that suicide is not a risk for young children. It would be comforting, I think, to tell myself this, because children understand death and suicide differently than adolescents or adults do, they cannot really engage in suicidal thinking or behavior. I could tell myself that children don't even really know that suicide exists. I could tell myself these things: I would be wrong. Children think about, attempt, and die by suicide for reasons very similar to those of adults: to escape pain and distress that they find to be intolerable and believe to be interminable and inescapable (Goldman & Beardslee, 1999; Luby et al., 2003; Orbach, 1988; Pfeffer, 1986, 2000). Although the absolute numbers of children who die by suicide is small, more children die by suicide than from all childhood cancers combined (Masecar, 1999). At some stages of cognitive and emotional development and because of their lack of life experience, they may be more vulnerable than adults to believing that even relatively transient difficulties will never end or cannot be resolved. One Canadian researcher reminds us (chillingly) that if we don't educate our children about suicide, television will do it for us (Mishara, 1998). Even before they begin to go to school, children are familiar with suicidal actions from watching cartoons—if not from other media exposure, the conversations of adults, or family experience.

Suicidal thoughts and behaviors are common among children who are receiving mental health treatment, and suicide rates in children age ten to fourteen have increased by 300 percent since 1950 (Pfeffer, 2006). Children who engage in suicidal thinking and behavior are likely to be at higher risk as they grow up (Pfeffer, 2000). When possible, it is ideal for children who are drawn to suicide to be treated by professionals experienced in child therapy under these circumstances (Pfeffer, 2000); but such expertise is not always available. What can we do to make a difference for very young people who are in so much pain that death seems like a solution?

HELPING YOUNG CHILDREN WITH SUICIDAL THOUGHTS AND ACTIONS

We often meet adults who confuse a child's intelligence with their ability to express themselves in words. (Berg & Steiner, 2003, p. 237)

A fundamental challenge in doing helpful therapeutic work with children is *finding a common language* (Masecar, 1999). For solution-focused therapists, this is a particular case of a general focus. All human beings, young or old, are both constrained and enriched as communicators by their individual life experience, their constitutional makeup, and their levels of cognitive, emotional, and physical development. The therapist's task is to find methods or languages that are mutually communicative and that fit with the client's views, preferences, and abilities. The story of Annie illustrates such methods.

Annie

Annie was eight years old when I met her, a sweet, shy girl. Her parents had brought her to the hospital clinic where I worked to meet with a colleague of mine. Although my focus was working with adolescents and their families, I ended up meeting with Annie and her parents because my child-therapist colleague took sick, no one else was available on a short-term basis, and the referral was considered urgent. The referral was made following an incident two days earlier in which Annie had run out in front of a school bus. She survived with only minor injuries because the bus was not moving very fast, and because of quick reactions by both the bus driver and a pair of teenagers loitering outside the school for an illicit smoke. Annie told her teacher, who had arrived on the scene within minutes, that she wanted to be dead and in heaven with her nana. The psychiatrist who saw the girl in the emergency department diagnosed her as "dysphoric" and referred her to my colleague for treatment.

The young parents looked strained and exhausted. They described a series of recent deaths in the family that had left them "stunned." The latest loss was the sudden unexpected death of Annie's maternal grandmother, 59, in a motor vehicle accident. "Nana" had been Annie's regular after-school caretaker since Annie's mother had returned to full-time work when Annie was four years old. What follows is part of my interaction with Annie, a few minutes into our first (and only) interview.

THERAPIST: [*Draws scale from 1 to 10 horizontally on flipchart page*] So if ten, here, stands for happy as can be [*draws happy face beside 10*], and one, here, stands for sad as can be [*draws sad face beside 1*], where are you today, Annie?

ANNIE: [*Touches scale at about 3*]

THERAPIST: Can you put a mark there for today? What color do you want for today? [*Offers box of markers*]

ANNIE: [*Chooses blue, makes a star near 3*]

THERAPIST: Oh, a star, so that's for today. What was your worst day?

ANNIE: [*Points to 1*]

THERAPIST: Can you put a mark there to mean the worst day?

ANNIE: [*Chooses black, makes a scribble*]

THERAPIST: What day was that?

ANNIE: . . . . day I almost got hit.

THERAPIST: Mmm. So today is a better day. . . . by this much? [*Spans 1 to 3 with fingers*]

ANNIE: Yes.

THERAPIST: What makes today better?

ANNIE: . . . Different things.

THERAPIST: Different things can help against sadness.

ANNIE: [*Nods*]

THERAPIST: So these different things would be more on the side of helping your happiness?

ANNIE: [*Nods*]

THERAPIST: Tell me one of the things that helps with your happiness.

ANNIE: Mum took me to MacDonald's.

THERAPIST: You liked that.

ANNIE: [*Nods, very slight smile*] She always says she doesn't really like it, but she eats it all.

THERAPIST: Oh, I see. So Mum taking you to MacDonald's, that's one thing against sadness and on the side of happiness. I wonder . . . how can we show happiness on here [*another flip chart page*]?

ANNIE: [*Draws smiling face with yellow hair, rainbow*]

THERAPIST: *Great.* And this smiling face . . . is that you?

ANNIE: [*Nods*]

THERAPIST: . . . and with a rainbow, this stands for your happiness?

ANNIE: That's right.

THERAPIST: That's an excellent sign for happiness. Can we put on this page some of the different things that are on the side of your happiness? Sort of like . . . Annie's happiness helpers?

ANNIE: [*Nods quickly*] I know another one. [*Picks up crayon, draws cat and writes "Bart" underneath*] My cat, Bart.

For this interview I had available some basic items to help Annie express herself with or without talking: crayons or markers, flipchart, paper or black/white board, clay, a few toys. (One advantage of some training in working with children, of course, is the discovery that such materials are useful not only with children, but with anyone.) The advantage in this particular interaction was that Annie—although not very talkative—turned out to be fluent in the languages of drawing and list-making. Perhaps, like many children, she enjoyed using a flipchart and markers—another small advantage for the stranger-therapist. Therapists more fluent than I in some of the other "languages" children speak use other tools: puppets, toys, stories, games, work with animal partners, and many other creative forms of expression (e.g., Ash, 2007; Berg & Steiner, 2003; Bertolino & Schultheis, 2002; Chang, 1998, 1999; Corcoran, 2002; Freedman and

Combs, 1997; MacLeod, 1986; Pichot and Coulter, 2007; Selekman, 1997; Shilts & Reiter, 2000; Steiner, 2005; Zalter & Ash, 2006).

Annie was also fluent with numbers and was able to use a scale as a vehicle for expressing her feelings. Scaling may be particularly useful with children to help track rapid mood changes, and as a communication tool between Annie and her team and among team members. (Annie's "team" included her parents, her teacher, the therapist who took over working with Annie and her family, and myself. It expanded to include a child psychiatrist, an uncle who was a critical support for both Annie and her parents, and the school social worker, who helped with Annie's reintegration.) At this point we were already aware that if Annie was at a "1" on her scale, she could be in danger of suicidal behavior, and one useful thing to find out would be where on the scale she is likely to be safe ("a little bit of happiness beginning?"). Until then, I suggested exercising special caution if she said she was at 3 or lower. Use of both the scale and the list of happiness helpers helped to provide continuity in the transition from my session with Annie to the therapist who provided ongoing treatment and between the therapist's office, home, and school. All of Annie's team members could collaborate with her in reinforcing, practicing, and adding to the items on her list.

Our initial plan for Annie was that if she was at 3 or below on the scale, a safety plan would begin, including: one parent to be with her at all times, provision of comforts (Bart?), and attempts to introduce one or two things from her list. One of the values of this plan was that it provided some structure for her overwhelmed parents, giving them clear ideas about their "jobs."

ADDITIONAL SAFETY ISSUES

Providing a safe environment is a foundation for recovery for any child. When suicide is an issue, there are additional concrete requirements: "Most important is the availability of guns and firearms. If present, such weapons should be removed" (Pfeffer, 2000, p. 245). Because family members often fail to follow through with therapists' recommendations for the removal or securing of firearms (Brent, Baugher, Brimaher, Kolko, & Bridge, 2000) or other possible weapons, and because they may underestimate children's ability to find

and use guns and ammunition that have been locked away, I follow up
on these suggestions both by telephone and at the next session.

MAKING OUR METHODS CHILD-FRIENDLY

A useful place to start—especially in working with children who
are in acute distress—is with the following assumptions.

Solution-Focused Assumptions About Children

We believe that all children want to:

• Have their parents be proud of them
• Please their parents and other adults
• Be accepted and be part of the social group in which they live
• Learn new things
• Be active and be involved in activities with others
• Be surprised and surprise others
• Voice their opinions and choices
• Make choices when given the opportunity (Berg & Steiner, 2003, p. 18)

The miracle question is at least as interesting to children as to
adults, and as valuable in the therapeutic process. Modifications of
the miracle question for children often involve the use of magic,
magic wands, or allusions to their favorite fairy tales or Disney stories. A child therapist who trained with colleagues of mine suggested
an adaptation that I have used often (Laura Champion & Brenda
Zalter, personal communication, November 4, 1996). A large sheet of
paper is divided into four quadrants, and the child is invited to draw,
paint, or write four scenes. The first is the problem, or "something
you wish was different." Second is the miracle, or magic, or "something *amazing*!" happening. The third scene shows what is different
after the magic. The fourth quadrant can be used in several ways, to
show the effect of the miracle on the client and/or the client's family,
a current exception ("one small thing that is already a little bit like the
miracle"), or a first step from now toward the miracle picture.

As I wrote the last paragraph I had a vivid mental picture of a family that I worked with, a newly "blended" family with five children

between six and fourteen years old. They dealt with a great amount of conflict, and the fourteen-year-old had been diagnosed with depression. I had used the four-quadrant miracle-question task with the younger children, intending to ask the question verbally of the older family members while the younger ones made their pictures. Instead, all of the family members helped themselves to paper and were soon on the floor together, drawing and passing the crayons around. We had time for only a quick debriefing of the pictures before they left. (This was hard on me, because I tend to be word-dependent, but the family seemed satisfied.) They came back to report considerable progress, building on the unexpected commonalities and the hopes and ideas for change they had found in their drawings. The parents told me that they liked my "technique" and had decided that drawing together in this format was a much better way to deal with family disagreements than "discussions" that inevitably turned noisy and rancorous. I had to agree.

Among the many child-friendly solution-focused treatment methods described by Berg and Steiner (2003) is a wonderful discussion of how to use stories—whether read from books, narrated from memory, created for the particular child, or co-constructed with the child's active involvement. One of their suggestions is to use a story as feedback for the child:

> After you finish reading the story, make sure that there is no discussion about it—just read the story and then end the session. There should be no discussion about what the story meant to the child; trust their intuitive ways to understand the meaning and to find useful ways to incorporate this story to their life situations. (Berg and Steiner, 2003, p. 82)

Bruce and the Family Story

Bruce was eleven, the youngest of three sons in a close, hard-working African-Canadian family. His mother and two older brothers had been assaulted and terrorized during a brutal home invasion, and the whole family was badly shaken. The middle brother, sixteen, made a suicide attempt by overdose that left him with renal damage. Bruce's mother, who had a history of childhood trauma, was dealing with flashbacks, nightmares, and intense anxiety. Bruce had been visiting relatives with his father at the time of the home invasion, and everyone felt that he had been the lucky one. As his family struggled and his home became a very tense place, Bruce's increasing withdrawal went more or less unnoticed. He had always been quiet, and his parents thought that he was "fine" until his father found his pistol missing from its locked hiding place. The gun was eventually found, loaded, in Bruce's mattress, and Bruce told his parents enough for them to suspect that he had planned to use it to kill himself. The family was already involved with our clinic, and I was asked to see Bruce.

Bruce was polite and answered all my questions—in his own way. No matter what I asked, he talked about his favorite television show, a family sitcom. He described the characters and their various trials vividly. I had never seen the show, but I learned from him that although it was a comedy, there was an underlying theme of family troubles being resolved through the strength of their connection and loyalty to one another. However rude or selfish these family members might sometimes seem, when the chips were down they always looked out for one another.

I continued to see Bruce despite my reservations about what he was getting—or not getting—from our meetings, because his parents and teacher were delighted with how much better he was doing since beginning "therapy." After three sessions, I finally found an opportunity to watch Bruce's show—*Married with Children*. I was shocked to see the disrespect, hostility, and even outright cruelty of the television family: could this be the loving group that Bruce had been telling me about? In our next session, I listened as Bruce transformed the episode I had just seen, identifying signs of caring and thoughtfulness where I had seen only negativity and narcissism. I realized that Bruce was indeed getting "therapy," and that I had been privileged to watch him provide it for himself. "Trust their intuitive ways to understand the meaning and to find useful ways to incorporate this story to their life situations" (Berg and Steiner, 2003, p. 82).

Chapter 8

Hope and Energy:
Preventing Adolescent Suicide

"Adolescents need here-and-now skills for finding solutions to problems that arise in daily living." (Jobes, 1995, p.152)

"Contrasting a potential positive future with the adolescent's suicidal state may diminish the adolescent's suicidal thinking." (Overholser & Spirito, 2003, p. 36)

SUSAN'S MIRACLE

In the general hospital where I worked for many years, the demand for adolescent and family treatment was high, and community resources were few. My team of three or four professionals operated on a triage model where we saw the most complex, under-resourced teens and families and referred the rest to the handful of other counselors available in the community. An exception to this rule occurred when we were training interns: we tried to begin their practice opportunities with adolescents and families whose concerns were likely to be (we thought) a little more straightforward. So, for Ned, a brand-new intern, we selected a family from the waiting list who might normally have been referred out. According to our forms, Susan, age fifteen, was in conflict with her parents regarding rules about curfew and school performance and attendance.

Ned had extensive training and experience in child therapy and some training, but very little experience, in working with families. He had not encountered solution-focused brief therapy before, but after watching my sessions for a week, reading *Becoming Solution-*

Focused in Brief Therapy (Walter and Peller, 1992), and role-playing some solution-focused questioning with the team, he was eager to experiment with the model. He began well, engaging with each family member—even Susan, who kept her head down and muttered her replies. Following some general discussion about what they wanted from treatment, Ned asked the family the miracle question. The mother and father replied at length, describing how after the miracle Susan would be coming home on time, working hard and doing much better in school, reconnecting with her old friends instead of the "losers" she wanted to be with now, and spending time with the family instead of holing up in her room. Then Ned asked Susan to respond.

NED: Susan, what would you notice after this miracle?

SUSAN: The main thing is that my parents would give me permission to kill myself.

Supervising this session from behind the one-way mirror, I was shaken: concerned for Susan and her parents in the face of this very serious statement, and also concerned for Ned, dealing with suicide risk in his very first family interview. In my head I went into full-blown catastrophizing mode: Ned will never want to work with families again, he'll certainly never ask the miracle question again.* I almost charged into the therapy room to save him. In front of the mirror, though, things went much better.

N: [*Pause, deep breath*] And . . . how would that be better for you?

S: [*Sitting forward, intense*] *Because then I would know that they are really listening to me.*

N: And what difference would that make to you?

S: A lot! If they really listened they would know how bad I feel all the time, they might understand instead of just being mad at me.

N: So . . . what would they be doing that would show you they were really listening to you?

S: I guess. . . well, they would ask how I was and wait for me to really answer before they started telling me what I did wrong that day.

---

*I had never heard Susan's answer to the miracle question before, nor since.

And suddenly the conversation was in very different territory: the territory of solution, the specific territory of setting goals for improving family communication, a much more familiar and comfortable geography for family therapists than the treating-suicidal-adolescents region. For me this session was a lesson in waiting mindfully for therapists, clients, and the solution-focused process to find a way, together, to utilize their strengths and hopes.

Notice that Ned's questions helped Susan focus on what she really wanted: to receive a different kind of attention from her parents. Suicide was the means to that end. Am I saying that Susan was not really at risk? No. Susan was at risk for hurting herself, perhaps at risk of death; she was at risk of all the pain, loneliness, and desperation that can arise from living with the kinds of thoughts she had just expressed; she was at risk of interpreting even her parents' real desires and efforts to make things better as part of a bad story about them not caring for her; she was at risk of making the idea or threat of suicide a solution to her problems. She may have been at risk of rehearsing the suicide-solution scenario in ways that would make it more likely over time. In response to Ned's questions, she was already moving away from that scenario, talking about family interactions that would be part of a better picture. Risk had taken a hit, and safety and hope for the future were gaining.

As the session continued, Ned and the family built a story about exceptions, times even very recently when the family had operated in an attentive, loving and supportive way. After that conversation, I think that Ned could have asked Susan more about her suicidal thinking without derailing the productivity of the session. However, it went differently. When he asked the family if there was anything else before he took a consultation break with the team, Susan's mother asked if Susan had really intended to kill herself, and Susan said that she had thought about it—thought about using painkillers and some of her dad's booze. She reassured her mother that this was not what she really wanted and that she would not act on those thoughts. Everybody cried a little, and her parents told her how much they loved her. When Ned gave them feedback, one of the things that he stressed was that they were now coming up with a "life plan." I tried to imagine how the conversation with Susan might have gone if Ned had responded differently (PN = "Pretend Ned" and PS = "Pretend Susan"):

PN: Susan, what would you notice after this miracle?

PS: The main thing is that my parents would give me permission to kill myself.

PN: . . . And . . . is that something that you have been thinking about?

PS: Yeah. A lot.

PN: For how long?

PS: At least the last year. Lately, all the time.

PN: And do you have a plan for how you would do it?

PS: Yeah.

PN: What is your plan?

PS: Well, I could get drunk on my dad's liquor, since he wouldn't even notice, and take a bunch of pills.

I think that if it continued in this mode for very long, this "pretend" conversation could create a different kind of risk. Instead of focusing on what Susan wants to be different, the session could divert to a sole emphasis on her likelihood for self-harm, with her parents as horri-

---

Solution-Focused Work from Two Points of View

The fifteen-year-old client:

> You were interested in the different ways I did things, always wondering what kind of benefit it had for me. I knew in advance that you would ask me 'what is different', and I wanted to have something different to tell you. Your curiosity made me want to change things quickly. (p. 216)

The therapist:

> [Suicide] must be taken seriously, not just by looking in detail into the method contemplated by the adolescent, the triggering episode, past history, or actions planned, but by engaging a teenager in conversation. This means taking the time to listen, respecting the suicide as a potential means of solution to difficult problems, and being curious about their thinking. Engaged conversation also means . . . trying to determine whether such goals might be achieved through some other means. (p. 211)

(From Berg & Steiner, 2003)

fied, disempowered spectators. One possible outcome is that the family walks away from the session overwhelmed by the magnitude and insolubility of their problems. Pretend Ned could of course move the conversation back to what Pretend Susan wants to be different ("What can happen here today to make it less likely that you will act on that plan?"). However, my experience is that it is more difficult to build positive solutions after intensive focus on problems than to build solutions first and then see how the building process has (already) affected the problems. In the latter option, the discussion about suicide is part of a conversation about change and "life plans."

WORKING WITH "ANGRY YOUNG MEN"

Many practitioners find angry youth challenging, which is one reason that I have included two cases that—although very different—fall within this category. Also, young men (in their teens through young adulthood) who display angry, aggressive, irritable, and impulsive behaviors are at greatly increased risk of suicidal ideation and behavior (American Academy of Pediatrics, 2000; Apter & Freudenstein, 2000; Conner, Meldrum, Wieczorek, Duberstein, & Welte, 2004; Greenhill & Waslick, 1997; Wolfsdorf, Freeman, D'Eramo, Overholser, & Spirito, 2005), especially when they are also engaging in substance abuse (Garrison, McKeown, Valois, & Vincent, 1993). Some researchers have suggested a genetic/neurochemical basis for these behaviors in relation to adolescent suicidality (Bernagie, 2004; Ruescu, 2004). How many of these young men are affected by fetal alcohol, and to what extent, remains an open question (Buxton, 2004). Many of them, if they come to the attention of professional helpers, are diagnosed with conduct disorder or oppositional-defiant disorder, or if a little older, with antisocial personality disorder. Equally fitting diagnoses of depression or posttraumatic stress are often missed in young people (American Academy of Pediatrics, 2000; Apter & Freudenstein, 2000; Pfeffer, 2000), and so aspects of their suffering are also missed—or dis-missed.

Joe: Not a Model Citizen

Joe was fourteen when he was referred to our clinic. He had been seen by a consulting psychiatrist in the emergency room after a group of friends intervened when they came upon him struggling to climb the parapet of a bridge near his home in order to jump. (They subdued him easily because he was falling-down drunk.) The psychiatrist diagnosed Joe as conduct disordered and suggested that follow-up counseling was not indicated because Joe would be unreceptive and was already involved with the justice system. He also evaluated Joe as at low risk for suicide. Joe's mother, however, insisted that he get therapeutic help, and so her son was seen, twice, for an initial consultation. In the first interview, he refused to speak at all. In the second, he was rude and sarcastic and left early after threatening physical harm to the counselor. At that point he and his mother were informed that no further treatment opportunities would be offered. Joe's mother intervened again, begging that his name remain on the waiting list, obtaining a new referral from their family physician, and calling repeatedly asking when he could be seen. The upshot was that when I had a cancellation one morning, the secretarial staff asked me to *please* see Joe so his mother would leave them alone (squeaky wheels . . .).

I had some advantages in my first meeting with Joe. First, I knew that my colleagues' (very reasonable) approaches—in particular, attempts to assess Joe's risk, give him their opinions or advice, or to solicit a "no suicide" contract—had not worked well, so I would do something different. Second, Joe had a court case coming up and his probation officer had strongly advised him to obtain documentation that he had been complying with a previous order for counseling (i.e., he had a "letter deficit," Berg, 1989). Third, my first job was in a correctional facility, so I am desensitized to certain kinds of verbalization and behavior. In fact, I have always enjoyed working with "angry" kids: I usually like their energy, and the fact that they lay things out on the table so readily. (Possibly I am just lazy.) Last, I had been learning and practicing the solution-focused approach to work with mandated clients, utilizing the perspectives of referring individuals while staying within the client's own frame of reference (De Jong & Berg, 2002; Osborn, 1999; Rosenberg, 2000; Tohn & Oshlag, 1996).

Joe, Session 1

HF: So, what brings you here today?

J: [*Sarcastic*] The bus.

HF: How can I be helpful?

J: Beats me.

HF: What were you hoping to get out of coming here today?

J: I was hoping to get people off my back.

HF: How will it be better for you when people are off your back?

J: Oh God, my mother bugs me all the time, moaning about stuff I say when I'm pissed, always nagging about my drinking and my fucking "state of mind"—like she had a clue about it! And my fucking PO, like it's not bad enough I have to go to see him in the first place, he's breathin' down my neck about "counseling." No wonder I want to check out. My girlfriend, I mean my *ex*-girlfriend, *everybody*'s bugging me.

HF: Sounds rough. What if all those people do get off your back? How will that be better for you?

J: I'll be cool.

HF: Cool how?

J: Not so pissed off all the time. I can do what I want, be with my friends without all this *hassle*.

HF: When you're not so pissed off, what will you be instead?

J: I'll be . . . better than now.

HF: What else?

J: I don't know.

HF: [*Waits*]

J: . . . happier?

HF: That sounds good. So to get to this point, what would it take to get your mother off your back?

J: I don't know! You're the fucking shrink!

HF: I don't have a clue.

J: Christ! *She*'s the one who needs to go to counseling, so she can relax. The woman needs to take a downer.

HF: How would that help?

J: She might stop worrying and hassling me all the time.

HF: What could help her with that?

J: How should I know?

HF: Well, I've never met your mum. You know her well. In your opinion, what do you think would help her to calm down?

J: . . . Maybe if she thought I was going to be all right.

HF: What will that look like?

J: Huh?

HF: How will she know that you're going to be all right? What would it take to convince her?

J: I don't know.

HF: [*Waits*]

J: You're just going to fucking sit there, aren't you?

HF: [*Nods*] I'm really interested in what you think about this.

J: [*Shakes his head*] *Jeez.* I suppose she'd have to see me not getting in trouble with the cops, going to school, not saying stuff to her about checking out.

HF: Checking out?

J: Killing myself. But I only said it when I was drunk.

HF: I see. What else?

J: Just being a fucking model citizen in every way. No, that would shock her too much. Don't want to kill her outright.

HF: Glad you're realistic. I'd like to ask you something else, to help me figure out where to go next.

J: Where to go next.

HF: Yes.

J: You have a lot of fucking weird questions.

HF: Yes I do. Kind of a specialty of mine.

J: [*Shakes his head*] Okay.

HF: On a scale from one to ten, if ten stands for "I would do anything to solve this problem," and one stands for "I wouldn't lift a finger," where are you?

J: I'm ten! I've got to get a break from all this!

HF: So you're determined to show her. What's the first small step you can take?

Joe: Risk and Resource

Risk. Joe exhibits a number of warning signs (Appendix C) for imminent danger of suicide: suicidal ideation ("checking out"), substance abuse, anger, recklessness. His chosen method is relatively available with high lethality. In addition, he has had a recent loss ("my *ex*-girlfriend") and is in conflict with important people in his life (his mother is one of the people "on his back"). He has made a previous attempt, is on probation and has had trouble with the cops, and isn't going to school. His father had been absent since he was an infant. He is a young Canadian male. His verbal style and reluctance to engage have made it difficult for him to receive available help.

Despite this rather daunting picture of suicide risk, Joe would probably not be viewed as in immediate danger by most assessors. For one thing, the impulsive and state-dependent nature of his suicidal behavior means that the timing of his appearance in an assessment situation would rarely coincide with his periods of highest risk. On the other hand, the impulsive and state-dependent nature of his suicidal behavior presents major treatment challenges.

Resource. Joe is energetic, articulate, and engaged. He swears a lot, but as conversation, not as a weapon: his language is a congruent expression of his opinions and feelings. He has a strong advocate in his mother, and he is strongly connected to her: doesn't want her to die outright, wants the relationship to be less conflictual, and is uncomfortably aware of her distress and her worry over him. He has friends, and they are important to him, an excellent indication that he is developmentally on track in this important way. In fact, a number of people care about his survival and want his life to change for the better—even his ex-girlfriend. Joe wants to be happier, he wants to be "cool," and he is able to envision what might contribute to these changes. He is able to set goals: getting people off his back and staying out of detention (i.e., doing what he needs to for me to write him a letter). He is highly motivated ("ten!"). He has a sense of humor, however sarcastic its current expression. He demonstrates, just by showing up and by talking responsively with me, abilities for self-control, and frustration tolerance. Paradoxically, the impulsive and state-dependent nature of his risk can be seen as a resource in the sense that for significant periods of time he is not engaged in suicidal thinking and planning, and those times may be a window of opportunity for building and utilization of more hope-friendly skills, resources, and connections.

Joe: Utilizing Resource and Reducing Risk; or, Getting People off His Back

I suggested that Joe investigate how much he could control his mother's excessive worrying and nagging by observing when she *was* off his back, what he was doing at those times, and how he could do more of whatever that was. (Although I might have capitalized on his high level of motivation to suggest a more active task, I was also aware that at other times and in other states—especially when drinking—his motivation was likely to be quite different. I wanted to suggest something that he could do successfully.) He also agreed that I could talk with his mother about his safety and how she could help without bugging him. He decided to come back for a second session in two weeks.

Because of time constraints (she worked two jobs, one a night shift), I never met face-to-face with Joe's mother Evelyn, although we had a series of telephone conversations and developed a plan. Evelyn invited Joe's closest friends over for coffee. This was a first: she had been suspicious of his friends because they were older and had been in trouble. She asked for their support of an agreement that Joe would drink only in their company. The friends had been alarmed by the bridge incident and understood the risk presented by his solitary drinking. They signed on readily, as did Joe. Evelyn also passed on to them information from me about where they could call or go with any questions or concerns. This harm reduction plan offered no guarantees—but it was something that we could do.

One of the unforeseen consequences of this plan was that Joe's friends began to drink a little more responsibly (e.g., choosing a designated driver so that someone was sober to watch out for Joe). One of them appointed himself volunteer liaison with Evelyn, and would call or sometimes drop in to let her know that Joe was okay.

I saw Joe for nine sessions over the next year. Although he reported that at first he continued to think about jumping when he drank, this diminished. The frequency of his drinking also diminished. Joe's friends (bless them) were vigilant; at least as important, he knew that they were watching out for him. The primary focus of our sessions was his increasing fascination with how much control he had over how people treated him, and his behavioral "experiments" with getting more of what he wanted in his relationships by acting differently himself. (His descriptions of how adults treated him depending on which way he wore his ball cap were perceptive, fascinating, and hilarious.) Our relationship continued to be a source of frustrated amusement to him: he often teased me about making him do all the work, and I agreed that it was a wonderful arrangement. Joe dropped out of school but decided quickly that even if the regimentation of academics was not for him, working in a fast-food "factory" wasn't for him either. He kept the job, but finished high school in an alternative program. In my last conversation with Evelyn, she told me that he had gone to Western Canada to stay with an uncle and learn welding.

Joe: What Worked?

In order to get Joe's attention and help him focus on setting and pursuing goals, it was useful to stick to the position that he was the expert on his own life, rather than joining a long list of people who were telling him what was good for him, with negligible or negative impact. We were able to find a mutually acceptable collaborative goal: getting people off his back. Collaboration was facilitated when I remedied Joe's "letter deficit" with a brief report to the court stating that he was coming to "counseling." Taking steps to keep him safe (i.e., working with his mother and the harm reduction plan) was essential. Evelyn's implementation of the harm reduction agreement with Joe and his friends had the side effect of creating a collaborative relationship ("Joe's team") among Evelyn and Joe's friends. Joe's active "experiments" increased his sense of personal and interpersonal efficacy. And, I liked him. Having surrendered any attempt to control his behavior, it was easy to appreciate Joe's energy, intelligence, and wit.

Dan: Mad at God

Dan was nineteen and had graduated from a vocational high school with a cooking certificate. I had first seen him five months before, when his family doctor referred him after Dan's closest friend died by suicide (see Chapter 13). In that session, Dan talked about the pain of his loss, about surviving his own thoughts of suicide with the support of his girlfriend, and about using alcohol as a "pause button" when he was overwhelmed with images of his friend's death.

Dan left town to start a new job immediately after our first meeting. He called for a second session ten months later, and came in looking pale, thin, and unkempt. He seemed very tense, clenching and unclenching his hands, shifting in his seat, speaking with intensity and sometimes half-crying as we talked.

Dan, Session 2

HF: Hi Dan, been a while. What's been different since we met last?

DAN: Nothing good.

HF: Nothing at all? Not one small thing?

D: Nothing I can think of. I'm mad at the world. Mad at *everyone*, *everything*. Mad at God. Him most of all.

HF: Mad . . . that's very different from last time. How long have you been feeling this way?

D: I don't know, this last week for sure. I've been sober six days, the longest time since I saw you last.

HF: Six days . . . how have you managed it?

D: Going to meetings every day, usually two or three. I'll probably go today after I leave here.

HF: How have the meetings helped?

D: I don't know if they have helped. I mean, they help me stay sober but being sober means no escape.

HF: So they help in one way.

D: Sure, I couldn't do this on my own. [*Shakes his head*] I've been on and off the wagon so many times since I saw you. Never lasted more than a day and a half.

HF: You tried a lot of times.

D: Yeah, and failed.

HF: That must have been really hard. And yet . . . you kept trying.

D: Well, yeah. Dr. Wilson told me I would die if I kept on like I was, and I believed him.

HF: You wanted to live.

D: [*Sarcastic*] You'd think so, wouldn't you?

HF: Mmm . . . something has kept you trying, Dan.

D: Damned if I know what it is. I'm living in hell more now than I was before. I feel like shit. I tried to kill myself four days ago.

HF: How did you survive?

D: I had the belt around my neck, I was ready to jump. [*Plaintive*] I was looking *forward* to it.

HF: How did you stop?

D: I didn't stop, I was *stopped*. [*Hands still, leans toward therapist*] This Big Loud Voice said, [*loudly*] "*What the* hell *are you doing?! Get down from there* right now *and get yourself some help!*"

Dan's statement presented me with a powerful invitation to speculate. I had many possibilities for speculative response, from asking him how long he had been hearing voices and exploring possible "psychotic symptomatology," to wondering about which aspect of himself had created this big loud voice.

However, Steve de Shazer's advice for therapists rang in my mind: "If you have a hypothesis about a client, take two aspirins and go to bed. With any luck it will be gone by morning." I managed to resist temptation, and focused on the fact that he stopped and how he had done that. Assuming that he had made a decision was a solution-focused reflex:

HF: Whoa! . . .and you decided to listen.

D: Well yeah. I mean this big loud voice . . . but now I don't know what to do. I feel like I lost my direction in life. I lost my girlfriend, I lost my job, I lost Mark. I don't seem to have any reasons for living. I'm working in a diner for God's sake. That's professional suicide if you want to be a chef.

I could easily focus on the impact of Dan's losses and his growing despair. However, there are other interesting aspects of Dan's statement. One is that *he* raises the importance of reasons for living. Working to increase or reinforce reasons for living is generally easier than trying to destroy or weaken reasons for dying. Also, in Dan's statement he says that he doesn't *seem* to have any reasons for living, which is quite different from a flat statement that he has none. He had disclosed that he is working and that he still wants to be a chef. This ambition is an idea about a better future. All of these are worth exploring, but first I return to the importance of the experience that helped him to survive.

HF: Mmm . . . and this big loud voice. A powerful experience.

D: God yeah. There's something out there that wants me to live. Something big.

HF: Something out there that wants you to live. [*Writes*]

D: Whether I want to or not.

HF: Something wants you to live, even at times when you aren't sure if you want to or not.

D: Yeah. I thought it might be Mark, but it didn't sound like him.

HF: Mark would want you to live.

D: Yeah. I think he would. But dying sure looks better from here.

HF: Reasons for living are important. And yours have been shifting around on you.

D: That's one way to put it.

HF: Okay. You said you want to be a chef. If I remember right, that's a long-standing plan.

D: Yeah. I thought maybe if I could keep going to meetings for a while I might go back to school.

HF: Really!

D: Yeah, go to college, get some better credentials so I could get a real job.

HF: You've figured out the kind of job you want.

D: Yeah, nothing like this burgers and gravy crap. Some authenticity.

HF: Authenticity. Now that's an interesting word to use . . . do you mean in the food, or the restaurant, or. . . . ?

D: Well, both. [*Sits up a little, hands still*] Like the Creekside, they never really made a go of it but they were sincere, the whole approach had congruence.

HF: These things make a real difference to you, don't they?

D: Yeah.

HF: . . . Just in your work with food, or in other ways also?

D: Absolutely in cooking. And yeah, other ways too. Nothing matters without those things.

HF: When was the most recent time that you experienced even a moment of authenticity, or sincerity, or congruence?

D: . . .There was this guy talking in a meeting last week. I almost didn't go that day, I had about had it.

HF: So, how did you get there?

D: Don't know. Just. . . walked myself there. Felt the whole time like I just couldn't do it.

HF: "Something out there wants you to live."

D: Maybe. Don't think I got there on my own.

I had no idea what authenticity, sincerity, and congruence meant to Dan in the context of cooking. The important thing was that those words meant something to *him:* he was focused, energized, and passionate as he used them. They were critical to his view of a life worth living: "nothing means anything without those things." Connecting these factors to someone he had met in his recovery program reinforced another positive connection. He had gone to Alcoholics Anonymous on a very bad day through his own agency: "walked myself there." And he was respectful of the Big Loud Voice. His decision to call me had come on the heels of that experience, an especially good sign given that he had previously been unwilling to seek help. Dan had also begun to talk in concrete terms about hopes and possibilities for his future. In thinking about feedback for Dan, I wanted to utilize and reinforce these factors.

Post-Break Message to Dan

HF: So, Dan, this has been a *very* difficult time for you. I am so struck by how, in spite of all you are going through, you have made some important decisions in your life: First, you decided to get sober— and that's never easy, for anyone. Then—and this is a big one— you decided to listen to that big loud voice. And to act on what it told you. Even without knowing, quite yet, what that voice is. And somehow, in all of this, you also figured out something critical to your future: a pathway to work with authenticity, sincerity, and congruence. You have even—and this surprised me—been able to notice some real-life examples of authenticity, sincerity, and congruence in people you are coming to know, people you have made a connection with and are actually going to see later today even.

I've written down a few things on this card—things you have said today that I think are important to remember and perhaps to remind yourself of from time to time. You'll know better than I would when that might be useful. It says: "Something out there wants me to live." And underneath: "Authenticity, sincerity, congruence." My suggestion to you is to keep doing the things that give you chances to experience authenticity, sincerity, and congruence in yourself and others; and to stay watchful for further signs that "something out there" wants you to live.

I think, by the way, that your idea about taking Dr. Wilson up on his offer to start going to his meeting is another good decision. When should we talk again?

Dan: Follow-Up

I saw Dan just once more, because he pursued his plans for going back to school and soon began a part-time course at a chef training school in another city. These plans were his main focus in our session. He was still sober, still going to meetings. He had discovered a long list of instances of authenticity, sincerity, and congruence, many of them at AA meetings and even one or two in his family. I wondered about his own recent actions and if the way he had chosen to respond to some of the hardships in his life demonstrated authenticity, sincerity, or congruence, and he acknowledged that they might and we talked about how. The Big Loud Voice had not spoken again, and Dan seemed to accept the Voice as an aspect of the spirituality that had been a core interest for him and Mark before Mark's death.

WHEN THE ANSWER IS "I DON'T KNOW"

A chapter on working with adolescents seems like a reasonable place to discuss the "I don't know" answer. Therapists can feel blocked, "resisted," frustrated, or protective when clients say they don't know. Clients' "I don't know" answers can sound like invitations for therapists to air their own good ideas about what clients should do. If they don't know, then we have to help them out—or do we? And how is taking over "their" therapy helping? Perhaps other ways of viewing this answer can help us to be more flexible in our responses to it.

Steve de Shazer once said that "I don't know" was his *favorite* answer, because it left so many options open (personal communication, August 20, 1992). "Our colleague, Dan Gallagher says that 'I don't know' means 'Be quiet—I'm thinking' (personal communication, 2000)" (de Shazer et al., 2007, p. 66). A psychodynamically oriented supervisor suggested that saying "I don't know" was a defensive posture adopted by adolescents as part of a normal separation process— so it means the young person is on track developmentally. A child therapist told me that when a teenager says "I don't know," he or she is then "off the hook" for having the right answer and is free to speculate or wonder or just try to respond. Gale Miller (de Shazer, Berg, & Miller, 1995) explained that saying "I don't know" violates one of the tacit rules of human conversation, that is, that conversation means taking turns, and that "I don't know" is not a complete turn. Therefore, if we just wait, most people will get uncomfortable and come up with an answer. A description of how conversations are structured among First Nations people living on the Warm Springs Reservation in central Oregon offers another angle:

> Answers to questions are not obligatory. Absence of answers merely means that the floor is open, or continues to belong to the questioner. This does not mean, however, that the question will not be answered later. Nor does it mean that it ought not to be raised again, since the questioner might reasonably assume his audience had time to think about it. (Philips, 1973, p. 81, in Ross, 1996, p. 109)

Sometimes even unanswered questions have a useful impact: "A mind that is stretched to a new idea never returns to its original dimensions" (Oliver Wendell Holmes, in Ross, 1996, p. 113). And finally, I wonder if "I don't know" may constitute really good news in some conversations about suicide. If the client has been very certain that nothing can change for the better and suicide is the only solution, then isn't "I don't know" a step forward?

Options for Responding to "I Don't Know"

- Just wait. (the number 1 option) If you can, wait mindfully.
- Wait, and tell clients to take their time.
- "Suppose you did know, what would you say?" This is obviously an absurd question, and the first time that I heard it asked (by Insoo Kim Berg), I was in awe at what a master therapist can get away with. Since then I have heard this question asked, and asked it myself, many times—and almost every time, have also heard it answered.
- "When you know, what will you say?" This is a different question from the last (present-focused) one, because it specifically invites clients to look toward a future in which they know more about solutions than they do now.
- "What will be your first step toward figuring out an answer?"
- "What will be the first sign that you have begun to figure this out?"
- "How will it be different when you do know?"
- "What would your best friend say?"
- "What needs to happen first so that you can have an answer?"
- "Of course you don't know, it's a tough question. What do you think?" (de Shazer, interviewing a client, 1998)

RELATIONSHIPS AND RELATIONSHIP QUESTIONS

Even for a person who has acquired the capability for suicide and perceives him- or herself to be a burden, there remains one "saving grace"—belongingness. In my view, if the need to belong is satisfied, the will to live remains intact. (Joiner, 2005, p. 117)

Many years ago I met a thirteen-year-old girl, Tanya, who explained to me (an ignorant adult) the various important social groups in her school: preppies, rock-ons, skinheads, etc. "And I" she said, with evident pride, "belong to the loser group." Tanya made it very clear that it was *belonging to the group* that mattered. To be a loser among other, companion losers was obviously very different than being a loser alone. It was a valuable lesson in the protective power of group affiliation.

The National Longitudinal Study on Adolescent Health in the U.S. surveyed 90,000 students in grades 7 to 12 and found that the number one protective factor against suicidal behavior was "a feeling of connectedness" (Schools and Suicide, 2006, p. 26). When adolescents are in trouble, they prefer to talk to friends rather than family members and family members rather than helpers of any kind (Chiarelli et al., 2000). In fact, male adolescents' first choice when asked, "Who would you talk to . . . ?" is "no one" (Chiarelli et al., 2000). One implication of these findings is that professional helpers need to look at how their services can be more "youth friendly." A second is the critical importance of working with most youth in a relationship framework, whether by actively engaging members of their social worlds as a helping team or by using relationship questions: "What would your best friend say?"

I find relationship questions to be valuable in virtually any helping conversation, but in conversations with adolescents they are found gold. "How will your friend know that you are doing better?" is often much easier for teens to answer than direct questions about their own thoughts, feelings and actions. This makes sense developmentally: even when adolescents are unsure about who they are, they *are* sure that the best friend bond is uniquely strong and significant, and that a friend could have something useful to say about them. And teens often spend considerable time thinking about how they are viewed by others, so relationship questions tend to get their attention. Also, the normal egocentricity of adolescence may contribute to close-mindedness about the impact of their actions—including suicidal actions—on others. Relationship questions, also known as "other—perspective questions" (Lethem, 2003, p.120) can penetrate that constraint. In some circumstances, it may even be useful to ask: "Who will suffer the most if you make yourself 'dead'?" (Metcalf, 1998, p.115), or "*How* will you being gone be better for your mother/pet/ teacher/ . . . ?" Almost always we can ask what difference it will make to a friend or family member to know that the young person is working on life goals instead of on dying.

Dan, Joe, and Susan all made progress that was shaped and made possible by their significant relationships. Adolescents who need help are more likely to get it, more likely to engage in treatment, and more likely to benefit if that treatment happens in a systemic context, or if we can tap into systemic resources by using relationship questions.

Chapter 9

Teamwork with Natural Systems I: Collaborating with Clients' Parents and Peers

PARENTS HELPING/HELPING PARENTS

One of Rudd and Joiner's (1998) evidence-based practice recommendations for treatment of adolescents who are suicidal is to "involve parents or guardians in the initial assessment, treatment planning, and ongoing suicide risk assessment process. Acknowledge their helpful contributions and empower them to have positive influences in their roles as parents and caregivers" (p. 444). In this approach they echo other leading practitioners and professional groups (e.g., American Academy of Pediatrics, 2000; Ashworth, 2001; Berman, Jobes, & Silverman, 2005; Borman, 2003; Donaldson, Spirito, & Overholser, 2003; Group for the Advancement of Psychiatry, 1996; Hazell, 2000).

In practice, however, the involvement of parents often amounts to using them only as factual informants; acknowledgement and empowerment of their positive influence is relatively rare. Furthermore, even if their children are in treatment, the parents may be excluded, perhaps because the treatment of choice is individual or group therapy for the child, because confidentiality requirements prevent therapists from sharing with parents, because the young person rejects family therapy, or because the family has to wait for that service. Even when family intervention does occur in a timely fashion, it may not address many of the parents' pressing concerns. (I would like to think that biased and inaccurate views of parents as responsible for their children's troubles do not also affect mental health treatment practice, but I know that such prejudices still exist—even among those who should know better.)

Whatever the reasons, excluding parents has two important negative effects. First, they are left without professional support and guidance in what is often a state of acute personal shock and distress. Second, one of the most valuable suicide prevention resources available in work with young people—the "frontline" intervention of informed parents—is wasted. Inability or failure to include such valuable resources impairs treatment effectiveness and may have tragic consequences (Trautman, 1989). There have been a few documented attempts in the literature to include parents in a timely fashion (e.g., Brent, Poling, McKain, & Slaughter, 1993; Hazell, 2000; Kruesi et al., 1999; Rotheram-Borus et al., 1996; Rotheram-Borus et al., 2000; Zimmerman, Asnis, & Schwartz, 1995). Research findings have demonstrated that parents readily acquire useful knowledge and intentions regarding suicide prevention (Maine, Shute, & Martin, 2001), and that engaging parents in the treatment process immediately after an adolescent child makes a suicide attempt increases the likelihood that the young person will follow through with treatment recommendations (Rotheram-Borus et al., 2000; Rotheram-Borus et al., 1996); but these efforts have yet to become mainstream practice.

Justice Michael Sheehan is a parent who lost a child to suicide, and is an eloquent and impassioned advocate for collaborative treatment efforts:

> Involving the family gives professionals additional sources of information. It allows them to get the whole picture at the outset. It allows the family to be "clued in" to the danger at had and to understand the reason and the importance of . . . the treatment . . . It allows family members to accomplish their role as primary supporters and to keep professionals informed . . . Involving the family allows professionals to "practice what they preach": that "getting help is a sign of strength, not weakness." (Sheehan, 2005, p. 6)

A Psychoeducational Group Program for Parents

> I believe that when all is said and done, all you can do is to show up for someone in crisis, which seems so inadequate. But then

when you do, it can radically change everything. Your thereness, your stepping into a scared parent's line of vision, can be life-giving, because often everyone else is in hiding—especially, at first, the parents. So you come to keep them company when the whole world is falling apart, and your being there says that just for this moment, this one tiny piece of the world is OK, or at least better. (Lamott, 1999, pp. 163-164)

In 1988, concerned about treatment waiting lists for adolescents who had made suicide attempts in the hospital where I worked, I decided to offer a psychoeducational group program for their parents as a way to facilitate a safer "holding environment" until the teens could be seen in treatment. My primary goals were to increase parents' information about suicide prevention, and thereby their ability to intervene appropriately and effectively, and to support parents in coping with emotional reactions that are very natural in the circumstances, but that might hamper their ability to act. Such reactions include paralyzing anxiety, helplessness, and denial. Denial can be very helpful in countering the overwhelming impact of a child's vulnerability, but could also increase the risk that critical warning signs might be overlooked.

I designed a three-hour, single-session evening program (Fiske, 19923, 1998b) in which I taught parents about risk factors and warning signs, how to recognize a crisis and what to do, the necessity of means restriction, the importance of finding professional help, and where and how to get it. I used an educational video, overhead transparencies, and lots of handouts (e.g., earlier versions of Fiske, 2004b).

My hope was that a single "educational" session would be less scary than a commitment for treatment, and that parents who might otherwise avoid mental health professionals could experience a relatively benign introduction to the system, and perhaps be more likely to engage in treatment and/or to support their child's involvement. I expected that parents might agree to attend most readily if we were able to make the referral in the immediate aftermath of a crisis. I wanted to emphasize that the long lists of "risk factors" were all things for which help was possible and available, and that modeling appropriate help-seeking was something they could do for their children. I thought that this point of view might motivate some parents to get help for themselves when they needed it. I hoped to help parents begin to focus on something concrete that they could do immediately that would make a difference. These various hopes and expectations were largely borne out over the twelve years that I ran the program.

I realized quickly that two factors were probably more potent than any information resources I could provide. The first factor was group identification. I could see the weight begin to lift from the shoulders of those parents as they met other good people who were in the same boat and who loved their children and were doing their best. The second factor was that I didn't have horns and fangs, was generally polite and kindly, and offered them a hot beverage and a cookie. Most of the parents had come to the program in considerable fear, fully expecting that I (the "expert") would be shaking my finger at them and telling them what they had done wrong to land their children in this mess.

And here is the remarkable thing: *they came anyway.* Not only did they come despite their anxiety and their expectation of blaming and chastisement, they walked through a door with a big sign that said: "Psychoeducational Group Program for Parents of Suicidal Adolescents." Aside from being unimaginative, that title was an unkind announcement and reminder of the ordeal those parents were experiencing. I decided to make some changes.

Getting to What Parents Can Do

I started by changing the title of the program to "Parents in Crisis"—still problem-focused, I think now, but more accurate in many ways, and the parents preferred it. I also began a practice of telling parents as soon as they arrived how impressed I was that they were able to show up, how it was a hard thing to do and that doing it said something important about their commitment to their child. I saw the difference that those words made immediately.

I was learning about solution-focused therapy by then, and as time went on the program was increasingly shaped by that learning. Pichot and Dolan (2003) suggest that the integration of solution-focused practice occurs in stages, from adopting one or two "techniques" to living and breathing the philosophy of the approach. I went through those stages as I put the program through step-by-step shifts, from being a package that I delivered to the parents to something more like a collaborative conversation with them about what could help their children.

I changed content: we still talked about risk factors and warning signs, but now we talked about protective factors and signs of progress too, and about what works, about good outcomes and how to support and maintain positive changes when they began. I scrapped my recommendations about how to cope and started to ask them for theirs. I prefaced all of the content by reminding them that they knew their child and their family and I didn't, so it was up to them to decide what applied or fit, and what didn't.

I changed format: the program began with questions about what they wanted from it, and ended with their evaluations. I stopped the educational video often and asked their opinions about what was or was not useful and how realistic the scenarios were. What would they do the same or differently? What would their child say?

I changed my language: from mostly statements to mostly questions, from "how you should handle this" to "how do you" and "how will you."

I *really* changed format: I presented it as a "menu" and asked parents for their selections. I started to do opening warm-up exercises in which they identified some of their strengths as parents, and some of their child's strengths (see Nelson, 2005, for ideas about such exercises). I encouraged them to develop "action plans."

When I left the hospital in 2000, the program was called "What Parents Can Do."

Generalizing

In many clinical situations we see parents on their own or in family therapy rather than in groups. We may see parents whose suicidal child is an adult. However, many of the interventions used in the group still apply, for example: complimenting parents on their commitment to their child in a difficult situation, and asking what they want from treatment, how their child will know that the parents are getting on track, and what will be signs of progress for their child. We can ask the miracle question, and use scaling to look for pre-session change and progress on goals. We can support parents' good ideas about helping and coping. Holding steady to assumptions that parents are resources for their children, and observing and reinforcing the ways in which that happens, is an excellent platform for helpful work with parents.

Assumptions About Parents

Until proven otherwise, we believe that all parents want to:

- Be proud of their child
- Have a positive impact on their child
- Hear good news about their child and learn what their child is good at
- Give their child a good education and a good chance at success
- See that their child's future is better than theirs
- Have a good relationship with their child
- Be hopeful about their child (Berg & Steiner, 2003, p. 17)

A final word: "When we see parents who 'sabotage' their child's therapy, it is most likely that the therapist has not given proper credit for the child's progress to the client" (Berg & Steiner, 2003, p. 234).

FRIENDS

When Lois Lane asks Superman, "Who are you?" he replies, "A friend." That makes him, above all else, a symbol of hope. In the face of adversity, hope often comes in the form of a friend who reaches out to us. (Christopher Reeve, 2002, pp. 158-159)

She was someone to hold the belief that my life was worth living. (DeQuincy Levine, in Bright Mind, 2006, p. 14)

I sometimes wince as I remember how many times over the years I found a client waiting for me with "a friend," and how many times I shook the friend's hand, exchanged a little small talk, and then went off to speak with my client—leaving that extraordinary resource just sitting there, untapped. I hate waste, and I was wasteful in not jumping on the opportunity to meet with and learn from anyone interested, caring, or curious enough to accompany a friend to the therapist's office! I did this even with adolescents, despite working with adolescents as much as I did, and knowing how important friendship is for them. I routinely worked with both adolescents and adults in groups because I wanted to tap into the positive power of affiliation, and in families because I wanted to tap into systemic strengths—and still I left those potential treasures in the waiting room time after time.

Research findings suggest that perceived social isolation is a risk factor for suicide (Joiner, 2005), that social/friendship networks are a protective factor for suicidal behavior (Bille-Brahe & Jensen, 2004; Evans, Smith, Hill, Albers, & Neufeld, 1996), and that we should facilitate our clients' development and use of such networks (e.g., Eagles, Carson, Begg, and Naji, 2003). Adolescents consistently say that they would be more likely to talk to a friend about something that bothers them, rather than a family member, teacher, or helping professional (Chiarelli et al., 2000; Hawton, Rodham, & Evans, 2006). Very few practitioners have reported on efforts to utilize supportive peer connections in work with troubled adolescents (e.g., Bertolino, 1999; Laszloffy, 2000; Selekman, 1993). Morrissette (1992; Morrissette & McIntyre, 1989) strongly recommends encouraging homeless youth to maintain their social networks and inviting their peers to planning meetings. Solution-focused practitioners have long advocated deciding whom to include in a therapy session "based on who shows up; whoever walks in the door is seen" (de Shazer et al., 2007, p. 5). Tom and his friends helped me to understand the value of putting these ideas more fully into practice (Fiske, 1992).

Tom and His Friends

In the session transcripts excerpted in the following section, Tom was seventeen and in his last year of high school. He had recently been seen in the hospital emergency room following a suicidal "gesture" of taking twenty acetaminophen. Tom admitted the overdose to his mother, who brought him to the hospital, where the consulting psychiatrist referred him for follow-up psychotherapy to treat negative body image and eating disorder symptoms seen as "underlying" his suicidal thinking and behavior. The psychiatrist also noted a family history of depression, bipolar illness, and suicide, which included the death by suicide of an older cousin and the recurrent, cyclic depressions experienced by his mother. My first two sessions with Tom were very positive. He wanted to "put that [the suicide attempt] behind me and move on." We talked about his hatred of school, of not fitting in, and of his hopes for the future. His miracle picture focused on moving forward in his aspirations to be an actor and on being able to tolerate disappointment and criticism in both his acting and his personal life without falling into a pattern of self-denigration and hopelessness. Homework suggestions consisted of observations and experiments related to his developing capacity to deal with negative emotions.

Tom, Session 3

HF: Hi, Tom, what's better?

T: Oh . . . I don't know.

HF: [*Waits*]

T: I'm not so good.

HF: Not so good?

T: Yeah. A lot of stuff has gone wrong, but I don't think that's it, mainly. I just feel like it's all too much and it isn't worth it. I keep thinking about dying and it seems like the answer.

HF: So there's been a lot of stuff . . . but right now it's just all too much.

T: [*Nods*]

HF: So much that right now dying seems like an answer.

T: Yeah.

HF: Has it felt so bad that you have thought about making yourself die?

T: All the time. I want to take my mother's pills with some gin that I have . . . I tried at first to think about something else but it just keeps coming back, I can't turn it off.

HF: So that thought has almost taken over. How much of the time is it there?

T: I don't know, maybe ninety percent of the time.

HF: How do you keep it out for ten percent?

T: I don't know. What do you mean?

HF: I mean that from what you said, this thought has taken over ninety percent of your thinking, but you have somehow managed to keep ten percent of your thoughts to yourself. How have you managed to do that?

T: I didn't want to give in completely, to just hate myself.

HF: So you really wanted to fight this self-hatred.

T: I guess. But I don't feel like I can. It's too strong.

HF: It feels really strong. . . . like it's already taken over ninety percent of your thinking and you're not sure how you can fight it?

T: Yeah.

HF: What could help?

T: I don't know.

HF: [*Waits*]

T: What do you mean?

HF: Well, what quality in you could help you fight this?

T: You mean, like, what are my good qualities? I don't see any.

HF: If you could see a quality in you that could help in the fight against self-hatred, what would it be?

T: . . . I guess . . . my creativity?

HF: Your creativity! How can it help?

T: Everyone says it's the strongest part of my personality. . . . Any time I have liked myself, it's usually been when I was being creative.

HF: Can you tell me a bit about that?

We talked further about his creativity, the experience of acting, his particular skills and ambitions, his enjoyment of drawing and painting. Tom was fully engaged by the creative process and so less vulnerable to despondency and suicidal thoughts.

[*Later in session*]

HF: Thank you for explaining that. I'm really getting a picture of how strong your creativity is and how it can be a real ally in the fight against self-hatred. I'm putting it at the top of my list. So . . . what else should be on here? What else can help in this fight?

T: I guess my friends.

HF: Whose name should go first?

T: Natalie. I can always talk to her.

HF: How does talking to her make a difference to you?

T: I just feel better when I tell her stuff and she still feels the same about me.

HF: Okay. Whose name should be next?

T: Justin.

HF: How is Justin an ally against self-hatred?

We continued to add "allies" to his list, and soon came to Tom's mother. I asked Tom if she was aware of how he had been struggling lately, and when he said no, whether she would want to know. He thought that she would want to and probably should know. We called her from the session to tell her what was going on with him, that he was doing a little better than at the beginning of the session and meant to continue resisting thoughts of self-harm. She was concerned but glad to be informed and to know that Tom was "working on it." We agreed that she would remove her pills from the home and check in with Tom on a regular basis until he had at least a week free of suicidal thoughts.

At the end of the session, I complimented Tom on his creative skills and activities, as well as on the important personal relationships he had developed, as seen in his list of "allies." I asked him to do something to "activate" his alliances, and we talked about options, co-creating another list.

Tom's List of Options for Activating His Alliances

- Go to friends' party on Friday night (he noted that this seemed very challenging right now)
- Call Natalie, Justin, or one of the other friends on his list
- Complete a drawing that he had begun the day before
- Listen to music by his favorite band (Red Hot Chili Peppers)
- Read script for play he hoped to be in next semester
- Read script for play he was in last semester
- Draw what he was feeling
- Draw what he was hoping to feel

Tom agreed to do something creative from his list and something to connect with one of the human allies on his list (in addition to his mother), and we booked an appointment for a few days later.

Tom, Session 4

When I saw Tom in the waiting room, I thought that he looked better: he was sitting up straight and his eyes were clear. He smiled and stood up when he saw me. But when I greeted him and turned to go back to my office, he cleared his throat and said "Um, actually there are six of us."

"*Six* of you!" I was amazed, and Tom was grinning at me, as were the three young men and two young women who had come with him. After our last session, he had called his friend Natalie, who immediately came to his house to see him. She called another friend, who also came over, and the network had taken on a life of its own from that point.

What follows is an excerpt from my conversation with Natalie. Natalie was seventeen, the same age as Tom, was in high school, and was also interested in visual arts and theater. This excerpt has been extracted from a more complex discussion within the group. Although I did ask each person, including Tom, a similar series of questions, more back and forth occurred than can easily be represented here. At this point in the session we had already discussed confidentiality. When I inquired about goals for the meeting, there was a brief pause, some looks of amazement (how *can* adults be so thick?), and then a chorus: "to help Tom."

As an exercise, try to "hear" this excerpt from Tom's perspective.

HF: Natalie, I'm very curious about your friendship with Tom. What is it about the connection you two have that made it possible for Tom to ask you to come here with him, and for you to agree?

N: We've always just been close, you know. I went out with his friend Jeff for a while and that was how we really got to know each other. But the bond we had, right from the first, it was like we could always talk to each other. About art, but other stuff too.

HF: What is it about him that makes that possible?

N: He's a guy, but he never pretended not to care about things like some guys do. His feelings are right there, and he's always real. And I know he is always there for me, too. If I had to call someone in the middle of the night and say, look, I can't tell you why, but I need all the money you have and a ride to Vancouver, it would be Tom. No question.

HF: How do you know that?

N: It's just who he is. Doesn't matter what's up with him, how bummed out he is about stuff in his life—and he gets really bummed out—but, he would want to know, to *really* know, what's going on with me. And if he knew, or saw, or felt that I was in trouble, well, that would matter to him. I've seen it.

HF: So even if he was really bummed out himself, he would be there for you.

N: Yup.

HF: How can you tell when he's bummed out?

N: Easy. If I see him, he's quiet and he looks sad and he's not all excited about his art or a role he wants. Sometimes he'll call and tell me about it and that's hard because he gets so down on himself, but it's good that he calls and tells me. And then usually we talk for a long time and later he feels better.

HF: So you are aware that talking to you is one of the things that gives him relief when he's hurting.

N: Yeah, he tells me that later and usually I can tell anyway. And I always make him promise me not to hurt himself.

HF: Good for you. So he has talked with you about wanting to hurt himself?

N: Yeah. And I know about his cousin, so when he's down, I know it's on his mind.

HF: How is that for you?

N: Scary sometimes. But I'd rather he tell me than keep it in. I can't help him if he keeps it in. Lately I've been worried that he might not be talking to me about stuff because he knows I don't like him using so much . . . uh . . . you know about that, right?

HF: Yes, I do.

N: Oh, good, well. . . . I want him to know I'm his friend no matter what.

HF: What do you want to do about getting that through to him?

N: I already talked to him about it, after he called and asked me to come here. I don't hate him just because I don't agree with something he's doing.

HF: So, do you think that got through to him?

N: I'm not sure . . . [*Glances at Tom*] . . . Did I? [*Laughs*] Not one hundred percent, I guess.

HF: What percent is it? What was it before you talked and what is it now?

N: Oh. . . . just ten percent before and maybe . . .sixty percent now.

HF: Wow! Big shift!

N: Yeah. It was a good talk.

HF: What would it take for the percentage to go up to seventy percent?

N: Well . . . maybe if he told me that he would call me or Mike or Justin if he wanted to talk.

HF: How possible do you think that is?

N: If he says he'll do it, he'll do it. Tom takes his responsibility to his friends seriously. I'll ask him.

HF: That's great. You know, you obviously have a very good understanding of something that I've been learning from Tom, and that is how helpful it is for him to talk things out when he is down.

N: Yeah.

HF: I'm wondering, what else do you think is helpful for him? You know him so well.

N: Well, just being with us sometimes even if he doesn't feel like talking. Just going to Tim Horton's for an hour makes a difference; you can see it in his face.

HF: Great. [*Writing*] What else?

N: Doing his art. You can't just jump on stage any old time, but sometimes when he's crabby we'll go find his sketchbook and he'll just draw and draw.

HF: Wow! I didn't know that. What else?

A participant in a training workshop, after observing a re-creation of the previous excerpt, said wistfully that he wished his clients had friends like Natalie. I agree; I wish that all my clients had friends like Natalie. The benefits for Tom are obvious, and my job would be so much easier! The thing is, some of my clients *do* have friends like Natalie. So do some of yours.

The next excerpt is from my conversation with Tom's long-time friend Justin. Justin is eighteen, a high school student and musician and not a big talker. Justin has heard the discussion with Natalie.

Again, as you read, try to "hear" the conversation from Tom's standpoint.

HF: So, Justin, tell me about your friendship with Tom.

J: I don't know, we're tight.

HF: . . . for a long time?

J: Yeah.

HF: [*Waits*]

J: We knew each other in grade four. But then I went to a different school until after junior high.

HF: And you connected again?

J: First day of high school. Man, I was glad to see him.

HF: Yeah? How come?

J: He's just . . . [*Shrugs, waves hands*] . . . It's *Tom,* man.

HF: And he's special to you because . . .

J: He's like my brother. No, that's wrong.

HF: That's wrong.

J: Yeah, I *wish* my brother and me were like Tom and me.

HF: So, he's more like you wish a brother was to you?

J: Yeah! Like, like . . . like a brother *should* be.

HF: That's a real tribute.

J: Yeah, okay, I guess.

HF: It's a very close relationship.

J: Yeah, it's hard to talk about.

HF: Mmhmm.

J: No one is like Tom to me, man, no one.

HF: You really want him to know that.

J: Yeah, I do.

Feedback Session 4

HF: I want to thank you all for being here, and Tom for arranging this meeting. This has been a privilege for me, having the opportunity to see friendships like this close up. It has really helped me to understand more about Tom and the qualities in him that are so important to each of you. I have also had the chance to observe the openness, honesty, humor, and caring that each of you brings to your friendship with him. I can see how these friendships are part of what has helped him in his dark times.

I especially appreciate the sharing of wisdom about what is helpful to Tom, and the additions that you have made to the list he and I are working on, a list of things that can help to fight self-hatred. Tom, here's a copy of the updated list. I also have those lists I promised each of you, of local resources and telephone numbers, and a brochure and my card.

And, finally, I have a suggestion for you. Given the importance of the connections among you, and the creativity that I know you all share, I want to ask you to think about what could serve as a reminder or symbol of this discussion for Tom, or for all of you. You know sometimes when a person is down it's good to have a reminder of positive things, something concrete to help connect with. So I'll leave that with you, and I'll be really interested to hear what you come up with.

Tom and His Friends: Coda

Tom arrived alone for his next session. He had been doing better in responding to mood fluctuations without giving in to hopelessness and self-hatred. He had managed this in part by maintaining regular contact with friends, even—or especially—on his "off" days. He was eager to tell me what the six friends had decided to do in response to my suggestion about a reminder or symbol. They had created a symbol of connectedness (to my eye it resembled a Celtic knot design) and all of them had it tattooed. Tom's tattoo was on his hand, which I found surprising, but he explained that he wanted to be able to see it every day. He could also draw or doodle the design to reinforce his sense of connection.

A few months after the joint session, Tom had his heart broken when a new romance broke up. However, he got through that period without becoming suicidal, and he deliberately used both his creative outlets and his friendships to help him do that.

A Perspective on Working with Friends of Adolescent Clients

> When an adolescent at risk has trusted someone, whoever it
> might be, it is much more efficient to fully exploit that relation-
> ship and "back-up" the person the suicidal adolescent is relying
> on than to try to refer him or her to someone else, even if the sec-
> ond person is supposedly an "expert." (Perret-Catipovic, 1999,
> p. 37)

Arranging to work with clients' friends can be cumbersome, especially if they are younger and parental consents are required for the
meetings. However, in my opinion, the effort required is eminently
worthwhile. I have heard objections to this practice because it is "too
much to ask" of adolescents, but adolescents do talk to their friends,
so those friends are bearing the load anyway—alone. Psychological
autopsy research has indicated that 83 percent of adolescents who
died by suicide talked about it in the week before their deaths—but
more than half spoke *only to their peers* (Pearsall, 2001). "This may
seem a large burden to place on adolescents, but clearly if they are the
main source of help for troubled peers then they need help in managing this important role" (Hawton, Rodham, & Evans, 2006, p. 128).
Is it not preferable that we engage the friends of youth at risk in a
helping team, where they know that they have backup?

OTHER APPROACHES TO TEAM-BUILDING

Wraparound case management (VanDenBerg & Grealish, 1996) is
an excellent system for client-centered team building. The wraparound philosophy recognizes client abilities, and the "team" constructed for a vulnerable individual consists of people in the client's
world who are identified *by the client* as potentially helpful. Team
members may be professional or volunteer helpers, family members,
teachers, friends, employers, neighbors, police, etc. All of them know
that their roles have defined limits, and know where to go when they
need help, information, or backup. Wraparound is highly compatible
with solution-focused practice (Handron, Dosser, McCammon, &
Powell, 1998), and can be adapted to clients of any age. King et al.
(2006) utilized a very similar method in studying the impact of
youth-nominated support teams for suicidal adolescents.

The Geneva University Hospital's suicide prevention program includes a professional telephone hotline consultation component available to anyone in the community who is in contact with a suicidal adolescent, in an effort toward "reinforcing the ability to help of all those people they are close to" (Perret-Catipovic, 1999, p. 37).

At S.A.F.E.R. Counselling Services in Vancouver, an innovative "Concerned Other" program provides psychoeducation sessions, telephone consultation, and brief counseling to individuals and families who have a friend, family member, or co-worker identified as suicidal (Popadiuk, 2005). The approach is collaborative and competency-based, offers both individual and group counseling, and includes coping and skill-building interventions, encouragement of self-care, and facilitation of caregiver support networks.

Mishara, Houle, & LaVoie (2005) reported on four programs for family and friends of high-risk suicidal men who did not seek help for themselves: an information session, an information session with telephone follow-up, rapid referral to mental health or substance abuse treatment, and telephone support. The family and friends who participated in these programs reported that the high-risk men in their lives showed significantly decreased suicidal ideation and attempts and fewer symptoms of depression. Family and friends also experienced less distress, coped in more positive ways, and viewed their communication with the suicidal men as more helpful. Such strategies can help us to build on the healing power of natural systems.

Chapter 10

Teamwork with Natural Systems II: Family and Couple Therapy

SUICIDE PREVENTION IN FAMILIES

One of the oldest human needs is having someone to wonder where you are when you don't come home at night. (attributed to Margaret Mead, in Eisen, 1995, p. 180)

The suicidal crisis can become a rallying point, mobilizing the resources of . . . the family in ways that did not seem plausible in the past. (Zimmerman, 1995, p. 8)

Some writers (e.g., McGlothin, 2006) have recommended that therapists evaluate which family members will be positive, helpful resources and which will not, and engage in treatment only those likely to have a positive influence on the person at risk. I go at this a little bit differently. While I do not issue blanket invitations to any family member that I come across, it would have to be an extreme situation for me to deliberately exclude a concerned relative from some role on a helping team, or from a place at the table in a family therapy session. (A separate issue is that a client may choose to be connected with some family members and not with others, and I would of course respect that.) I have worked with family members whose major contribution—and it *was* in fact a major contribution—was as a negative example. (Remember Ashley, in Chapter 6, not wanting to end up a lush like her mother?) I have also worked with more family members than I can count whose history with the person at risk included less-than-positive, or in some cases, downright negative aspects—and who made critical contributions to that person's chances for recovery, sometimes at considerable personal cost or sacrifice, sometimes just with a steady determination to do what they could. I have seen brothers who voluntarily went for addiction treatment, and uncles and grandmothers who sent a postcard every week or an e-mail every day, and estranged mothers who worked two jobs to pay for a child's treatment. I believe in the possibility of change, but I do not fool myself that it is easy or even common. The desire to do something to help a beloved person who is at risk of death by suicide can be a powerful change motivator. Witnessing such change in people and relationships, or just noticing that someone is trying to help, can make a difference for clients who have been caught in feelings of hopelessness and perceptions of isolation and helplessness.

The bottom line: I would not ask "Should this family member be part of the team?," but rather "*How* can this person contribute to the team?"

Jobs for Everyone

September 11, 2001, was a Tuesday. Tuesday is my private practice day. (Stay with me, this is relevant.) When I heard about the World Trade Center and the Pentagon, I was already getting ready to go to work. Instead of watching CNN, I had a job to do—for me, a saving grace on that terrible day. There were people in trouble who needed my help, and I knew how to help them. Most people don't know how to help a family member who is suicidal—or think they don't, or imagine that ordinary gestures of caring and comfort have no place in such a serious matter. Many are discouraged from helping by a pervasive cultural mythology about suicide that says "there's nothing you can do" (Miller, Azrael, & Hemenway, 2006). If those family members can walk away from a family therapy session with an understanding of *what they can do to make a difference*—their "jobs"—then we have probably done something useful.

Sonya, Mary, and Devon

I first saw Sonya, thirteen, and her mother Mary for five joint sessions initiated by them because Sonya was binging and purging on a daily basis. Sonya had complained that she was ugly and that no one liked her. Despite severe learning disabilities, Sonya was a highly conscientious and successful student in a special education program.

She was also a friendly, engaging girl with a strong connection to her parents, her dog, and even her "perfect" older sister, a college student. Our treatment plan had three aspects: (1) identifying a list of healthier alternatives to binging and purging that Sonya could use at vulnerable times, (2) proactive planning for Sonya to spend time with two girls who she thought could be her friends, and (3) recording in a special notebook when she did these things and anything else that worked for her that day. Sonya showed considerable initiative with these goals: for example, she conceived and arranged two special outings with potential girlfriends. (The three plans and the notebook were copycat strategies adopted after Sonya explained how a planning notebook was one of her "best things" at school. The three plans were on the first page so that she could reread them to "stay on track" and refer back to them in making her daily notes.) Recording both plans and progress in writing was a key element. It seemed that for Sonya the old maxim of "what gets written gets done" was literally true.

As Sonya began to have more days free of bulimia and more positive peer interaction, she became more talkative, and her natural warmth and humor emerged. After three good weeks she confronted her mother in a session about her mother's "secret" drinking problem and Sonya's fears that her mother, already disabled by multiple sclerosis, would die of alcoholism like Mary's own parents. As a direct result of Sonya's intervention, Mary went through detoxification and began to attend Alcoholics Anonymous. Soon after, they ended treatment, saying that everything was going well. The frantic telephone call came six months later.

Mary called to say that Sonya was in crisis. In recent weeks her daughter had become increasingly unhappy, waking early, crying, and not wanting to go to school (we learned later that one of Sonya's two friends had moved and that she was being bullied by a group of girls in her class). Mary had taken her to the family doctor, who diagnosed school phobia and depression and recommended antidepressant medication. Mary and her husband Devon were uneasy about Sonya "being on drugs," so they did not fill the prescription. A few days later, Sonya refused "in hysterics" to go to school and told her mother that she didn't want to live. At that point, Mary called me. In our telephone conversation, Mary confided that she was "at wit's end" and that she thought the stress was endangering her sobriety.

Session 6 with Sonya and Mary*

As you read through the transcript excerpted here, notice the following:

- how information emerges about the problem and about risk factors and warning signs for suicide;
- Sonya's reasons for living; and
- how the previous treatment relationship is utilized.

HF: So, Sonya, Mary, it's been a while.

M: It must be a few months.

S: It was in April, last time, right before the school fashion show.

HF: That's right! I remember you telling me about it. You were helping with the music . . . how did that go?

S: Good.

M: Better than good! Everyone said that the music made the show; she did a wonderful job.

HF: Wow! Good for you! I hope you felt proud.

S: [*Small smile*] Yeah, I guess so.

HF: What else has been good?

S: Mum's still going to AA and she's doing really good.

HF: [*Stands up, shakes M's hand*] That's *great*. How is it for you?

M: It's wonderful—seven months last Wednesday. I go to at least two meetings a week, and Devon goes with me on Friday nights. Sonya's come a couple of times as well.

HF: So everyone in the family supports you.

M: [*Nods*]

HF: I'm curious about how this ongoing commitment of your mum's makes a difference for you, Sonya.

S: Helps a lot. . . . I don't have to worry about her so much, and it really helps me feel like if she could do it, I could do it . . . like with the throwing up, I haven't done it again at all.

HF: [*Stands up, shakes S's hand*]

S: [*Smiles, giggles, covers mouth and looks down*] Thanks.

---

*This case has also been described in Fiske, 2001.

HF: What do you think that says about you, that you have been able to overcome a tough problem like the throwing up?

M: I think it says—

HF: [*Holds up hand*] I'm really interested in your thoughts, Mary, but first I want to hear Sonya's ideas.

S: I guess . . . I guess maybe that I can be strong.

HF: [*Writing*] *Strong.* Yes, I agree—sure looks like good evidence to me, that you're strong. What else?

S: I guess . . . that I can change?

HF: What a valuable thing to know about yourself, that you can change. Mary, what do you think?

M: I agree one hundred percent. She's right; she's a strong person. She's been through a lot, and she's a lovely girl.

S: Still doesn't help with how I feel now!

HF: Mmmm . . . things are tough right now?

S: *Awful.*

HF: Tell me about it.

S: I feel awful. I cry all the time, even at school, and that's so embarrassing. And I hate going to school. Everyone looks at me and I'm so ugly and nobody likes me. I just want to stay *home*.

M: She's so upset, and she wouldn't go to school at all most of last week . . . I try to encourage her but I don't know how far to push, she was in such a state and so *desperate*. She's really hurting.

S: [*Sobbing*] I never felt this bad, even when I was throwing up, and that was disgusting.

HF: Has it been so bad that you have thought about killing yourself?

S: Yes.

HF: How far have you gone with those thoughts?

S: I thought it would be better to be dead, I wouldn't have to go to school or worry about failing if I don't go.

HF: [*Waits*]

S: I thought about hanging myself.

M: [*Gasps, covers mouth*] Oh Sonya, *no.*

S: I didn't do anything, Mum.

HF: How did you stop yourself?

S: I knew I'd hurt Mum. I knew we were coming here.

HF: Anything else?

S: It sounds stupid but . . . Jessica sleeps with me and I knew she would miss me.

HF: That's right, dogs really like their people to be around. Sounds like you and Jessica have a special relationship.

M: They do. If Sonya is late, Jessica is in a terrible mood, just whines and gets underfoot. [*More elaboration about Sonya's importance to Jessica and Mary*]

[*Later*]

HF: Sonya, you also mentioned coming here.

S: It helped before. This seems worse, but I know things were pretty bad before too.

HF: So the success you had before, helped you think that this could make a difference now?

S: Yes, I guess.

HF: Even though you weren't sure how yet.

S: Yes.

HF: So, how do you think I can be helpful this time?

S: . . . I think talking is good

HF: [*Waits*]

S: I still feel bad and I don't know how to fix everything, but . . . it's kind of a relief.

HF: How's that?

S: Well, my dad just doesn't understand and I don't want to upset them so much.

HF: You worry about them too.

M: Oh honey! [*To HF:*] I feel bad about that, I've always encouraged her to talk to me, but it's hard to find answers and I just get so tired. . . . it makes it hard to focus on my recovery.

HF: That's a tough balance, to encourage Sonya but not push too hard, to support her in a tough time but still stay focused on your own recovery.

M: Yes. It seems selfish sometimes.

S: Mum, it's not.

HF: You both know, Mary, your recovery is one of the ways you *do* help and support her.

S: Yes, I couldn't stand it if that fell apart.

M: Honey, I won't let it.

HF: So you're really letting me see how making your support system bigger right now was a good idea. Because there's a lot of stress on you both at the moment. Good timing, to use extra resources right now.

S: M: [*Both nod*]

HF: So, how can I be helpful?

M: What do you think, honey?

S: . . . Maybe I could talk to you sometimes myself, now, and sometimes still with Mum?

HF: I think that is an excellent idea. We can set that up today. What else?

S: [*Clouding over, becoming tearful again*] It's just *school*. I can't stand being there, and I don't know what anyone can do.

HF: So let's work on that. Your mother said something about that a while ago that really got my attention. [*Looks through notes*] She said that you were out of school *most* of last week.

S: Yes. I only went Monday morning and Thursday.

HF: So what I want to know is: How did you get yourself to go half of Monday and all day Thursday?

S: Well, on Thursday I only went because I made a plan with Mrs. Smith—she's my counselor—because she called me the day before.

Sonya: Risk, Reasons for Living and a Plan

Risk. Sonya seemed to be experiencing acute pain and perturbation. In terms of other warning signs for imminent danger (Appendix 3), she exhibited suicidal ideation; anxiety, hopelessness, and a sense of being trapped with regard to school; withdrawal from school; and mood changes. She had a suicide plan with relatively available and lethal means. Also, there was a family history of suicide, mood disorder, and alcoholism. Her primary support, her mother, was distressed. Based on overt physiognomy, the developmental and family history on file, and her learning disabilities, I thought that Sonya was probably affected by fetal alcohol.

Reasons for Living. Sonya had strong positive relationships with her mother, father, sister, and of course Jessica. She had at least one positive ally at school, the counselor. She wanted therapeutic involvement and had concrete ideas about what might help. Her attitude about treatment was positive, and she had a past experience of success with a tough problem (it was especially noteworthy that in her recent distress she had not relapsed). These were hope-inducing factors. She knew that her actions affected the people in her family—after all, she was instrumental in her mother's sobriety—and she had told her mother that she would not harm herself. She wanted to achieve in school, and had had considerable academic and extracurricular success.

Feedback and Planning

I did not see Sonya as in imminent danger of suicide at the time of this interview. That opinion was complicated by a feature of fetal alcohol effects that appeared to be characteristic of Sonya, which was difficulty learning from past experience. This raised a concern that her ability to respond positively in a treatment session might not generalize to her behavior in other situations, especially if she were in distress. The primary treatment implication was the need to intervene at an *environmental* level. Systemic intervention with Sonya—working with her family and with the school—was one aspect of this. A second aspect was using concrete reminders (like her notebook) of positive plans and supports, to anchor and reinforce Sonya's awareness of them in a variety of situations.

Mary was also on my mind, because Sonya was much affected by her mother's well-being, and also because Sonya saw her own strength and capacity to change as so connected with her mother's. Therefore it seemed important to support Mary's stability and in particular her continuing recovery from alcoholism. It seemed likely that Mary would do better if other people had clearly defined helping roles with regard to Sonya, so that Mary did not feel she was carrying the entire load.

By the end of the interview, we had developed a mutually acceptable plan with a number of components that were written down and photocopied for Mary, Sonya, Devon, Mrs. Smith, and myself:

- Sonya and I were to begin individual treatment, and had booked our next appointment.
- Both Mary and I were to call the guidance counselor to find out what supports were available for Sonya at school.
- Sonya agreed to meet and talk with her counselor.
- Building on what had been helpful before, Sonya began a list of supportive people she could go to when she felt sad or overwhelmed, and also a list of helpful activities. As before, these plans would be in the front of her notebook, and she would write down each day how she used them.
- I would facilitate a consultation with a psychiatrist so that the family could get more information about the pros and cons of a medication trial.
- I spoke with Devon on the phone and asked him to conduct an environmental safety check of their home to remove or modify ropes or long cords and hooks or bars that could support a hanging body, "blocking the exit." I also emphasized the importance of him continuing to accompany Mary to AA meetings. He also volunteered to arrange his schedule so he could drive Sonya to school in the mornings, an idea that I strongly reinforced.
- Mary agreed to find an AA sponsor, something she had not done so far, as an additional support for her own recovery program.

Sonya: What Happened Next

The guidance counselor arranged a modified school program that eased some of Sonya's immediate distress. After consultation with the psychiatrist, Sonya and her parents decided to try antidepressant medication. Within two weeks on an SSRI antidepressant, Sonya experienced noticeable relief. Sonya and I worked primarily on the identification, reinforcement, and practice (practice, practice) of coping skills. Her parents, her school counselor, and her main classroom teacher actively supported and applauded her coping. Sonya had some further suicidal thoughts, but was able to utilize her coping skills and support network. She met with me for another five sessions, and also participated in a ten-session therapy group. I had further telephone contact with her parents, and had one case conference with Sonya, her mother, school personnel, and myself. At that time a referral to an alternative school program for the following year was decided on, and that placement worked out well. Mary followed through on her commitment to get a sponsor, and continued to attend AA with Devon's support. Jessica did her job too.

SUICIDE PREVENTION WITH COUPLES

> What Dana said made living seem possible, because I felt the depth of her love and commitment. (Christopher Reeve, 1998, p. 28, on committing to life after considering suicide)

There is considerable literature to suggest the usefulness of couple treatment for depression (Denton & Burwell, 2006; Yapko, 2006). The case of Jim and Sahinder illustrates how solution-focused questioning can help a couple to focus on immediate, accessible alternatives to suicidal thinking.

Jim and Sahinder: A Good Moment

Jim, fifty-six, and Sahinder, fifty-eight, had been married for thirty-eight years when they were referred by their family doctor for "marital therapy." The doctor had been treating Jim with medication for depression. The session began with chat, mostly between me and Sahinder, and a brief discussion about confidentiality, informed consent, and the structure of the session. Sahinder cried on and off for the first few minutes.

HF: So, what I am wondering now is, if we suppose that, say in six months' time from now, you talk about this meeting and you think that it turned out to be useful, it was a good thing that you came, how will you know that?

S: In six months?

HF: Yes.

S: Well, I don't know what he thinks, but for me, just that we are both still here, together. . . . [*Crying*] just to know that he will be here.

HF: Just that, just for you to know that he will be here and you will be together. That's important to you.

S: [*Nods*]

HF: So that's one thing that will tell you that this meeting was a good idea. What else?

S: [*To Jim*] Dear? What do you think?

J: How would I know?

S: Well there must be something. *Something* that would be important to you.

J: Okay, we'll both be here.

S: You don't really mean that.

J: [*Rolls his eyes, folds his arms*] You tell her then.

HF: [*To Jim*] You said that you would both be here.

J: Well, I'm not sure that would be a good thing.

HF: What *would* be a good thing?

J: I don't know.

HF: [*Waits*]

J: She could be happier.

HF: Ah. Sahinder could be happier. How will you know that she is happier?

J: She'll stop crying.

HF: Okay, she'll stop crying. And what will she be doing when she isn't crying?

J: Ask her.

HF: Oh, I will. But first I'm curious about how you see that.

J: She's the one who wanted to come here.

HF: Thanks, that's useful to know. I appreciate that you chose to come also. Now getting back to Sahinder not crying, what is she doing when she isn't crying?

J: Huh. She's busy, she works and she takes care of the house.

HF: Oh, she *is* busy.

S: Well Jim drove a truck and he worked long hours. No overnights though.

HF: That's great, he didn't do long-haul.

S: Not after the kids. He said that you have to be with your family to have a family. He saw too many truckers end up divorced.

HF: That makes a lot of sense. Not many guys figure that out ahead of time though.

J: Huh.

HF: How did you put that together?

J: Like she said. You can't be a family man if you're not with your family.

HF: And you're a family man.

J: Thought so.

S: [*Forcefully*] Very much so!

J: They have their own lives now.

HF: What are your children doing?

S: Our oldest is married and lives in Edmonton with her family. The middle one is here, he works for the city. And our youngest is in college in Halifax; he wants to be a teacher.

HF: Mmm. Sounds like you two have done a great job. (to Jim) So, you both said that one positive thing that could come out of this conversation would be for you to still be here.

J: Yeah.

HF: How will you still being here be better?

J: That's the question.

HF: Okay. How will it be better?

J: Can't say I really think it will be.

HF: [*Pause*] So that is a question for you.

J: Yeah.

S: He told Dr. Singh that he was going to kill himself with the car exhaust.

HF: You had a plan for doing that?

J: I thought about it.

HF: Things looked that bad to you?

J: I guess.

HF: Mmm. You're how old?

J: Fifty-six.

HF: And you've been married how long?

J: Thirty-eight years.

HF: Thirty-eight years! [*Writes*] And raised kids, so that they have their own lives now, and worked hard, I imagine.

J: Yeah.

HF: And been through a lot in those years, I would think.

J: Yeah.

S: You have no idea.

HF: Right . . . so for you to be thinking that way, that's saying that lately things must have looked *really bad* to you.

J: Worse.

HF: Worse than really bad.

J: Yeah.

HF: That bad. And yet . . . even feeling that way, worse than really bad, you still want for Sahinder to be happier. And you chose to come here today with her.

J: Well, yeah.

S: He promised me he would try.

HF: Oh! You did?

J: Yeah.

HF: Try to . . . ?

J: [*Pause*] Live, I guess.

S: And get better.

HF: Live, and get better. [*Writes*] How did you manage to make that promise to Sahinder, even feeling as bad as you did?

S: I told him I still need him, and the kids need him too, just not the way they used to.

HF: Ah, you need him. [*Writes*]

S: Yes.

HF: And the kids?

S: Yes! They adore their dad, and they look up to him. They couldn't stand to lose him, and especially not *that way*.

HF: By suicide.

S: Yes. [*Crying*]

J: Sachie . . .

HF: So, Sahinder has very strong feelings about this. She wants you to stay alive, and get better, because she needs you and the kids need you.

J: I guess.

HF: And you, even feeling as terrible as you have been, you somehow could see that this meant a lot to her.

J: I don't want to hurt her. Or the kids.

HF: Good for you. You really are a family man.

J: Yeah.

HF: Even now, in maybe the worst pain of your whole life, you care about them.

J: Yeah. Yeah.

HF: So, I'm getting some idea about what Sahinder wants to have happen. What about you?

J: I don't want her hurt.

HF: Ah. And that is important to you. [*Writes*] You don't want her hurt.

J: Yeah.

HF: And to lose you would hurt her.

J: Yeah.

HF: No two ways about it.

J: I thought she would be better off.

S: I will never be better off without you. How could you think that?

HF: [*To Jim*] That's the way you thought about it then. I see. But now . . .

J: I guess not.

HF: So how do you see it now?

J: I guess I have to keep going.

HF: Keep going. [*Writes*] Okay. So, what can happen here that could help you to keep going?

J: I don't know.

HF: [*Waits*]

S: Dr. Singh gave him Zoloft.

HF: Okay, thanks, I'll come back to that. What could happen here that could help you keep going?

J: I need to believe that I'm good for something.

HF: Ah! Of course you do. [*Writes*] Of course you do. I would like to ask the two of you this strange question, to help me to get as clear an idea as possible about where you want to go. This might take some imagination. How are your imaginations?

S: Okay.

J: [*Shrugs*] Whatever.

HF: Suppose that, after we finish this conversation and you leave here today, you two go home and carry on with the rest of your evening. Eventually tonight you go to sleep, and it happens that tonight you both have a very deep, restful sleep. . . And while you are sleeping, a miracle happens. . . And the miracle is, that these problems that have brought you here today are solved. It's a miracle. *But* because you are sleeping, you don't know that this miracle has happened . . . So, tomorrow morning, after you wake up, what's the first small thing you will notice that will tell you, something has changed?

S: That's easy.

HF: Really?

S: Yeah. Jim will be up before me and he will bring me my tea, like he used to.

HF: What difference will that make to you, when he is up and brings you your tea?

S: He has always done that in the mornings, since right after our daughter was born.

HF: What a lovely thing for him to do. And what difference will it make?

S: Just that he is himself again.

HF: Himself again. How will that make a difference to you?

S: It was just so kind for him to do that, I don't know any other men who do that for their wives day after day. [*Blows her nose*] It was always this good moment, even if I had been up all night with a sick baby.

HF: Even after a bad night, a moment like that, Jim bringing you your tea, stood out.

S: Yes.

HF: You knew that was special, that kindness, that not all men do that.

S: Yes.

HF: So after he brings you the tea, then what?

S: I sit up and thank him.

HF: [*To Jim*] And what do you do then?

J: I always kiss her on the forehead.

HF: Oh! You always do that? All those mornings?

J: Yeah.

HF: And what does she do?

J: Well, she smiles.

HF: She smiles. I see. So after this miracle, when you bring her the tea . . . and she thanks you . . . and you kiss her on the forehead . . . and you see her smiling at you . . . what difference will that make for you?

J: I like to see her smile.

HF: Ah, you like to see her smile . . . she's smiling a little right now.

J: Haven't seen that for a while.

HF: So just thinking about you bringing her tea and kissing her on the forehead brought on that smile.

J: I guess.

HF: I can't think what else it could be.

J: I guess it was.

S: It was. I have always loved that moment of the day.

HF: So, after this miracle, what difference will that moment make?

Everyday life is the path. (Zen Master Nan-Sen, in Mars, 2002, p. 78)

Chapter 11

Teamwork with Unnatural Systems: Collaborating with Our Colleagues

Networking is an interpersonal operation. Struggling and organizing among and on behalf of people is an emotional process. The anger, disappointment, and frustration of rebuff, the jealousy and competitiveness driven by funding allocations, and the soul-searching that accompanies surrender to the group purpose are examples . . . Yet, opening a new community shelter, developing a needed outreach program, or signing a written agreement to expedite referrals of suicidal adolescents are the tangible rewards for the effort. (Aaronson, Bradley, & Cristina, 1990, p. 151)

ALL MY RELATIONS

"All my relations" is the English equivalent of a phrase familiar to most Native peoples in North America. It may begin or end a prayer or a speech or a story, and . . . is at first a reminder of who we are and of our relationship with both our family and our relatives. It also reminds us of the extended relationship we share with all human beings. . . . More than that, "all my relations" is an encouragement for us to accept the responsibilities we have within this universal family by living our lives in a harmonious and moral manner (a common admonishment is to say of someone that they act as if they have no relations). (King, 1990, p. ix)

My immediate family is small, but my extended family network is large and complex—as my friend Martha would say, "rich." It is further enriched by traditions of adoption and fostering. The network is replete with close relatives, whose doings are of consuming interest and importance to me even though I rarely see them in person; and distant relatives, some whom I know surprisingly well and many whom I have never met. All of them are made real and important to me by the fabric of history and anecdote (and let's face it, gossip) woven with telephone, e-mail, snail mail, and too-infrequent meetings. The weaving is supported by common threads of identity and of love and loyalty to our elders, both here and gone. Further strengthening comes from common projects and rituals, some joyous, some deeply poignant. And of course are the precious conservators, who do the work of connecting that keeps the fabric vibrant for us all. All of this makes us a perfectly ordinary family.

We are ordinary as well in that the fabric, while rich, is patterned with thin places and rips and patches and mendings. I do not always like or agree with every member of my family (!). (Even more surprising, they do not always like or agree with me!) We have wide variations in emotional climate, with periods of storm and frost that can last far too long. Still, similar to Tom's friend Natalie in Chapter 9, if I have to call someone in the middle of the night and ask for all the money they have or a drive across the country, I know that I am covered. I have always been able to act and to think of myself as independent, as making my own decisions and choices for my own reasons—because I have always been able to take my backup in life for granted. What a gift this is.

You who work to help people struggling with pain and hopelessness, who strive to prevent suicide and to reduce its painful impact, who do what you can to support another human's reasons for living, whose work gives me the backup I cannot do without—you are all my relations. I can take you for granted. What a gift this is.

THE CHALLENGE OF COLLABORATION

I take you for granted. I forget what a gift this is, how the work that you do allows me to do the work that I do. I think that you are so problem-focused, or so hierarchical, or so pessimistic, or so . . . *not like me*. You think that I am so unscientific, or so full of psycho-babble, or so naively optimistic, or so . . . *not like you*. The differences seem to matter more because we care about our clients and the work we do,

and so we want things done *right* (my way). We focus on and cultivate our differences and soon the gulf between us has become a
chasm. We open a gap in the "safety net," and clients fall through.

MEETING THE CHALLENGE

As Harry Korman says, "Solution-focused therapy is so simple—
and so damn hard" (2006). Learning to apply it in my work with clients is still a challenge after many years. Applying it with my colleagues is a much bigger challenge. Somehow it seems easy to leave
all these useful habits and skills of relating and communicating at the
therapy office; they don't come along to meetings. (And I don't think
that this is true only for me—or only for solution-focused practitioners.) Still, the shortest and easiest route to real collegial collaboration seems to lie in utilizing with one another techniques that we already know how to do, and practice with clients every day.

BORROWING A FRAMEWORK

Lance Taylor (2005) has developed a "thumbnail map" for SFBT
that highlights the shift from the language of problems to the language of solutions (and fits on a handy wallet card) (See Table 11.1).
Table 11.2 shows an application of Taylor's ideas and format to
helper systems.

TABLE 11.1. Thumbnail Map for Solution-Focused Brief Therapy

Language Shift	Line of Inquiry
What I *don't* want → What I *do* want	What is the goal?
When things go *wrong* → When things go *right*	When do little pieces of that happen?
Forces *beyond* my control → Forces *within* my control	How do they do that?
I'm *stuck* → I'm *progressing*	What good things result from that?
More *troubles* to come → Positive possibilities	What's next?

Source: Adapted from Taylor, 2005.

TABLE 11.2. Thumbnail Map for a Solution-Focused Approach to Helping Systems

Language Shift	Line of Inquiry
What we don't want, or What one of us wants and the other doesn't → What we both/all want	What are our common goals?
When things go wrong → When things go right	When do little pieces of that already happen?

Forces beyond my control or beyond your control →
  Forces within our control together, or
  Forces within my control with your help (or v.v.)
	How do we do that?
	How do each of us contribute?

We're stuck → We're progressing	What good things result from that?
More troubles to come → *Positive possibilities*	What's next?

Source: Adapted from Taylor (2005).

APPLYING THE FRAMEWORK: QUESTIONS AND EXAMPLES

What We Want: Common Goals

One method for focusing on common goals that is readily available in many agency settings or interagency groups is the regular review of mission statements. O'Brien (2006) suggests that integrating such organizational review with discussion of staff members' individual mission statements can "support a more coherent and compassionate work environment. The process of sharing values, purposes, and objectives . . . could enhance the sense of shared goals and community" (p. 28).

I like to read the following "vision statement" (from the Ontario Suicide Prevention Network) out loud to myself occasionally: "We envision a world in which life is always supported and encouraged to achieve its fullest potential." There is something very powerful about being part of a diverse group who share such a vision.

Finding common goals can happen through many kinds of formal and informal goal-setting conversation, including use of the solution-focused questions in the following "Examples of Questions for Finding Common Goals" exhibit. It can also happen through our deliberate attention to the common ground that brings us together. Once we begin to notice or remember the common goals and values, it becomes much easier to introduce them into conversations with our peers and to acknowledge and reinforce them when they are identified by others. Notice the differences in tone and outcome of conversations that begin with an acknowledgement of commonalities.

Sometimes it is enough just to say: "I know that we are all here because we want the best possible outcome for our clients." In fact, sometimes it is enough just to say this silently to ourselves and to carry that attitude into a conversation or meeting with colleagues.

Examples of Questions for Finding Common Goals

- How will our clients know that we have done a good job here today?
- How will we know that our conversation has been helpful to our client?
- What can happen in this conference call so that all of us will say it was helpful?
- Suppose a miracle happens and a tragedy like the one that brought us all here today is prevented. This miracle may happen very quietly, bit by bit, so that we hardly even notice at first some of the changes that will make this difference in our community. What will be the first small signs that this miracle is happening here?
- Suppose a miracle happens and we all really look forward to coming to this meeting. Next time we get together, what will be the first small sign that you will notice that will tell you something is different?
- Imagine that while you are asleep tonight, a miracle happens. The miracle is that this [agency] is the best place to work that you could imagine in spite of [specific or general challenges]. However, because you are sleeping, you don't know that the miracle has happened. So, when you wake up tomorrow morning and come to work, what will be different that will tell you that a miracle has happened and this is a great place to work? (adapted from Pichot & Dolan, 2003)
- What will our mutual client be doing that will show you he or she has made progress?

Finding Common Ground: An Individual or Group Exercise

The task is simply to watch for and make note of anything another person says that you agree with. You can make it more challenging by choosing to listen in this way to people whose opinions you expect to be very different from your own. In meetings where many people will be speaking, you can challenge people to find something they agree with for every speaker. Or you can make a rule that every new speaker has to begin by stating some aspect of his or her (genuine) agreement with the previous speaker. Be warned: this exercise is much easier than it sounds. Common ground is surprisingly easy to find when we look for it, when we use what Matthias von Kibed (von Kibed & de Shazer, 2003) has described as the "eyes of connection"—eyes ready to notice what works, what helps, and what relates in preference to the "eyes of separation"—eyes ready to analyze, break down, and discover flaws, faults, errors, and differences. Defining the common ground in useful ways is facilitated by solution-focused habits of using the other person's "language" (words and concepts) in order to increase positive connection. "One can speak French without becoming French" (Insoo Kim Berg, quoted in Pichot & Dolan, 2003, p. 130).

A suggestion: Once you have found some common ground, put your foot on it. Stand. Get your balance. Look around. This is a wide and beautiful country. Plan to visit often, and perhaps to move in.

When Things Go Right

When was the most recent time that the safety net we wove held fast, and supported a vulnerable person? What was working? Identification of current "exceptions" to the problem situation of intercollegial or interagency noncollaboration is a critical step. Conveners of meetings or case conferences can make a practice of beginning with concrete examples of success. Communicating with one another about such exceptions can be hope-inducing and can provide information about how better linkages occur and can be enhanced. Communication about what is going right includes voicing our appreciation for what our colleagues do that makes such exceptions happen.

What if at the outset of a staff gathering we spent a few minutes turning to our colleagues and speaking to them directly about one aspect of their work or character that we've been influenced by, that we appreciate, or that inspires us in our own work. This can occur as a go-round at the outset of a meeting, with each person present speaking in turn to the person to their right or to their left, until all in the room have been included. Would the practice of speaking about our respective contributions to, and influences on one another, serve to renew and energize us, as well as lay the foundations for attending to one another in a manner that weaves a richer tapestry to our work culture? (O'Brien, 2006, p. 29).

Examples of Questions About What We Are Able to Do Together

- How many urgent referrals have been fast-tracked by the inter-agency program?
- How many crisis calls from the distress center were we able to follow up on?
- What difference is our joint tracking form making for clients?
- How has the tracking form improved our follow-up?
- Whose idea was the tracking form? Thank you!
- What referrals have happened this week among the people at this meeting?
- You convinced that family to agree to treatment? Wow!
- How has it been helpful to your clients when you utilize the services of colleagues in the organization/our partner agencies?
- How has the information the crisis worker sent about the client been helpful?
- What would the client say was useful for her about the way that we worked together?

Within Our Control

How exactly do we apply existing skills and practices, or develop new ones, to improve collaboration? What do we say and do, and how? What do each of us do to contribute to what works? One of the many helpful aspects of going to the Brief Family Therapy Center in Milwaukee for training was listening to Insoo Kim Berg returning telephone messages. In every case, she began the conversation—

before the other person could say anything—with compliments. "Thank you so much for being so persistent trying to reach me! You are really dedicated!" I have learned from her example that a conversation can go very differently if I begin it with a sincere compliment. This has been tremendously helpful in working with client's family members and invaluable with colleagues. Of course the compliments have to be genuine or they will not work. This means that I have to think about what I value in the work that my colleague does, even—or especially—if we are in disagreement about some aspect of a case. As in the "common ground" example, this is surprisingly easy. And I suspect that my focus on what is helpful in my colleague's approach has other positive effects, for example on my tone of voice. Conversations that begin with such comments are much more likely to result in shared views and goals and in an appreciation of our common interest in what will help the client.

Pichot and Dolan (2003) describe solution-focused case management as "interagency diplomacy" (p. 129) and emphasize respectful consulting about the other helper's views of what can make a difference for the client. In particular, they suggest that inquiring for specific behavioral criteria (what the client will be doing differently) often helps "solution-focused" and "problem-focused" practitioners get to common ground and common language. Assuming that helpful change can happen in many different ways, and noticing the "common threads" even in diverse practice (Ellis, 2000) is a useful basis for this kind of collaboration.

Examples of Questions about How We Work Well Together

- What do you think was helpful for this person/family/program?
- How did you convince that family to agree to treatment?
- What is your experience of how this kind of collaboration has worked most effectively? What else have you noticed? What else?
- What have clients said about how this collaboration is making a difference for them so far?

Making Progress

What are my colleagues doing that I value and appreciate? What have we accomplished together? And how are we acknowledging and celebrating our positive efforts?

To capture and build on the progress we are making, we have to develop habits of watching for it—and celebrating it when it comes. For some years I was part of a regional suicide prevention council, a group of remarkably dedicated and talented people who worked hard to support and enhance the capacity of their community to prevent youth suicide. We were all volunteers, and sometimes we just got bogged down. The magnitude of the task and our intense desire to make a difference meant that our focus was always on the work yet to be done. Over time we realized that in order to sustain our efforts we needed to pay regular attention to our accomplishments. This could be as simple as making a list of what we had done so far this year—an exercise that inevitably produced a sense of satisfaction, renewed energy, and hope. We learned the importance of including "partial" accomplishments on our lists, that is, steps already taken toward our larger goals. And of course as we reviewed our progress, we noticed what worked for us and were more likely to repeat it. The more that such regular review and acknowledgement of steps forward is included in routine practice, the stronger the collegial bonds and the more enduring the joint effort. Initiatives that include these practices as an integral part of suicide prevention planning (e.g., Masecar, 2006) offer sustainable models for collaborative work. Of course we need to do more than notice: we can amplify and enhance the progress we make by showing our appreciation and giving credit wherever it is due.

My husband told me a story about a much-anticipated speech on fund-raising given by the chair of a commission of the American Bar Association (A. Hill, personal communication, November 5, 1998). After dinner and lengthy introductions the guest of honor took the podium and said that when someone does something that is helpful to your organization, say thank you publicly, give the person a plaque, and take a photo. Then he sat down. In under one minute he had provided a cogent reminder of something that all of us know, but often forget to apply: how important it is for good efforts to be appreciated sometimes, and the practical differences in goodwill, commitment, and cooperation that often follow.

In 2000, the Canadian Association for Suicide Prevention decided to offer an annual Media Award in recognition of responsible, ethical reporting on suicide. Instead of focusing on the (many) dangerous, inaccurate stories, or counting up failures to abide by established media guidelines for reporting on suicide (e.g., American Foundation for Suicide Prevention and Centers for Disease Control and Prevention, 2001; Canadian Association for Suicide Prevention, n.d.; World Health Organization, 2000), the CASP board has chosen to highlight those accounts that provide responsible, nonsensationalized information and preventive education, and to publicly thank the reporters responsible.

Insoo Kim Berg found myriad ways to show appreciation and distribute credit. What follows is part of a Web-based conversation about how to deal with situations in which parents and/or professional helpers find it difficult or impossible to accept even very clear, major positive change in a troubled young person who has been the recipient of multiple kinds of help. Insoo was responding to Nick Triantafillou:

> Think about how many people have tried to help the child, in their own ways. . . . recognize that we did not do it all and therapy or placement is only a small part of a child's life. The parent's nurturing, love, and many years of hard work is just bearing fruit and we just provided an environment in which these good influence[s] and learning[s] have a chance to show . . .

> Not only is this a respectful way to work with these other professionals, but they also need to know that what they have done . . . [has] some part in the child's success. This is a very collaborative stance . . . and also, advocating for the child so that their relationship with these people will remain positive long after we are out of their lives. (Triantafillou, n.d.)

Verbal acknowledgement of other helpers' contributions makes a sometimes startling difference in our collegial conversations. Expressing our appreciation in more concrete ways further reinforces the positive impact. As the ABA commissioner said, we can give a plaque, or a certificate run off on our home computer or written up by hand. We can send appreciative e-mails, or write letters to our colleagues or to their supervisors or administrators. We can have dough-nuts with morning coffee, or lunch, or dinner, in special recognition of good work done. And we don't have to wait for a special occasion, or the end of a project, or the annual review: small acknowledgments of ongoing contributions—"A" for effort, always—are rocket fuel for collaborative work.

Examples of Questions About Seeing and Celebrating Our Joint Progress

- What have we done this week? . . . this month? . . . this quarter? . . . this year?
- What client feedback have we received that tells us we are doing something right? What else?
- How have each of us contributed? What else did each of us do that made a difference?
- What difference have our efforts made? What difference will they make in the future?
- What should others know about the work being done here? How will we let them know?
- How will we mark this accomplishment? Whose contribution shall we acknowledge first? What would be a way of saying thank you that would be meaningful to that person?
- How should we celebrate our teamwork?

Positive Possibilities

All of us need "courage for the journey." Effective collaborative work, especially when acknowledged and celebrated, feeds that courage.

Examples of Questions about Positive Possibilities

- What is our next step?
- How can we approach this using the team approach we have al-ready developed?
- How can I support the good work your agency is doing?

(Continued)

(Continued)

- What will clients see that will tell them we are working well together?
- What needs to happen first? Which of us can do that?
- Who should take the lead with part A? Part B? How can the others provide back up for that effort?
- What have we learned from our previous experience about how we can back each other up this time?
- How can we continue to build on what has worked for us so far?
- What do we do together that benefits our clients most—and how can we do more of that?
- Suppose clients understood how the system works, what would they advise us? What would they tell us to keep doing because it works? What would they suggest we change?
- How can we ask clients directly?

CONCLUSION

Part of the healing process involves showing lost, hurt and frightened people that relationships built on respect and care are *possible*. (Ross, 1996, p. 147, emphasis in original)

You have to involve them in processes built on real-life manifestations of respectful relationships, not simply talk about them. . . . the healing process must involve a healthy *group* of people, as opposed to single therapists. (Ross, 1996, p. 150, emphasis in original)

Question: What do we call an unnatural system, or even a group of unnatural systems, whose members share common goals, work together on common projects, recognize one another's value, and treat one another with respect and esteem?
Answer: A community.

Chapter 12

Teamwork in Communities

Most of the work of suicide prevention must occur at the community level, where human relationships breathe life into public policy. (David Satcher, 2001, p. 2)

Being a member of the CASP here has opened my eyes to see that we can all do a little bit to help someone. (Helen, elder and survivor from Tuktoyaktuk, Northwest Territories, speaking at the plenary session of the Canadian Association for Suicide Prevention, Toronto, Oct. 27, 2006)

David Masecar, former president of the Canadian Association for Suicide Prevention and tireless suicide prevention advocate, tells a poignant story about a small fly-in aboriginal community in northern Ontario in which eighteen people, most of them teenage girls, died by suicide over a two-year period (1998; personal communication, Oct. 29, 1997). The community was shattered by these traumatic losses, and local efforts at postvention response were overwhelmed by continuing tragedies. The method used by most of these young people (I am sorry to share this graphic detail, but it is necessary to the story; please skip the rest of this paragraph if you prefer) was to tie a cord around their necks, attach the other end to a closet rod and lean forward. However, "one of the crisis workers suggested . . . installing . . . 'breakaway' closet rods" (Masecar 1998, p. 251). So a group of local men set out with their tool boxes. They knocked on every door and installed breakaway rods—strong enough to hold clothing on hangers but not strong enough to bear the pressure of a human body without snapping—in every house.

Of the many things about this story that amaze me, first is the courage and determination of those men, who overcame grief, trauma, and a pervasive atmosphere of helplessness to do something that was within their power in order to protect their families and their neighbors' families. Then there was the practical ingenuity of the crisis worker who paid attention to what was possible. I am also struck by how clearly their efforts demonstrate that everyone can play a role in preventing suicide: "Suicide prevention is everybody's business" (Ontario Suicide Prevention Network, 2005).

My colleague Peggy Austen once gave a speech called "Must we 'bake-sale' our way to suicide prevention?" (Austen, 2000), an eloquent and impassioned plea for suicide prevention on a larger scale. I share Peggy's belief that suicide prevention should be shaped and supported by planning and investment at the regional and national level, and yet I also think that the answer to her question is "yes." I want everyone who bakes cookies or knits socks or wears a T-shirt or joins a swim-a-thon for other good causes to know that they can also do something to prevent suicide. I think that when grandparents are baking cookies for suicide prevention we will have come a long way toward dispelling the myth of helplessness that stops good people from picking up their toolboxes and making a difference, and the safety net will be immeasurably stronger.

How exactly is this related to solution-focused conversations about suicide? Systemic resource utilization is a powerful helping tool, and for clinicians like myself it is easy to be myopic, focusing on the individual and family and neglecting community resources or community participation that may make an important difference to clients. And it is not just individuals or families who may need help: "Where the loss of hope affects whole communities, . . . [the] individualized approach may be woefully inadequate" (Kirmayer, Fletcher, & Boothroyd, 1998, p. 207). To broaden my thinking I try to pay attention to stories, research, and client experiences that illustrate the potential positive impact of community engagement. I want to "flex the muscle" of thinking at the community level. As I work on this, I notice how many successful efforts—like the closet rods—are characterized by beginning where people are respecting local expertise, utilizing existing capacity, setting constructive goals, taking small first steps, and then continuing to build on what works. What follows is a series of diverse (and I hope, heuristic) examples of community strengths making a difference for individuals, families, and whole communities who are at risk. Several of these examples come from

First Nations or Inuit communities, where the role of whole-community factors and responses seems to be better understood and utilized. Their application of this more relational world view (Cross, 1998; Ross, 1992, 1996) provides important examples for other communities.

NOTICING EXCEPTIONS

Wisdom is to be found in the communities. (Kral, 2003, p. 4)

Death by suicide is tragically common among First Nations and Inuit* peoples in North America (Advisory Group on Suicide Prevention, 2003; Lester, 2000; May, 2003; Royal Commission on Aboriginal Peoples, 1995). The elevated rates have been described as an outcome of the historical legacy of acculturation and loss of traditional knowledge and practice (Conners, 1996) or more pointedly as an aspect of "cultural genocide" (Sinclair, 1998, p. 167). Despite popular perceptions of suicide as a traditional way of death, particularly among Inuit, suicide—especially youth suicide, the most serious current problem—has not always been common (Kirmayer et al., 1998). Nor is suicide equally common among all tribal councils and language groups, or even from one community to another (Lester, 2000; Chandler & Lalonde, 1998). Two British Columbia sociologists, Michael Chandler and Charles Lalonde, noticed this disparity among First Nations youth suicide rates in their province and asked a wonderful question: What is different about the many communities with no youth suicides? The study they developed (Chandler & Lalonde, 1998, 2000) looked at a range of potential differences between communities with very high rates and those with a rate of zero. They identified six factors that made unique contributions to differences in suicide rates.

Their findings showed that in those communities characterized by all six factors, there were *no reported youth suicides* during the five-year study period. Communities that had fewer of the six factors had correspondingly higher numbers of suicides.

---

*In characterizing groups of people, I have used language that is considered respectful in the time and place where I live and work. I am aware that different terminology may be preferred by other people and in other times and places, and I hope that readers will be tolerant of my choices.

Factors That Differentiate First Nations Communities with High Youth Suicide Rates from Those with No Youth Suicide

- Securing title to traditional lands (either achieved or being attempted)
- Achieving a degree of self-government
- Developing some community control over education
- Developing some community control over health
- Developing some community control over police and fire services
- Establishing recognized "cultural facilities" for preservation and enrichment of their cultural lives and heritages

Source: Adapted from Chandler & Lalonde (1998)

Chandler and Lalonde (1998, 2000) used the theoretical framework of *cultural continuity* to explain their findings. They suggested that for individuals who were struggling through the challenges of adolescent development and identity formation, cultural continuity could provide a stabilizing sense of connectedness and permanence, a link to a personal future. Their work provided empirical support for observations about the importance of community-based interventions in First Nations communities (e.g., Connors, 1996; Levy & Fletcher, 1998; Mussell, 1997; Ross, 1992, 1996) and supports ongoing efforts toward systemic, community-wellness-based suicide prevention initiatives (Dechant, 2005; Idlout & Kral, 2005; Wieman, 2006; White & Jodoin, 2004). One telling indicator of this shift in orientation is the renaming of the Nunavut "suicide prevention" coalition: it is now the "Embrace Life Council" (Levy et al., 2005).

Although research on community factors is limited, evidence suggests that it is not just among First Nations people or among youth that community strengths are protective factors. For example, a Rhode Island study of adolescents who had attempted suicide showed that even with depression and socioeconomic status controlled, those who lived in neighborhoods with stronger social networks were less vulnerable to hopelessness than those from neighborhoods with weaker networks (Perez-Smith, Spirito, & Boergers, 2002). Simple participation in a social support system can sometimes reduce suicidal ideation, with or without improvements in stress management and self-esteem (de Man, 1991, reviewed in Breton et al., 1998). Social supports are most likely to be helpful when individuals at risk perceive the quality of the relationships as positive (Spiece, Duberstein, Conner, Eberly, & Conwell, 2004). I wonder about Motto's postcard study (Motto & Bostrom, 2001) and the extent to which that minimal but effective intervention may have provided patients who received postcards with an affirming sense of connectedness to a hospital community. *Social integration* (in contrast to *social fragmentation*) is strongly associated with lower suicide rates (Congdon, 1996). Community cohesiveness protects against suicide among immigrant groups (Trovato, 1998). "Ethnic density" is a contextual protective factor (Neeleman, Wilson-Jones, & Wessely, 2001), that is, members of a minority ethnic group are less likely to attempt or die by suicide when they live in larger rather than smaller local ethnic communities. Johnston, Cooper, & Kapur (2006) have recently suggested that the construct of *social capital* may be useful in describing area characteristics that are protective factors for self-harm. (Social capital is a composite index that includes ratings of physical features; home, work, and play environments; public services; sociocultural features; and area reputation.)

EXAMPLES OF COMMUNITY RESOURCE UTILIZATION

Another story from David Masecar (personal communication, November 12, 1999) concerns a massive plant layoff in a one-industry town. Within a short time, local health, social service, and police personnel began to notice an increase in personal and family problems, including suicide threats and attempts. One pragmatic protective response to this situation was the development of a volunteer program at local schools, in which out-of-work parents provided a wide range of programming: teaching, coaching, and tutoring students in everything from basketball to snowmobile maintenance. Not a perfect or universal solution, perhaps; and yet, something to provide a focus, and a sense of purpose, usefulness, and connection—all antidotes to negativity and suicidal thinking.

In New Mexico, where deaths by suicide among young people on reserves are distressingly high, most suicide prevention initiatives and therapy programs transplanted from nonaboriginal communities have failed to generate positive results—or even to get the young people identified as at risk to show up. However, some positive gains have been made using "arroyo therapy," that is, working with young reserve members *literally* where they are—in the arroyos, the dry river beds that form a network of gullies in the dry earth and provide a secluded place for hanging out and partying (May, 2003).

Attorneys are six times more likely to die by suicide than members of the general population (Hill, 2000). The Ontario Bar Assistance Program, which assists members of the legal profession with mental health and addiction issues, has developed an innovative peer volunteer mentoring program (Hill, 2000). As an example, a lawyer who has not been working in the aftermath of a depression-related suicide attempt could be matched with another lawyer who would offer the first one advice, information, and support in the processes of returning to work; explaining his or her absence to co-workers, clients, and court officials; and getting a functioning law practice reestablished. Whenever possible, the volunteer is someone who has rebuilt her or his own life and practice after going through something similar to the client lawyer's current distresses. The mentoring support as a fragile person reintegrates into the professional community is invaluable.

Perhaps the clearest examples of community resource utilization come from "natural helper" or "community helper" programs (Austen, 2003; Dunne-Maxim, 2000; May, Serna, Hurt, & DeBruyn, 2005). These programs are based on sociometric findings that in most communities—neighborhoods, schools, workplaces—a handful of individuals are identified by large numbers of people as someone they would talk to if they were in pain or in trouble. These individuals are rarely professional or volunteer helpers; they may be the waitress at the local coffee shop, the school crossing guard, a bus driver, a teacher, the guy next door. Natural helper programs involve seeking these people out and offering them, first, recognition and appreciation, and second, information, training, and professional backup so that they can continue doing the good work they already do for their communities in an even more effective way.

> The program becomes a key mechanism for capacity building as it highlights the existing strengths in a community and not what is missing. The *Community Helpers Program* does not *create* volunteers to work with youth, but finds a way to *discover* the community members, the "natural helpers," who youth already

relate to when they have a mental health problem. Not only is the glass always viewed as half full, but there are many people in the community who can top up the glass. (Austen, 2003, p. 22)

CLIENTS CONSTRUCTING COMMUNITY/COMMUNITY SUPPORTING CLIENTS

I used to think that for therapists the community aspect of the job was helping clients to discover, tap into, connect with, and utilize community assets that might be helpful to them. I now see this approach as a narrow one, utilizing only one aspect of the complex interactive process between community and individual that can be constructive and sustaining for both. Communities develop further by serving as resources to their members, and community members create community as they interact, and, perhaps especially, as they "give back," becoming a support to the resource that supports them. I think about homeless individuals I know who serve as volunteers in the shelter and food-bank systems, and of the good things that derive from that service: a social network, personal pride and satisfaction, and the strong sense of being part of something important. *Reasons for living.* I think about the practice (which I learned from Yvonne Dolan) of suggesting to clients who cannot pay therapy fees that they contribute time to their communities in exchange for what they receive, and of the changes in those clients as they begin to see themselves as people with something to offer, people who can make a difference and who participate in something larger than themselves (Duvall & Rockman, 1996).

Mostly, though, I think about James.

Learning with James

We are all works in progress . . . We expand understanding of how many ways there are to be a human being." (Feinberg, 1998, pp. 1-5)

James was born Jill. The youngest child of an immigrant family, Jill thought of herself as a boy from earliest childhood. When we met, Jill was forty years old, married, and the mother of four teenagers, and had recently come out for the first time, to her family physician, whose wise support and compassion provided the safety she needed. In our sessions Jill struggled with basic questions of identity: Am I a man, or a woman, or a woman who thinks of herself as a man? What do I wear? What do I call myself? Who do I tell? *Are there words for what I am?* She had never met another transgendered individual or even heard the word, and had spent thirty years thinking she was "crazy" and feeling profoundly hopeless. A referral to a gender identity clinic yielded a description of gender dysphoria and a diagnosis of gender identity disorder but no related counseling or follow-up because Jill was not interested in full gender reassignment surgery (also known, perhaps more fittingly, as gender confirmation surgery). Instead, she simply yearned for a quiet, celibate life as a man. And although she was only a short distance by car or train from a large city with a vibrant and diverse transgender community, Jill lived on an extremely limited income, had no Internet access, did not drive, and resided in a suburban area with no services or supports, formal or informal, for female-to-male (FTM) transgender people.

Eventually, Jill decided to be herself—that is, himself—"James," with a small number of people, while continuing to live most of the time as Jill. Wearing men's clothes and a short haircut and giving up any pretense at "womanliness" helped him to live out this difficult compromise. It was the best solution James could find in trying to balance his own wishes and emerging sense of himself, his strong sense of responsibility to his children, and his appreciation for the loyalty and true friendship that was the foundation for his marriage.

Most of the available literature and much of the limited public understanding assumes that transgender means transsexual, and that such individuals have unitary goals of changing from their "original" gender to the opposite one: FTM or MTF (male-to-female). In fact, many people, similar to James, live somewhere in between, for their own good reasons. For some this is a compromise between desire and possibility; for some it is a developmental way-station on the path to a more comprehensive change; and for some a more "mixed" status is the closest approximation of who they are. Researchers who have studied this population without limiting either/or preconceptions have suggested continuous rather than categorical understandings of gender, or "gender-blending," as appropriate models (e.g., Denny, 2004; Ekins & King, 1997; Eyler & Wright, 1997; Lewins, 1995). For most individuals with "gender-variant" identities, whatever diffi-

cult choices they make about self-expression also bring social challenges:

> There is most certainly a privilege to having a gender. Just ask
> someone who doesn't have a gender, or who can't pass, or who
> doesn't pass. When you have a gender, or when you are per-
> ceived as having a gender, you don't get laughed at on the street.
> You don't get beat up. You know what public bathroom to use,
> and when you use it, people don't stare at you or worse. You
> know which form to fill out. You know what clothes to wear.
> You have heroes and role models. You have a past. (Bornstein,
> 1994, p. 127)

And you have a community; in fact, most people who enact gender
in socially expected ways have a number of communities in which
they feel a sense of belonging, of comfort. Lack of or loss of community is a pressing issue for many transgendered individuals. (In recognition of this, the Gender Identity Project at the Gay and Lesbian
Community Service Center of New York has built its treatment program around a community empowerment model [Warren, Blumenstein, & Walker, 1998].)

James's experiences of belonging or fitting in—being part of a
community—had been rare and unsatisfying his whole life. As he acknowledged his gender identity, the need to feel that he was not alone
became intense. For a time he attended a local lesbian support group,
which required a one-and-a-half-hour, three-bus trip each way. Being
able to relate to feeling different and to the fears and disappointments
associated with "coming out," along with his natural kindness and
sense of humor, allowed him to connect with other group members.
In time the group recognized his participation by changing its name
to "Lesbian, Bisexual, Transgendered Support Group."

An avid reader despite limited formal education, James devoured
books and articles about anything related to transgender or transsexual people, especially anything with a personal or social dimension
he could relate to. He watched the press, celebrating when coverage
of transgender issues was sensitive, positive, and balanced, or when
"good news" came, such as government approval for transsexual
treatment costs or the acceptance of a transgendered youth in school.

These fragments of connection were James's only access to a sense
of community as a transgendered adult. This was the context in which

he and I decided to prepare a paper for a professional conference. The catalyst for our academic collaboration was an unexpected find: I stumbled across an out-of-print transgender text that I had been trying, without success, to order, at a yard sale in a fishing village in Newfoundland. When I brought the book back and told James where I had found it, his reaction mirrored my own: he wondered about who in that very small, isolated place had wanted to read about being a "gender outlaw," and how that individual would manage alone if facing troubles similar to James's own. What support and understanding would be available to the unknown Newfoundlander? James knew that I sometimes presented at suicide prevention conferences, because my travel schedule occasionally disrupted our appointments. He began to ask me about transgender awareness in the mental health community. I had to tell him that it was very limited. He persisted: given the statistics that we had both read, and the difficulties, including suicidal behavior, that transgender individuals faced (Cole, O'Boyle, Emory, & Meyyer, 1997; Harry, 1994; Lev, 2004; Ramsay, 1996), wasn't it likely that most practitioners would see some people "like me" in the course of their careers? I admitted that it was. Well, then, shouldn't they be better prepared? Yes, they should. Well, you already give these talks—who better than you to do it? Hmmm. You and me, together.

I put together a package of information about what it is and what it means to be transgendered, and James reviewed it carefully and gave suggestions, especially about the importance of language. (In fact, he gave so many suggestions about language that we decided to include a separate glossary.) We tried to convey a "trans-positive" or "trans-affirmative" disposition to counseling (Carroll, Gilroy, & Ryan, 2002). The centerpiece of the package was a letter that James wrote about his experience and what he had found helpful so far.

The package with James's letter was the basis for a workshop and several poster presentations (e.g., Fiske & "James," 2002, 2003). Be-

An Open Letter from "James"

I am a person who has GID (gender identity disorder). I am transgendered (a person who believes they are in the wrong body), not a transvestite (a person who just enjoys dressing up in the opposite sexes clothes) or a transsexual (a person who has had a sex change operation).

It is hard being transgendered. You think that you are the only one, you also believe that you are not normal, but what is normal? Normal for different people means different things. You want to die sometimes because you are different. It is lonely sometimes being transgendered. I managed to find a support group for lesbians who would accept me for what I was. The name of the group then changed to Lesbian, Bisexual, Transgendered Support Group. You really need a support group where you are welcome to talk and get your feelings out in the open.

I wanted to kill myself some days because you get depressed over who you are. You also think people are looking at you even though they are not. You have to come out to yourself before you can come out to other people. That may only be 10 percent of your comfort level but it helps. Choose carefully who you are comfortable coming out to. Always tell them the truth and give them the chance to ask questions and always answer them no matter what the question is. I still cannot come out to my mother or sister because they would not be comfortable with my being transgendered.

Make sure you have a good doctor who can help you. In my case I am lucky I have two wonderful doctors who are very supportive. Friends may drop you because they are uncomfortable with who you are; it hurts, but then they are not true friends if they don't understand you or want to understand you. Comfort level with yourself can vary. Some days you are more comfortable being you than others. But always remember you don't have to answer to anyone but yourself.

cause James could not be present to share the credit and see the impact of his work, I always provided sheets of paper with the heading "Feedback for James" and asked participants to let James know how the material was helpful. The feedback was diverse, but uniformly appreciative. Some examples:

- Thank you for sharing your story with us. Your willingness to talk about your feelings and experiences is quite a gift. It is important that we hear from people directly instead of make assumptions. Your courage and altruism are special!
- Thank you so much! Blessings for your work to put together this presentation, for your own transition, the courage you have.
- My own lover is FTM as well. I wish you find more support soon in your life.

- There is much you can teach my program and our members. I appreciate and value your courage. Just in myself, I have moved to more understanding and empathy and less fear.
- Thank you for your openness.
- Thank you for your voice to help people understand your experience—it enriches our practice.

These responses—which he read over and over—did not in themselves create a community for James. However, they did reinforce the slow accumulation of "belonging" experiences, as well as providing deeply satisfying confirmation that he has something valuable to say, that his experience is meaningful to others. And in some small, isolated place, a transgendered young person is gathering courage to speak to a local professional—a professional who will be ready to help because he has heard James' voice.

CONCLUSION: VOICES OF EXPERIENCE

> The Inuktitut name Kamatsiaqtut means "thoughtful people who care." (Levy & Fletcher, 1998, p. 355)

The beginning, development, survival, and impact of the trilingual (English, French, and Inuktitut) Baffin Crisis Line, Kamatsiaqtut, is a fascinating story of determination in the face of limited resource and extraordinary challenge. This 100 percent volunteer, community-grounded program serves people in distress across the vast region of Nunavut and Nunavik (Arctic Quebec), and has become a model for other, similar lines. In a 1998 article, two of Kamatsiaqtut's founders, Sheila Levy and Errol Fletcher, shared some of their hard-earned wisdom:

> Kamatsiaqtut's model is "Helping Others to Help Themselves." . . .

> Ownership, control, and responsibility are our thesis statement and motivating belief . . .

> Belief in the ability of people to change is essential. . . .

Foster co-reliance, not dependence, in individuals and within families, groups, and communities. Assisting people, not rescuing them, is the objective. An effective program involves the people for whom it is developed. . . .

When planning, look not at what doesn't work, but find the successes and explore what did work, even partially. Build these ingredients into projects and programs . . . (pp. 358-363)

Chapter 13

Survivor Wisdom: News of a Difference

Postvention can be viewed as prevention for the next decade and the next generation. (Shneidman, 1973, p. 41)

Every story is a story about death. But perhaps, if we are lucky, our story about death is also a story about love. (Humphreys, 2002, p. 50)

Grief is love, I suppose. Love as a backward glance. (Humphreys, 2002, p. 50)

David Satcher is one of my heroes. He is probably a hero to many people. There's that tall, handsome, deep-voiced man-in-a-uniform thing, and that, after an already distinguished career, he became the sixteenth surgeon general of the United States. Then as surgeon general—one of the most powerful public health figures in the world—he said that suicide was a public health problem, and that he would fight it using public health resources. The U.S. National Suicide Prevention Strategy, and the direction and resources that go with it, are direct outcomes of his call to action. These are all good reasons to consider someone heroic. But David Satcher is a hero to me for another reason: because of how he *listened*.

Mainly, because he listened to some nice people from Marietta, Georgia: Gerry and Elsie Weyrauch. In 1987 the Weyrauchs lost their thirty-four-year-old daughter, Teri, a physician, to suicide. One of the things that they decided to do in the aftermath of that terrible loss was to establish an association that would help survivors organize to lobby policymakers in support of suicide prevention efforts. The Weyrauchs founded the Suicide Prevention Action Network (SPAN). They sent letters and petitions to elected representatives and attended hundreds of meetings to ask other people to send letters and petitions. They sold bags and bumper stickers and gave away pens to support and publicize the effort. They stood in front of a big white building in Washington, DC, with cardboard signs, whenever they had the chance. I stood there with them once, in the rain—I think it was 1998—and it seemed like a well-meant little effort, more meaningful to us standing there than to anyone in the big white building.

More than ten years and 575,000 letters after SPAN began its campaign, a tall, good-looking man in a uniform came out of the big white building and looked at the Weyrauchs and their friends standing there patiently with their placards. He asked: "Who are you people, and what is it that you have to tell me?" And then he listened.

Actually, I have no idea if that's how it happened. Although I can picture that scene very clearly, probably in reality an assistant made a call to Marietta and set up a meeting. The number of letters, though, is a fact. The listening and the action that followed are facts. The vision and unyielding dedication and sheer hard work of the Weyrauchs are facts. The grassroots support that the Weyrauchs had in their work, mostly from other survivors finding a way to make meaning out of loss, or helping the Weyrauchs to make meaning out of theirs—is a fact.

David Satcher isn't the only hero in this story.

The word *survivor* causes the field of suicide prevention no end of headaches, because it is so easily misread as meaning someone who attempted suicide and survived, instead of the intended meaning of someone who has survived the death by suicide of someone close. As a person who has always thought parsing fun (i.e., I'm a language geek), I sympathize with complaints that this terminology is confusing and ambiguous; and yet, if somehow a consensus developed to change the term, I would miss it. *Survivor* has acquired such power for me. When I think "survivor," I think of the Weyrauchs and what love and determination can do.

I think of Bonny Ball's annual presentations at the Canadian Association for Suicide Prevention on Survivors Making a Difference or Survivor Success Stories (e.g., Ball, 2003b, 2005a), one story after another of survivors putting their painfully won knowledge into altruistic action to provide research, education, and resources for their communities, of survivors thriving after loss. I think of Anne Edmunds, after losing her twenty-seven-year-old son Richard to suicide in 1982, putting her empathy and remarkable verbal skills to use by writing and speaking about her experience (e.g., Edmunds, 1998) and by training to become a survivors' support group leader, and then putting her experience and the skills from her teaching career to use by training other leaders all over North America (e.g., Edmunds, 1994, 2000). I think of her husband Hugh Edmunds, supporting Anne's efforts in silence until 2003, when he joined a panel in Iqaluit to finally talk about the experience of grief as a man and how he had survived and found some hope (Fiske, Ball, Edmunds, & Hill, 2003; Edmunds, 2006). I think of dedicated professionals like John McIntosh and Frank Campbell teaching about the importance of therapist-survivors finding help and support for their own losses (Hill, Fox, Campbell, & Fiske, 2004; McIntosh, Allbright, & Jones, 2002). I think of the Baton Rouge Crisis Intervention Center's active postvention program, in which trained volunteers who are themselves survivors work as a team with professionals and first responders to provide immediate supportive outreach to survivors at the scene of a suicide, and in so doing provide both a lifeline to further help and "an installation of hope" (Campbell, Cataldie, McIntosh, & Millet, 2004, p. 30).

I think about the hundreds or thousands of support groups and newsletters and meetings that tell survivors they are not alone. I think about the love, acceptance, and support that my husband Adrian and our whole family received from the other survivors in our lives when his mother, my mother-in-law Frances Hill, died by suicide. I think about the recently bereaved survivors at every suicide prevention conference or gathering, and how the more seasoned survivors show them, through simple human comfort and their own steady example, that there are ways to make the journey and lives worth living on the other side.

Bonny Ball, who lost her twenty-one-year-old son Reid to death by suicide in 1994, is a passionate survivor-advocate, and has worked hard to inform the public, challenge stigma, and to forge fruitful partnerships among researchers, clinicians, and survivors (e.g., Ambrose, Ball, & Fiske, 2001; Ball, 2005b; Ball & White, 2005). She is insightful and articulate about the role that her activism has played in her own healing. However, she recognizes that not all survivors want or need to become involved in suicide prevention advocacy. There are many paths to healing. In a Listserv posting to a recent survivor, Bonny said:

> The very first step in suicide prevention is to take care of your-self. I am quite serious. Suicide survivors, like you and me, are statistically more vulnerable to suicide, or to otherwise crash-ing. The good news is that with work and luck the loss of fam-ily/friend can actually be "transformative." While the loss is always there/honoured for most of us, many of us also find new meaning in our lives and/or address issues that had long been festering. It is rather amazing! (Ball, 2003a)

Like other humans who go through profoundly difficult and pain-ful experiences (Nolen-Hoeksma, 2000; Tedeschi, Park, & Calhoun, 1998; Weisel, 1958/2006), survivors can eventually thrive (Ball, 2005a).

> Do you want to find a way to stay hopeful when trying to help people after someone they love has died by suicide? Hang out with survivors. We are a community of resilient and empathetic men and women, passing on our insights of hope and endurance to each other along with whatever wisdom we may have picked up along the way. (Carla Fine, survivor of her husband's death by suicide, in Myers & Fine, 2006, p. 180)

CHALLENGES

> We just cannot assume to know which are the intense issues for any particular client until we find out the hard way—by listen-ing. (Butler & Powers, 1996, p. 246)

The raw, visceral power of loss is one of the most universal human experiences, and also completely individual. One of the difficulties helpers face is empathic overload, the possibility of being emotion-ally overwhelmed by the grief and trauma of clients. Another is find-ing ways to stay hopeful; in this essential effort, personal and profes-sional experience with people thriving after profound traumatic loss is invaluable. However, the challenge that I encounter most com-monly in my day-to-day work is the problem of *knowledge*. The knowledge problem is twofold: On the one hand, there is the effort to ignore what is known or expected about the experience of surviving the suicide death of a loved one, in order to focus mindfully on individual experience. I have heard many times how much survivors want other people, however well-meaning, to stop prescribing formulas and timelines for their grief. Some survivors struggle with an added burden of perceived failure because they think or are told that they aren't doing their grief right: talking too much, or not enough; "still" grieving after a "whole" year—or "already" moving on after "only" one year. On the other hand, survivors tell us that they want helpers to know about suicide bereavement and how it is different from other kinds of loss (Grad, Clark, Dyregrov, & Andriessen, 2004). Familiarity with professional literature and personal stories about survivors is useful in helping us to appreciate some of the things that survivors may go through, for example, being treated as murder suspects by the police, and in keeping us from making assumptions based on information that is inaccurate or distorted.

Suicide postvention is in general a neglected area (Clark, 2001; Jordan & McMenamy, 2004), the "poor cousin to prevention" (Grad et al., 2004, p. 134). Much of the available research has consisted of attempts to define a "survivor syndrome" (McIntosh, 1997, p. 48) with associated DSM diagnoses. The sudden, unexpected, and violent nature of suicide death has been cited to explain higher rates of complicated grief (de Groot, de Keijser, & Neeleman, 2006; Letofsky, 1998; Mitchell, Kim, Prigerson, & Mortimer-Stephens, 2004, Mitchell, Kim, Prigerson, & Mortimer, 2005; Rando, 1996), which in turn is the diagnosis most predictive of suicidality (Latham & Prigerson, 2004). Survivors are also vulnerable to intense emotional reactions and posttraumatic stress, especially if they find or see the body (Brent, Poling, McKain, & Slaughter, 1993; Callahan, 1997; Rando, 1996). Some reviewers (e.g., Ellenbogen & Gratton, 2001) have concluded that limited empirical support exists for differences between people bereaved by suicide and people bereaved in other ways. However, others (e.g., Jordan, 2001) review the same evidence and cite quantitative and qualitative differences in the grief process and content, the survivors' social environment, and the family systems impact. Clark and Goldney (2000) suggest that even if "rigorous comparative studies" do not show that suicide bereavement is more difficult than other kinds of bereavement, survivors of suicide deal with "difficult emotional themes and questions which are different in many respects from those resulting from other modes of death" (p. 481). Despite these concerns, reviews of treatment interventions for suicide survivors have found a sparse literature (Clark, 2001; Jordan & McMenamy, 2004), with little available evidence to suggest what can be helpful, and indications that at least one group treatment model *increased* symptoms of posttraumatic stress in male participants.

Systematic observations by therapists (e.g., Clark & Goldney, 1995; Worden, 2002)—and, more important, contributions by survivors themselves (e.g., Alexander, Klein, Gray, Dewar, & Eagles, 2000; Bolton, 1983; Grad, Clark, Dyregrov, & Andriessen, 2004)— suggest that reactions that are common in suicide bereavement include shock and disbelief; a pressing need to understand the *why* of the death; fears that other family members, friends, or oneself might attempt or die by suicide; strong feelings of grief and anger; and struggles with social stigma, internal shame and guilt, and interpersonal blame. These observers also offer suggestions about what helps survivors to heal: the creation of meaning, finding something positive, support for taking whatever time they need, openness to talking about the death in spite of the possibility of misunderstanding or prejudice, and, perhaps most important and certainly most reiterated, connections with other survivors.

THE HELPING CONNECTION

uffda (OOF-dah) Swedish

A word of sympathy used when someone else is struggling in pain.

There is pain and struggle in being human. . . . When we say *uffda* to people, we simultaneously acknowledge their pain, and express sympathy, joining them in their suffering. (La Cerva, 1999, March 9)

The collected wisdom can be condensed into a single sentence: Postvention practices for suicide survivors should not be prescriptive but instead should empower the survivors to find their own paths . . . We should not give the survivors rules, but should let them find new goals. (Grad et al., 2004, p. 139)

However difficult the grief experience, there is the possibility to successfully adapt to a bereavement. (Clark, 2001, p. 106)

When I meet with a survivor in my role as therapist, my first task is to set aside my experience with other survivors and discipline myself to mindfulness: what is important to *this* survivor, today? As in other solution-focused conversations, I am interested in what this client wants, what will make a difference. Language is of course important; for example, the idea of being "on track" in one's grief process (Walter & Peller, 1994) allows us to ask about positive change without making inappropriate or insensitive assumptions about "resolution" or "getting over it." I do ask the miracle question and other future-oriented questions with survivors, and often the answers, while endlessly varied in their details, contain elements of peace with the loss, and of reconnection and renewed appreciation for life. Such answers may come even when survivors are devastated by a recent death; I am often surprised at how pervasive and transcultural is the awareness that loss and grief can bring transformative gifts.

Opportunities to talk about the dead person with a receptive listener are important for many—but not all—survivors. I sometimes see mandated grievers, individuals who have been pushed to seek help because someone in their lives believes that therapeutic discourse will help them to grieve. Such pressure is founded on assumptions (1) that someone who is not expressing grief in words is not grieving, and (2) that everyone needs to grieve, and ideally soon after a loss. However, people grieve in myriad ways, with and without words; gender, developmental, cultural, and, most important, individual differences exist in the extent to which oral dialogue is part of grief expression. Pacing and readiness are critical: people have many good reasons why they might need or choose to delay aspects of grieving, or to grieve in and through action. In such cases it may be helpful for us to utilize professional authority and give the person permission not to grieve, or not to grieve *now,* or to grieve differently.

In discussing rituals and observances related to the death, a useful position to take is simply to be curious about how these events or actions were helpful. Sometimes asking about what else could have been more helpful for the individual survivor can open a conversation about alternative or additional rituals—whether culturally available, "borrowed," or idiosyncratic—that can help the survivor move forward—or stay still—in a helpful way. Facilitating contact with other survivors through groups, reading, or online forums is useful for many survivors.

Solution-focused questions about the future, about specific, achievable goals and steps toward those goals, may be part of an "adaptive" mourning process, as described by hope theorist C.R. Snyder (2000):

> Hope theory offers three touchstones. First, the survivor may establish new goals that bring meaning to his or her daily life. Second, the mourner can attend to pathway thoughts about how to get to those goals. Third, this individual may become energized to use the pathways for the new goals . . . The three components of hopeful thinking—goals, agency, and pathways—are so intertwined that the elicitation of any one should ignite the entire process of hopeful thought. (pp. 139-140)

Useful Questions in Suicide Bereavement

When Survivors are Struggling with "Why"

- What needs to happen first—before you can understand?
- What is helpful about not knowing yet?
- What would [someone important to client] say?
- How will it make a difference for you to have an understanding of what happened?
- "What do you think is the most useful way to look at it?" (Dolan, 2002, p. 5) or
- . . . the most useful way to look at it for now?
- How do you explain it to yourself? (Dolan, 2002, p. 5)
- How do you want to explain it to yourself?
- How do other people look at this? How much of that view is useful to you? What would make it more useful?
- What *do* you understand about the person [who you lost]? What else?
- (When the person is very negative or self-blaming in their beliefs about "why") What is another way of looking at/thinking about that? And another?

(Continued)

(Continued)

Navigating the Loss

Imagine that while you are asleep tonight, a miracle happens. The miracle is that even though you have lost the person most important to you, you know that he will always be a part of you and have a powerful impact on your life. However, because you are asleep, you don't know that the miracle has happened. So, when you wake up tomorrow morning, what will be different that will let you know that a miracle has happened and that your friend will always be a part of who you are? (Pichot & Dolan, 2003, p. 200)

- How do you remember ____ (the person)?
- How do you want to remember ____?
- How will you honor your memory?
- What will the person's legacy be in your life?
- How will you know that you are on track in your grieving?
- How will [someone important to the person] know?
- What steps have you already taken to be on track?
- What will tell you that you are doing what is right for you?
- "What has helped you in the past after a death or trauma? What do you need to help you through this? What would [the name of the person who died] say you need to help you through this?" (Rynearson, 2001, pp. 69-70)
- How have you coped so far?
- "How did you know that it was worthwhile to survive the loss?" (Lelonkiewicz & Lelonkiewicz, in Fiske & Zalter, 2005)
- On a scale from 1 to 10, if 10 stands for, "I am moving through this in the way that is on track for me," and 1 stands for the opposite of that, where are you right now?
- What tells you that you are at a 4?
- What can you do to begin to move toward a 4.5?
- How will you know that you are ready for that step?
- What will be important to keep doing in the meantime to hold steady at the 4?

It is important in bereavement to let people go through whatever emotions they need to rather than generating alternatives to loss too quickly, but clients will let you know when they are ready to move on and these questions can be useful in helping them recast their lives. (Hawkes, Marsh, & Wilgosh, 1998, p. 24)

"THIS OTHER JOURNEY"

Dan was nineteen and had just finished a chef training course when we met. He came to the session "under duress" because his mother and his girlfriend had pushed him to follow through with his doctor's recommendation. Dan's best friend, Mark, had died by suicide a month before. The two had been close since childhood, and in recent years shared a strong interest in yoga and spirituality. Dan told me early in the session that since Mark's death he had felt "like a cipher."

Dan, Session 1*

HF: Like a cipher?

D: Yeah, like a big nothing. Except for the pain. So then I turned to alcohol to kill the pain.

HF: And how did the alcohol help?

D: Well, I didn't hurt as much. It was like a "pause" button.

HF: You could pause the pain.

D: Yeah. But the drinking got to be a problem too.

HF: So having a "pause" button helped with the pain, but . . .

D: I got down, I started thinking about suicide. I wanted to be with Mark. It was like I would go into this hole. It was the first time in my life I even contemplated something like that.

HF: Thoughts like that hadn't been part of your life.

D: No.

HF: How much are they part of your life now? All the time, some of the time, rarely?

D: Well, I still sometimes have just this flash-in-the-pan kind of thought. But I cut back on my drinking and those feelings really went down.

HF: Cutting back helped you to reduce the suicidal feelings.

D: Yeah.

HF: What else helps you to reduce those feelings or thoughts?

D: . . . I went down to Buffalo for the memorial service. It was just last week, it took all that time for them to release the body. I saw this

---

*Dan part 2 is in Chapter 8.

outpouring of absolute grief, his mother, his brother ... [*Shakes his head*] ... I made a promise to him and myself not to do something stupid just because I was in pain. So many people were just ... it was awful. I know a lot of people and, just the emotional impact on me ... I wouldn't do that to anyone else.

HF: So altruism saved you.

D: Huh. I suppose so. And the promise I made.

HF: So, caring for others, and the promise you made. You said you made the promise to yourself, and also ...

D: I made it to Mark.

HF: ... to Mark. And you are honoring your promise.

D: So far. I had to mean it when I promised him.

HF: It was important to make the promise to Mark?

D: Yeah. Maybe I just don't want to believe he's gone. It's umimaginable. I'm not willing to let the thought of him disappear.

HF: So, promising him ... is part of keeping him in your life?

D: Yeah, I know he's there. ... Another friend died just a month before Mark. Car accident.

HF: I'm so sorry. So, you were already grieving that friend when Mark died.

D: Yeah. And especially with Mark, I just never would expect him to do something like that, at all. Any time either one of us had a problem we would get together and things would be okay. The *one time* he didn't call, this happened. I feel responsible. I'm not talking *fault* ...

HF: Not fault ... "if only"?

D: Not even that. I know I could have saved him if I had just made a call, but because I'd seen him the day before ... I can't kick it, can't get rid of the bad thoughts. And this visual that goes with them, repeating in my head, he's in that casket. When I saw the casket I knew it was real.

HF: What are your other images of him?

D: Image is the word. I think about us, memories, just hanging out together. But the casket image comes in again. I don't know how to make it go away, it keeps rewinding.

HF: Does it change at all?

D: No.

HF: How do you want it to be different?

D: I'd like it to be not that image—something else with him in it, not a problem. I know there were good times.

HF: You do know that.

D: Yeah.

HF: How do you remember that there were good times?

D: I talk about him with my girlfriend. She's the steady thing in my life right now. Mark and I were kind of falling in love with Buddhism when he died, and she's like the right-action part of my life now. My parents and Mark's parents were really good friends, and none of them is much good for anything right now.

HF: So you can talk about Mark with her—what's her name?

D: Suki.

HF: And she helps you to focus on right actions?

D: Yeah. She blew the whistle on my drinking. And she said that I should think again about going to this big new age fair. I would have gone with Mark, and being there without him was the weirdest thing. I brought his picture with me but it just didn't feel right.

HF: So it didn't feel right—and yet in some way it was right action.

D: I thought—it's something I enjoy as well, not just because of being with Mark. You could call it selfish, but if he was here, he would be there and he wouldn't want me not to go.

HF: He would want you to go, and it was a good thing for you as well.

D: Yeah. I think so.

HF: How did you figure out to take his picture?

D: I knew I'd be thinking about him, and I didn't want the casket image. But I didn't really need it, the image stayed away.

HF: I wonder if you helped to keep it away by having the picture with you.

D: Huh. Like a shield.

HF: Yeah, exactly, like a shield.

D: I don't know, maybe . . . Maybe.

HF: Maybe something to keep in mind.

D: Maybe.

HF: How was it helpful to go to the event?

D: It sort of seemed to get me going a bit, instead of being stuck in a rut. He still occupies my thoughts every day. I haven't been able to go to work, I had this job lined up in a really good place, but I couldn't do it.

HF: What were you going to be doing?

D: The most junior of junior sous-chefs, but I don't care, if you get in somewhere good and you do a good job you can work up.

HF: That's what you want, to get in somewhere good and work up in that field?

D: Yeah, I love cooking.

HF: You do!

D: Yeah. But lately I can't even get myself to make the calls.

HF: So, is that something you want to get to? To be able to make the calls about getting started on work?

D: Yeah.

HF: That would be one small sign that you are beginning to be on track?

D: I guess.

HF: I'd like to ask you this sort of strange question, to help us see a little more about this. Okay?

D: Okay.

HF: Suppose that, after we finish this conversation and you leave here today, and you go on with your day—will you see Suki later?

D: Yes.

HF: Good. And eventually tonight you will go to sleep. And while you are sleeping, something mysterious, almost miraculous happens. And because of this happening, whatever it is, you will be doing what you need to do to get through this in the right way, in the way that honors your promise and your beliefs . . . But because you are sleeping, you don't know that this mysterious thing has occurred. So tomorrow morning, after you wake up, what will you notice that will tell you this change has happened?

D: . . . I don't know . . . Not a big change. Not very much. I mean, I would like for it to mean the pain goes away, but I don't think that's it.

HF: You would like to feel less pain.

D: God yes. It's like physical pain, all the time. Ever since it happened I've had to swallow this feeling at the top of my stomach . . . But—I don't really want it to go away.

HF: You don't?

D: I don't want to forget. [*Cries*]

HF: [*Waits*]

D: I mean, I should feel pain, right? He's not here. I don't want to lose everything, all the memories and the stuff we believed, and re-membering hurts.

HF: So—you don't want to let go of the pain if it means letting Mark go too.

D: Yeah.

HF: What you really want is to keep your memories of Mark, of all the things that you believed.

D: Yeah.

HF: What if you could keep the memories and the pain could gradually ease?

D: I guess that's what I hope. That Mark could be in dreamtime and I'll be on this other journey, just with the elapsing of time. A process.

HF: So, how will you know that you are going through a process that is right for you?

CONCLUSION

One of the most important things we can do in helping survivors is to *stay out of the way:* to respect natural healing cycles and refrain from interfering.

> Bereavement is not a maladaptive process to be ignored or hurried. Instead, it is a crucial process that prepares people to hope again. (Snyder, 2000, p. 140)

Chapter 14

Walking the Talk: The Hopeful Therapist

Like the expert surfer, . . . while you cannot control the waves, you can control how you meet them and attune yourself to their energies. So too each person can do little to change the major (and many of the minor) events that shape their lives—but each bears a responsibility for developing and using all the skills that can keep them afloat. (Ross, 1996, p. 76)

Happiness lies in the absorption in some vocation that satisfies the soul. (Sir William Osler, in Eisen, 1995, p.73)

If I am suicidal, I want a therapist who believes I'm going to live, not die. Even if I am chronically suicidal and have only a smidgen of ambivalence left between me and a lethal attempt, I don't think I need a healer who has already quit on me psychologically to show me the fatal door with an "I told you so." I don't need more treatment, I need a new therapist. (Quinnett, 2005, p. 4)

There are many days when the privilege of doing work that I love and value is a clear and present joy. And then there are other kinds of days, days when clarity and joy are obscured by the volume of e-mail and the unwritten reports or chapters or handouts and the calls to return and the workshops to organize and the shortchanged family time and the unwalked dog and the neglected friends and the unread, enticing novels gathering dust on my shelf. I get tired and discouraged and, well, *grouchy*. Sometimes when I am feeling that way, I mutter to myself "rich, rich." This eccentricity is a gift from my friend and colleague, Martha LaCasse. On the too-seldom occasions when we talk, she is sometimes greeted with a list of complaints about all the things

I am trying to do in an unlikely time frame. She listens and murmurs and then in her lovely warm voice she says, "Oh Heather, your life is so rich!" And I pause in my complaint, and feel surprised, and I think "*Rich!* You think my life is *rich?!* . . .Well . . . yes. It *is* rich." In just that space, with that word, said by that person in that way, my list of impossibilities becomes incontestable evidence of *richness*. Thank you, Martha.

I don't talk to Martha very often. Sometimes I can get myself back on track with the incantation of "rich." Sometimes stronger medicines are required: I go for a walk, I call my parents or my sister or my friend Ruth, I play with my dog, I look at my children's pictures, I make tea, I write that report and am amazed and humbled by what that client has accomplished, I talk to my colleagues and am infected with their hope and enthusiasm, I breathe and stretch and laugh and am restored. I shake my head at myself and remember what my husband says about moody people: "just another one of God's children, doing the best she can."

By now perhaps some of you are saying, yeah, yeah, very nice, self-care blah blah, we get it. I agree with all "motherhood" statements about the importance of self-care in the lives of helpers. "Never confuse having a career with having a life" (Sign attributed to Eddie Bauer in store window, Halifax, 1998). We all know what we need to do to care for ourselves, and I will not lecture you about it (much). Therapists are well-advised to pack their own "emotional emergency kits" (Dolan, 2002) and to keep them available. As for what to put on your list, one place to start would be with your answers to Gillian Aykroyd's question: "What are you doing to feed your spirit?" (Aykroyd, 2003). But self-care is only part of the issue, one aspect of a larger need: staying hopeful. For anyone who works to prevent suicide, staying hopeful is an essential, constant responsibility. "Believing in anything less than a favorable outcome is to flirt with tragedy" (Quinnett, 2005, p. 4).

The risks of losing our connection with the value of the work we do, and the hope that supports it, are very real, both for us and for our clients. Much has been written about compassion fatigue, burnout, and secondary or vicarious trauma among helpers (e.g., Figley, 1995; Pearlman & Saaktvine, 1995). An essential point about these devastating conditions is clear in the following definition of vicarious trauma:

. . . the transformation in the inner experience of the therapist that comes about as a result of empathic engagement with clients' traumatic material . . . [characterized by] our strong reactions of grief and rage and outrage which grow over time and also our sorrow, our numbing, and our deep sense of loss which follows those reactions. *It is an occupational hazard* and reflects neither pathology in the therapist nor intentionality on the part of the traumatized client. (Pearlman and Saaktvine, 1995, p. 151, emphasis added)

So trauma, like other kinds of suffering, is catching: we are vulnerable to vicarious trauma because of our empathic connection with people in pain. That is, sometimes this terrible trouble happens because we are doing our jobs *right*. More than that, sometimes doing our jobs right is part of healing from such hurts:

In order to transform vicarious traumatization, you must love your work or some aspect of your work . . . This work is too difficult and too personally demanding to do without a sense of mission or conviction . . . your work must be meaningful to you. Then, paradoxically, your work itself is part of your antidote. (Saaktvine & Pearlman, 1996, p. 72)

A similar understanding is found in many kinds of healing traditions: "The common ingredients in struggling against loss, pain, and cruelty are hope, help, and meaning" (Young-Eisendrath, 1996, p. 64). Working closely with people who are confronting loss, pain, and cruelty can serve to remind us of this necessary balance: "The more I study suicide the more focused I am about what it means to be alive" (Jobes, 2006, p. 87).

As with suicide survivors, some helpers find healing in addressing their work at another level, for example, through writing, teaching, or social action. Such activities can both invoke and support our hopes for institutional, community, or social change. For many, including myself, such work provides an important balance. More than the forums or systems in which we work, however, I think that our hopeful ness is elicited and maintained by the approach that we take and the tools that we use every day. This seems to me to be one of those areas where technique does make a difference. I suspect that some approaches and some tools are more "hope-friendly" than others for the therapists who use them.

HOPE-FRIENDLY PRACTICE?

> If you focus only on what isn't there, what's missing that one would rightfully expect to have in their life, what happens is profound despair, not just on the part of the client, but on the part of the therapist. (Yvonne Dolan, in Duvall & Rockman, 1996, p. 83)

> We have found that the best way not to feel hopeless about a client's prospects is to tell ourselves that there is always another side, and then set about exploring it. (De Jong & Berg, 2002, p. 228)

Any therapeutic stance outfits its users with lenses through which to view clients and their stories. A solution-focused "lens" can function to keep therapists hopeful—*realistically* hopeful, because our lens and the questions that we ask focus on evidence for strength, resource, and resiliency, and for withstanding, overcoming, coping, doing one's best. The more we look through such lenses and ask such questions, the more evidence we encounter, and the more evidence we encounter, the more attuned we are to such evidence and the more likely we are to perceive it, even when problems loom large.

One of my clients, whose spouse has struggled with suicide, recently brought me a wonderful example of this kind of evidence, from an anthology of writing by and about people living with various illnesses. The writer's wife has made many attempts to die by suicide in the years that she has been diagnosed with bipolar disorder:

> From this first attempt at suicide through to others, I see the will to live. I see that spark struggling against terrible odds not to be stamped out. I see a gigantic battle going on within. If such heroism doesn't inspire, not much on earth will. . . .

> How small the petty annoyances of life become as we endure this trial by fire. What a victory it is to be here, to be together, to be frustrating the beast. (Morris, 2002, pp. 137-138)

One has to celebrate and cherish the kind of achievement represented by this perspective, and also the achievement of my client in searching out and valuing the affirming words of his or her fellow-traveler. The privilege of the work we do is in seeing such love and courage, close up, day after day. The challenge is in maintaining awareness of that privilege to sustain us in darker times.

Dolan (2006a) suggests that we "try borrowing Milton Erickson's stance of imagining that something very pleasing is going to happen in today's session and communicating this to the client nonverbally through your tone and facial expression." Given the connections between doing and feeling and thinking, such small disciplines are also likely to affect the therapist in a positive way. Similarly, discussing the details of a better future for the client can make such possibilities "real" for us as well as for them. Stressing the minutiae of progress, the efforts and struggles to change, keeps us as well as our clients focused on possibility.

Other aspects of solution-focused practice can contribute to therapists' hope, including the assumption that the client is the expert: "It's easier to be an interested and compassionate companion for someone on the road to change when you don't feel burdened with the responsibility of their change" (de Shazer et al., 2007, p. 236). On the other hand, it *is* a discipline, and sometimes a very difficult one, to maintain that position:

> I think that therapists have to be very brave . . . it would be easier to talk about something trivial sometimes than to wait for the answer to the miracle question . . . but I am disciplined to believe and behave in way that implies something good will happen. (Y. Dolan, in Malinen, Cooper, & Dolan, 2003 p. 7)

CONCRETE REMINDERS

Cornelia Wieman is a psychiatrist and a leader in both research and practical implementation of health/mental health programs for First Nations communities. One of the ways that she maintains her clarity and optimism about the purpose of her work is to carry a copy of *Choosing Life: Special Report on Suicide Among Aboriginal People,* by the Royal Commission on Aboriginal Peoples (1995). How does this help? Does she read it? No, she puts it on the table in front of her at every meeting. On the cover is a photograph of a group of laughing aboriginal children. They keep her grounded.

Lance Taylor tells a story about a child welfare worker who was assaulted while on the job. When he asked her "how she was able to continue positively and effectively . . . she said that this was a low-light in a job that also had highlights, and . . . she 'keeps these high-lights close at hand'" (Taylor & Fiske, 2005, pp. 84-85). That worker is wise. I wonder *how* she does that, keeping her highlights close.

You already know about some of my highlights, and about the re-minders I use to "keep them close at hand" (Kay's and Ashley's paintings in my office). I have other, more portable reminders. Per-haps when we meet I will show you my narwhal and tell you that story. And what about you? What are your highlights, and how do you keep them close at hand?

CONCLUSION: MY FAVORITE STORY

Like most good stories, this one exists in various forms in many different traditions. I heard it for the first time in Iqaluit, Nunavut, at a suicide prevention meeting. A young man named Rory spoke to us about the suicide deaths in his community and in his own family, and about his personal struggle to find reasons to carry on. And then he told his version of this story, for which I thank him.

This is a story about a young man confiding in his grandfather. The young man is telling his grandfather about his despair. He says that he has nothing—no job, no skills for getting a job, and the girl he loves has left him. Half of the young people he grew up with are already dead by suicide. Most of the rest are out there in the dark right now, stoned out of their minds. He is out there too, most nights. Why go on?

The grandfather listens quietly for a long time. Finally, he says, "Your despair is a wolf. This wolf is very powerful. This wolf will kill you, and it will eat your soul. But hope is also a wolf, just as powerful, and it will fight the wolf of despair for you." And then he stops. (The elders do that, with their stories. They don't always wrap it all up neatly like Aesop with a little moral at the end. They want you to fig-ure some things out for yourself.)

But the grandson cries, "Grandfather, please! I need to know! Which wolf wins the fight? Which wolf survives?"

And his grandfather says, "The one that you feed."

Conclusion

TAKE THIS STORY

The Peacemaker . . . looks at, and listens to, each party to a dispute, then turns from the parties as individuals to consider the kind of relationship that exists between them. The Peacemaker does not ask of it is "good" or "bad," given the absolute nature of those declarations. Instead, the Peacemaker wonders, "Is it *hashhkeeji* (moving toward disharmony) or is it *hozhooji* (moving toward harmony)?" The emphasis, then, is still on the movement that all things demonstrate . . . value judgments thus appear to be relative things, not absolutes, applied to the *direction* in which things appear to be moving—toward or away from harmony. (Bluehouse & Zion, 1993, in Ross, 1996, p. 123)

Therapists cannot save people who are struggling with suicide. We *can* pay careful attention to their own good reasons and ways for saving themselves. Solution-focused brief therapy offers both a philosophy and a technology, a way of listening and talking, for helping people to save themselves. I trust that you will utilize or adopt that philosophy and technology in whatever ways will enhance your own practice and the experience of your clients.

I hope that the story I have been telling in these pages has been of use to you. I have tried to tell it in a *hozhooji* way, to honor the dynamic relationship, the movement and change that is part of all human stories. This is hard to represent on the page, but I have faith in your imaginations. I began this book with a quotation from Thomas King's wonderful series of lectures, *The Truth about Stories,* and I close with another.

Take . . . [this] story. It's yours now. Do with it what you will. Tell it to friends. Turn it into a television movie. But don't say in years to come that you would have lived your life differently if only you had heard this story.

You've heard it now. (King, 2003, pp. 28-29)

Appendix A

Solution-Focused Brief Therapy: The Basics

WHAT IT IS

Solution-focused brief therapy (SFBT) is a respectful, collaborative, client-centered approach to helping people make changes that was developed by Insoo Kim Berg, Steve de Shazer, and their colleagues at the Brief Family Therapy Center in Milwaukee, Wisconsin. SFBT is often described as "strengths-based," because solution-focused practitioners routinely help clients utilize their existing strengths and resources in the service of achieving their particular goals. A key practice is the orientation of clients toward the possibility of a different and better future, and the detailed exploration of that possibility. Solution-focused work is "brief" not because it limits the number of sessions but because practicing in this way tends to mobilize clients' capacities, resulting in more rapid progress. The usual rule of thumb for treatment duration is "as many sessions as are needed—*and not one more.*"

The "essence of solution-focused brief therapy" has been summarized in five therapeutic intentions:

- To work with the person rather than the problem
- To look for resources rather than deficits
- To explore possible and preferred futures
- To explore what is already contributing to those possible futures
- To treat clients as the experts in all parts of their lives (Ghul, 2005, p. 171, based on George, Iveson, & Ratner, 1999)

In *More than Miracles: The State of the Art in Solution-Focused Brief Therapy,* a group of leading solution-focused practitioners offer a succinct description:

SFBT develops solutions by first eliciting a description of what will be different when the problem is resolved. The therapist and client then work backward to accomplish this by carefully and thoroughly searching through the client's real-life experiences to identify times where portions of the desired solution descriptions already exist or could potentially exist in the future. This leads to a model of therapy that spends very little or even no time on the origins or nature of the problem, the clients' pathology, or analysis of dysfunctional interactions. . . . a true paradigm shift. (de Shazer et al., 2007, p. 3)

HOW IT WORKS

Therapeutic Stance

Insoo Kim Berg has described the competent helper as listening with "respect and curiosity" (1994, p. 13). Our curiosity demonstrates our respect: We ask many questions because we do not assume that we understand what is best for clients. Solution-focused therapists try to take a "not-knowing" posture: clients know what they want and what solutions will work for them.

The "Central Philosophy"

The "central philosophy" consists of three maxims that are the pragmatic core of SFBT:

1. If it ain't broken, don't fix it.
2. If it's working, do more of it.
3. If it isn't working, do something else.

Assumptions

- *Clients are the experts*. The therapist's task is to help clients pay attention to the knowledge and resources they already have that will help them make desired changes. There is very little room for the therapist's ideas in SFBT practice.
- *People are always changing*. Therapists can work with or against the direction of change; working "with" is easier and more effective. To collaborate with clients' change processes, we need to start where clients are—not where we want them to be or think they "should" be.

- *Small changes lead to larger changes.* It doesn't matter where you start, and the most useful place to start is generally with something that is salient, relevant, and important to the client.
- *Clients have strengths and resources that can be utilized in building solutions.*
- *Clients have good reasons for what they do, say, and feel.*
- *Developing a clear, detailed picture of a better future helps clients set solution-focused goals.* It is difficult to move forward without direction or motivation; activating the possibility of a better future can provide both.
- *The first rule of brief therapy is "go slow"* (John Weakland). We are most helpful when, instead of rushing toward solutions, we keep to the client's pace, and "unpack" the details of desired changes, better futures, coping, and progress on goals.

Tools

(Selective) Reflective Listening

People need to tell us their stories, and to know that they have been heard; respectful, reflective listening is the heart of helping. All talk therapists are selective in terms of which aspects of clients' stories they notice, highlight, and reinforce. Solution-focused therapists attend especially to evidence of clients' strengths and resources, their histories and potentials for coping and changing.

Opening Questions

Opening questions are variations on "What do you want to be different as a result of coming here?"

Exception-Finding

No problem happens 24/7; there are *always* exceptions to the problem. (So exceptions are not, in fact, exceptional!) Often we discover exceptions as we listen to clients ("So you did make it to work last week"), but we can also ask about them directly:

- When doesn't the problem happen?
- What about times when you see your friends without getting drunk?

Exceptions provide opportunities for learning about what clients are already doing that works.

Coping Questions

Coping questions are a variant of exception-finding questions and take the general form of "How are you able to do *x* (something positive or helpful) in spite of *y* (problems)?" Questions about coping are useful when clients are finding it difficult to see anything positive or hopeful; we can commiserate about their troubles and wonder how they cope.

Presession Change Questions

These questions may take various forms, for example:

- What is different since you made the decision to get some help?
- What has already begun to change between the referral and this appointment?
- How have you already begun to work on making changes?

Questions about what has already changed before the treatment or the session began have two important advantages:

1. They convey to clients that the process of change is *their* process, not a function of being in therapy or talking to a counselor.
2. They are supported by research showing that finding positive answers to these questions, or sometimes just being asked, is associated with better treatment outcomes.

Miracle Question

The miracle question invites the client to look ahead to a time when the problem(s) of the present are no longer present, and to describe how life will be different without the problem:

> Let's suppose that after we talk here today you leave and you go do whatever you usually do on a day like this. Then as the day goes by you continue doing whatever you usually do. Then it gets late, you get tired, you go to bed and you fall asleep. Then during the night . . . while you're sleeping . . . a miracle happens. (pause). And not just any miracle. It's a miracle that makes the problems that brought you here go away . . . just like THAT. But since the miracle happens while you are sleeping, you won't know that it happened. So . . . you wake up in the morning. During the night a miracle happened. The problems that brought you here are gone. How do you discover that things are differ-

ent? What is the very first thing you notice after you wake up? (de Shazer et al., 2007, pp. 42-43)

This is an unusual, attention-getting question, and it helps to ask it with confidence, expecting that the client will have or construct a useful answer. It also helps to introduce the miracle question before beginning, for example, by saying, "Is it okay if I ask you a strange question?" and to continue only after the client gives permission (e.g., by nodding). We then go on to develop the "miracle picture" in as much detail as possible, using concrete descriptions and examples from the person's daily life ("videotalk"):

- What will happen next? And what difference will that make?
- What will you do differently as a result of feeling more confident?
- Who will notice that you are behaving differently? What difference will that make to your boss?

Clients often say that something unpleasant will *not* be happening; in this case we can ask what will be happening instead, since we are looking for the presence of something helpful rather than just the absence of something hurtful. Descriptions that include what the person will be feeling, thinking, and doing after the miracle are useful because they help to make the miracle picture "live." The use of *relationship questions* (what will your best friend notice?) helps to anchor the miracle picture in the client's social world.

When the client has provided sufficient detail to make the miracle picture vivid, we can ask, "When is just a small piece of your 'miracle picture' already happening?" This question begins the process of connecting the client's here-and-now to aspects of the miracle picture.

De Shazer et al. (2007) suggest four reasons for asking the miracle question:

1. As a way of creating therapy goals
2. As a "virtual" or emotional experience of a better future
3. To establish a context for noticing exceptions
4. As part of creating a "progressive story" about change for the better

Goal-Setting

Developing concrete goals after asking the miracle question means that the focus can be on what clients want (solution-building) rather than what they don't want (problem-solving). "Well-formed" goals

- are important to the client;
- specify an interactional context;
- are specific as to place and setting;
- describe the presence of desirable behaviors rather than the absence of problems;
- focus on beginning steps rather than final results;
- clarify the client's role in change;
- are realistic (do-able); and
- are described in concrete, measurable, behavioral terms (De Jong & Berg, 2007)

Scaling

The general format for scaling questions is:

"On a scale from one to ten, if one stands for (least desirable option) and ten stands for (most desirable option), where are you in terms of (issue)?"

The advantages of scaling questions include the following:

- *Versatility:* they can be applied to a wide range of issues; the numbers on the scales are not fixed, externally defined absolutes, but are "self-anchored," that is, they are relative to the client's perception and life context (my 3 is not your 3 on the same scale); and they can be presented in a variety of formats: verbal, graphic, sculptural, pictorial, action.
- *Simplicity:* they can be used with anyone who understands basic number or hierarchy concepts, including children, relatively nonverbal clients, and those with cognitive limitations.
- *Usefulness:* scaling questions can operationalize problems and goals, even when verbal descriptors are vague; readily summarize divergent views, for example, in a couple, family, or group; and allow for negotiation and observation of small, reasonable changes.

Among the diverse applications of scaling questions are the following:

- Goal-setting:
  —"On a scale from one to ten, where are you now [with regard to your goal]?"
  —"Where do you want to be?"
  —"What will be the first small sign that you have moved up even a little on the scale—say, from two to two point five?"

- Evaluating motivation:
  —"On a scale from one to ten, if ten stands for 'I would do anything to solve this problem,' and one stands for 'I wouldn't lift a finger,' where are you?"
  —"What would help you to move up even one point on the scale?"
- Evaluating optimism:
  —"On a scale from one to ten, if one stands for 'I don't believe that this will ever change,' and ten stands for 'I am certain that I will reach my goal,' how hopeful are you that things will improve?"
  —"What allows you to be (even) that hopeful?"
  —What would help you to move up even one point?"
- Evaluating treatment effectiveness:
  —"On a scale from one to ten, if one stands for 'not at all helpful' and ten stands for 'extremely helpful,' how helpful was this conversation?"

Compliments

Compliments direct clients' attention to their own strengths, resources, efforts, and successes. (Solution-focused therapy is not about "turning negatives into positives"; it is about finding *real* positives.) Compliments will be more potent and more readily acceptable to clients when the compliments are genuine, sincere, and honest; "anchored" in concrete evidence; and stated in the client's language. They may include the following:

- Acknowledgement of the difficulty of the problem and the hard work required
- Recognition of obstacles overcome
- Identification of qualities that will be helpful in reaching clients' goals
- "Positive blame," that is, credit for "assists" with other people's successes
- Reinforcement of efforts or qualities that prevent relapse or worsening, or that help to maintain previous gains

Indirect compliments may be more readily accepted by clients who find accepting positive feedback difficult, and may include the following:

- Nonverbal expressions of surprise, wonder, or pleasure
- Verbal "punctuators," such as "Wow!" "Really?!" or "Ahhhh"
- Questions such as: "How did you figure that out?" "How did you *do* that?" "How did you know that this . . . would work? . . . would make a difference?" "What does this tell you about yourself as a person?" and "How would Joe say you were able to do that?"

Solution-Focused Messages

Solution-focused messages are usually given by therapists toward the end of a session, following a short break to think or consult with a team (if this is available). Planning to give a structured feedback message is useful because

1. it helps the therapist to stay quiet during the session;
2. clients generally listen very carefully; and
3. the break offers therapists an opportunity to carefully construct a take-home message that can have useful impact.

Solution-focused messages typically have three important elements:

1. Compliments, including statements about how difficult the problem is
2. A suggestion or homework task
3. A "bridge" between (1) and (2), which provides a rationale for undertaking the task that will make sense to the client. The bridge may be as simple as using the client's language or ideas, or may include statements such as: "I agree that it is time to try something specific," "Because you have shown me how much you want to change things," "Since it is clear that what you are already doing is making a difference" or "Since you don't feel that what you are doing so far is working . . ."

Homework tasks (or suggestions, or "experiments") are geared to the client's readiness for change, and may be passive and reflective or more active. General examples of more reflective or observational tasks might include the following:

- Notice what you want to have continue
- Notice when things are going better
- Mentally rehearse the changes that you want to make

More active tasks could include the following:

- Do more of something that has worked for you already
- Pretend that you have made the changes you want to make.
- Do one thing different

Approach to Second and Later sessions: EARS

Elicit positive change: "What's better?"
Amplify positive change: "What happened as a result of that? What else?"
Reinforce positive change: "Wow! How did you know that would work?"
Start over: "What else is better?"

Language Use

The language of solution-building is different from the language of problem-solving:

- Solution-focused therapists use presuppositional language to convey expectations for positive change, for example, "What's better?" rather than "Is anything better?" and *"When* you have met your goal . . ." instead of *"If* you meet your goal . . ."
- They use the language and concepts of the client rather than rephrasing or reinterpreting or teaching the client a new, therapeutic language.
- They prefer "how" questions to "why" questions
- They invite positive speculation: *"Suppose* you find a way to deal with this differently . . ."

Putting it All Together

In SFBT, the next question is almost always built on the client's last answer. This is what makes the therapeutic conversation a conversation rather than an interrogation or an interview.

SFBT: RESEARCH SUPPORT

SFBT is "a highly disciplined pragmatic approach rather than a theoretical one" (de Shazer et al., 2007, p. 1). Solution-focused method is the result of years of scrupulous observation, application, and refinement of what works in psychotherapy: SFBT rests on "practice-based evidence." Thus, "from the outset the development of solution-focused brief therapy by the Milwaukee team was research-based in the sense of being driven by feedback from clients as to which elements of therapy were effective in increasing goal attainment" (MacDonald, 2003, p. 12).

Given currents demand for models of therapy that demonstrate an evidence base, it may be useful for new practitioners to know that although SFBT is a relatively new model and has particular methodological challenges in its evaluation (see Appendix B), a growing body of effectiveness research exists. Several reviews of the available studies on solution-focused process and outcomes have been published (George, Iveson, & Ratner, 1999; Gingerich & Isengart, 2000; MacDonald, 2003, 2007; McKeel, 1996, 1999), many more studies have been published since the last review was written, and still more are in process (Research Committee of the Solution-Focused Brief Therapy Association, 2005).

Appendix B

Notes on the Evidence Base: Toward Communities of Curiosity

THE SPECTER OF EVIDENCE-BASED PRACTICE

What do we do in the face of empirical uncertainty? (White, 2004)

Most therapists are accustomed to working comfortably with individuals whom other people might find scary, to giving other humans the benefit of the doubt, and to applying their skills in the negotiation of what might be considered very difficult communications. But some of us—myself included—may run screaming at the suggestion that some outside body of "objective, scientific evidence" will determine the validity of our practice. Given that solution-focused therapists are strongly aligned with ideas of accountable practice, this may seem like a perplexing response.

Certainly some potential pitfalls exist in the implementation and impact of EBP. The primary focus of controversy has been a report by the American Psychological Association's Division of Clinical Psychology (Task Force Report on Promotion and Dissemination of Psychological Practices, 1993), which provided a roster of "empirically validated treatments" (EVTs). Saunders (2004) and Leenaars (2006a,b) cite views of this report as unnecessarily rigid and as biased in its recommendations toward the very behavioral and cognitive-behavioral treatments practiced by most of the division's members, bringing accusations of "methodolatry" (Leenaars, 2006a, p. 309) and pseudo-science. Fears abounded, especially as managed-care providers and government funding agencies began to pay attention, that psychological therapies would become restricted to a handful of models that "were psychological analogues to drugs and fit within a medical framework" (Saunders, 2004, p. 13) and that flexibility and innovation in psychotherapy practice would be finished. Research supported therapists' concerns that "manualizing" of treatment approaches—a necessary step in the process of acquiring EBT or EVT status—had a negative effect on therapeutic relationships and outcomes (Duncan & Miller, 2005). Models for rating therapies as more or less "evidence-based" favored efficacy (tightly controlled experimental design) over effectiveness (real-world application) research, and RCT evidence over therapist expertise. Client expertise did not appear to be a factor.

However, advantages to an EBP approach also exist, starting with the idea that it is reasonable to want to find out what works and then do more of it. Other "pros" for EBP include encouraging therapists to consider supported methods from alternative models and facilitating clear description of therapy procedures (Paul, 2004), and providing improved public information for consumers. Calmer and more reasonable voices have entered the lists. For example, a widely accepted definition of EBP is "the integration of best research evidence with clinical expertise and patient values" (Sackett, Strauss, Richardson, Rosenberg, & Haynes, 2000, p. 1). The emphasis is on collaboration and a "constantly evolving state of information" (Thyer, 2004, p. 168). Five steps are recommended for practitioner implementation of EBP:

1. Convert one's need for information into an answerable question.
2. Track down the best clinical evidence to answer that question.
3. Critically appraise that evidence in terms of its validity, clinical significance, and usefulness.
4. Integrate this critical appraisal of research evidence with one's clinical expertise and the patient's values and circumstances.
5. Evaluate one's effectiveness and efficiency in undertaking the four previous steps, and strive for self-improvement (Thyer, 2004, p. 168).

The five-step process as described sounds time-consuming and still far from client-centered—but not unreasonable or even unduly threatening.

Furthermore, the controversy surrounding EBP has served to focus attention on issues of acute interest to practitioners, such as the multiple meanings of *clinical significance* or *clinical utility* (Kazdin, 1999):

> Clinical significance refers to the practical or applied value or importance of the effect of an intervention—that is, whether the intervention makes a real (e.g., genuine, palpable, practical, noticeable) difference in everyday life to the clients or to others with whom the clients interact. (p. 332)

The attention and resulting debate has resulted in increased recognition of the importance of including client perceptions of "outcome," and understanding that "the value, significance, and impact of a therapeutic change of a given magnitude may vary considerably" among individuals and contexts (Kazdin, 1999, p. 337). It has also stimulated renewed interest in single-case research (Goldfried & Wolfe, 1999). And it has sharpened awareness of the role played in psychotherapy process and outcome by "common therapeutic factors" (Asay & Lambert, 1999; Lambert, 2004; Maione & Chenail, 2000) and/or "general change mechanisms" (Gassmann & Grawe, 2006; Smith & Grawe, 2005).

A number of leading suicidologists have recently emphasized the importance of including the client's voice in evidence-based practice research, calling for qualitative and especially phenomenological work as an adjunct or partner to quantitative research that can further our understanding of client views and needs (e.g., Links, 2004; Platt & Hawton, 2000). Links (2004) reported on research into crisis service utilization by suicidal men, using qualitative methods to "bridge the gap between scientific evidence and clinical practice." Leenaars (2006a,b) makes an impassioned plea for therapy and research that is person-, patient-, or client-centered rather than technique-centered.

In navigating the ups and downs, pros and cons of life as a therapist in the age of EBP, I hope to become more "multilingual" in the manner of Milton Erickson, as described by Tom Strong (2002): "While he could speak the language of contemporary psychiatry, his mind wasn't held to its tracks" (p. 81).

SUICIDE INTERVENTION RESEARCH: CHALLENGES AND LIMITATIONS

Hoyt: I think that when some people get nervous, they want to replace imagination with precision.

Berg: That's right. Or the illusion of precision.

Hoyt: Control.

Berg: There's no precision in life, right? (Hoyt, 1996, p. 83)

In addition to the formidable challenges that face all applied research, studies on interventions to prevent suicide are complicated by some particular issues:

- The "low base rate" problem (Goldney, 2005), that is, that death by suicide is rare enough that it is difficult to study without massive numbers of research participants (and generally, massive expense). This means that interventions that might actually make a difference are difficult to validate, because with more realistic sample sizes, effect sizes do not reach statistical significance.

- "Even given a well-defined treatment for a specific disorder, the inclusion of moderator and mediator variables in the equation quickly multiplies the number of potential predictors . . . the number of subjects required to conduct a simple study rapidly escalates" (March & Curry, 1996). Suicide is not a specific disorder, and the potential moderator and mediator variables are legion.
- For ethical and/or legal reasons (Mishara & Weisstub, 2005), many efficacy trials for treatment of suicidality exclude high-risk participants (e.g., 45 percent of trials evaluated in Comtois & Linehan, 2006).
- An even higher proportion of trials for treatment of depression exclude high-risk-for-suicide participants (88 percent, according to Beasley et al., 1991). This is a problem since, in the absence of more specific data, findings from these studies have been used to formulate practice guidelines for people at risk of suicide.
- Exclusion of high-risk individuals may also diminish the statistical power of the findings, that is, these may be the very people who would benefit most.
- "Only a minority of patients actually take up treatment" that is offered or recommended, which limits the interpretive utility of "studies evaluating treatment of attempted-suicide patients" (van Heeringen, Jannes, Buylaert, & Henderick, 1998, p. 215).
- Definitional obfuscation. (Huh?) Different researchers mean different things when they use terms such as *suicide attempt* or *self-harm*.
- Although suicidal ideations and behaviors are much more common than death by suicide, and therefore more amenable to RCT (randomized controlled trial) research, findings are difficult to interpret because of (1) definitional obfuscation, and (2) the often weak and tangled relationships among suicidal thoughts, suicidal actions, and death by suicide.
- The number of studies examining the impact of therapeutic interventions in this area is relatively small; the number of well-controlled studies, smaller still (Comtois & Linehan, 2006; Hawton, 2000; Hawton & van Heeringen, 2000; Linehan, 1998, 1999a,b, 2004; Rudd, Joiner, & Rajab, 2001).

RESEARCH ON SOLUTION-FOCUSED BRIEF THERAPY: CHALLENGES AND LIMITATIONS

As with any relatively recent model, more research is needed. Accumulating data on this topic presents challenges. Some of these challenges are related, again, to the general difficulties of applied clinical research, and some to the problems associated with testing outcomes in a client-centered model. For example, although many solution-focused practitioners (myself included) work at least part of the time in a medical-model environment and speak diagnostics as a second or third language, solution-focused work with a "depressed" person can proceed effectively without ever assessing symptoms and making a diagnosis. Goals of SFBT treatment are idiographic and relate to what is salient, important, and relevant for a unique individual. This means that "manualization" of the model is not easy, and also that assessment of progress is not ideally measured by, for example, changes on standardized tests of depressive symptoms or suicidal thinking. Such measures can still be applied to evaluate solution-focused practice, and frequently are. This application is important in allowing for comparisons with other models, and no therapy should be assessed only through its own lens. There is a definite role for increased use of assessment tools that are more congruent with SFBT practice. In particular it would be essential to include clients' feedback as an integral aspect of any research on SFBT, and to do whatever can be done to contextualize research methodology and findings.

MODEL FOR A COLLABORATIVE, PRACTICE-FRIENDLY EVIDENCE BASE

Janet Bavelas (2006) has provided a clear, collaboration-friendly structure for a broader base of evidence in psychotherapy research. She suggests four "cornerstones" on which to build a case for EBP, that is, four kinds of research that are relevant for psychotherapy:

1. Traditional outcome evaluation = Randomized, controlled trials
2. Microanalysis of communication = Examining what the therapist does in a session
3. Experimental tests of key techniques that therapists use in practice = Using non-therapeutic tasks and populations
4. Experimental tests of assumptions that guide therapeutic pracitce = Tests of underlying principles (Bavelas, 2006)

A body of evidence based on such diverse investigative strategies would encompass differences in research setting, focus, and purposes, providing converging evidence, generalizability, and evidence relevant to practitioners as well as to clients and to organizations who select services (Bavelas, 2006).

Process research is also important for practitioners (Links, Bergmans, & Cook, 2003), and cornerstones two, three, and four address therapeutic processes rather than outcomes. Microanalysis of communication (Bavelas, McGee, Phillips, & Routledge, 2000; McGee, DelVento, & Bavelas, 2005; Tomori & Bavelas, 2007), or discourse/communication analysis (Couture & Sutherland, 2004) is of particular interest to many of us, because "the methods used . . . can be used by practitioners in their own practice, thereby erasing the dividing line between research and practice" (Couture & Sutherland, 2004, p. 13). Adaptations of experimental design, including single-case and qualitative/ethnographic methods, may be better "fits" with SFBT and provide greater clinical utility.

AN EXERCISE IN PRACTICING MY PREACHING

"How do you develop a therapy that is not applied, but practiced? . . . that is created by the people creating the therapy, by the therapist and the client together" (Audience member 3, in Hoyt, Miller, Held, & Matthews, 2001, p. 87)

Common Ground

What is the common ground among researchers, providers, and receivers of therapy, and their supporters—whatever their preferred models, theories, and orientations?

- We want working and workable links among practice and research.
- Our overall goal is for psychotherapy clients to benefit.
- We want psychotherapy to be accountable.
- We want psychotherapy to be both effective and efficient.
- We want our contributions to be meaningful.
- We want our contributions to be appreciated and respected.
- We want to appreciate and respect the contributions of others.
- "Just more of God's children, doing the best we can."

Useful Questions for Collaborative Efforts

- How are our views similar, and how is that useful?
- How are our views different, and how is that useful?
- How can your view of your approach inform what I do?
- How can your view of my approach inform what I do?

A THERAPIST'S RESEARCH WISH LIST

I have always thought that there ought to be a productive tension between theory and practice, and that they ought to fructify each other. (Shneidman, 1993, p. x)

My understanding and clinical practice would be enriched by any of the following:

- More carefully controlled, clearly described case studies, in particular those that incorporate transcripts or, even better, taped sessions (actual or reeenacted)
- Much more information on the subjective experiences of first voices and survivors in helping relationships: what works?
- Microanalysis of therapeutic conversations about suicide, including solution-focused conversations, looking at elicitation and reinforcement of client statements about reasons for living, hope, the future, etc.
- Tests of underlying principles of SFBT, for example, that solution-focused therapists select solution-focused formulations in conversation with clients
- Further investigation of the common factors and general change mechanisms in psychotherapy, specifically in suicide intervention studies, and as facilitated by different methods of therapy, including SFBT
- Further investigation of "client-directed, outcome-informed" protocols, specifically in treatment of suicidal thinking and behavior (e.g., building on Jobes, 2006)
- Research on the relative cost-effectiveness of client-centered versus standardized therapeutic methods
- Laboratory-analogue validation studies of solution-focused tools
- Discursive collaborative research (Ungar, 2004) on resiliency, pathways to hope, and reasons for living among individuals who have thought about or attempted suicide
- RCTs showing the general impact and the specific impact on suicidal thoughts and behaviors of (1) timing and sequencing of assessment and treatment interventions; (2) reasons-for-living versus reasons-for-dying content in therapeutic conversations; (3) future-oriented talk, including the miracle question (also the impact on, and interaction with, future-directed thinking); (4) SFBT as a treatment modality versus TAU or other treatment models; (5) positive emotions and cognitions in psychotherapy sessions; (6) psychotherapeutic methods and "behavioral activation," or the extent to which clients utilize ther-

apy in their real lives; (7) solution-focused scaling questions (an idiographic measurement tool) versus standardized methods (nomothetic tools) or a combination of the two; (8) presession change questions; and (9) utilization of existing client competencies versus introduction of new skills.

CONCLUSION

Jennifer White is a collaborative researcher-practitioner who regularly reminds her colleagues that statistical studies are just one form of valuable evidence (2004, 2005). I am struck by her ideas about the development of *communities of knowing,* in which relevant knowledge is co-created in nonhierarchical ways (White, 2004). Perhaps another way of thinking about this is to look for and build "communities of curiosity," diverse groups that share an interest in what works and whose ways of asking answerable questions can both inform and support one another's efforts.

Finally, because research on suicide prevention is so very difficult . . . we certainly cannot pronounce with confidence about the effectiveness of our approach. . . . However, just as our patients sometimes make a suicide attempt because they feel that they "have to do something!" about difficulties that confront them, so also do we, with a far more productive intent, feel that we "have to do something" that might help when given the chance, even without research data confirming effectiveness. We even dare to think that what we do does help. Sometimes. And that's what we're trying for. (Dulit, 1995, pp. 104-105)

Appendix C

Warning Signs of Imminent Danger
for Suicide

EXHIBIT C.1. Is Path Warm: A Warning Signs Mnemonic

Ideation
Substance abuse

Purposelessness
Anxiety
Trapped
Hopelessness

Withdrawal
Anger
Recklessness
Mood changes

Source: Adapted from A. Berman, cited in Rudd (2006).

The list in Exhibit C.1, in the mnemonic form suggested by Dr. Alan Berman (Rudd, 2006), condenses the most reliable and valid information available. It is the outcome of an American Association of Suicidology consensus panel on warning signs (Rudd, Berman, et al., 2006). The panel's goal was to agree on a brief, evidence-based list of proximal warning signs for suicide that could be used to promote public awareness and in screening and decision making. Validation results to date have been positive (Van Orden et al., 2006; Rudd, Mandrusiak, Joiner, Berman, et al, 2006).

The presence of any of these factors should alert helpers to the possibility of self-destructive thinking or plans, the need to inquire, and the possible need for safety planning. Practitioners should also apply an understanding of more distal or background risk factors, including aspects of personal and psychiatric history such as psychiatric diagnoses, past suicide attempts, and experiences of abuse, loss, or marginalization, and access to lethal means.

My hope and recommendation to the panel would be that they reconvene to consider the literature on protective factors and to distil that information into a similarly succinct and useful tool, perhaps "Signs of Resilience" or "Survival Signs."

Appendix D

Reflective Questions

The following questions provide a possible structure for solution-focused case review when suicide is a concern.

REFLECTIVE QUESTIONS FOR CASE REVIEW

- What can I do to increase this client's safety?
- What can ease this client's pain and perturbation even by the slightest amount?
- How can I facilitate that?
- What can I do directly?
- Which other people does this client see as potentially helpful?
- Who would this client choose as a helper?
- What can I do to involve others in a helping network or team to maintain this client's safety?
- Who else can I involve as part of a team for this client?
- How can my expertise be helpful to others so that they can (1) provide helpful support, (2) set appropriate and necessary boundaries and limits, and (3) focus on what they *can* do?
- What is one telephone call that I can make right now that might be helpful?
- What does this client say will be helpful?
- If nothing will be helpful in this client's view except dying, *how* will that help?
- What is the goal or function of the suicide wish?
- What would be alternative ways to meet this goal or function?
- How can I help this client get even a little bit more of what he or she wants other than by suicide?
- If a pattern has been identified that has led in the past to suicidal behavior, what can interrupt the pattern?
- What has interrupted it in the past?

- Looking at the pattern, what is one small, concrete change that would make a difference? (e.g., a contact, a comfort, a new skill, a contract)
- What behaviors/cognitions/emotional skills does this client say will be useful? (e.g., "to be able to walk away when I'm angry," "to drink and have fun without getting depressed," "to not care so much when my boyfriend or girlfriend seems to like someone else")
- What is realistically and conservatively possible for me in terms of availability to this client (e.g., only scheduled sessions? telephone calls—scheduled or as needed? day/evenings/weekends?)
- For occasions when I am not available, what support *is* available?
- How can I work with this client to make these alternative connections real, useful, and more likely to be accessed and utilized?
- With whom will I debrief this case?
- How am I modeling self-care?
- What am I doing to keep my hope alive?

References

Aaronson, S., Bradley, J., & Cristina, P. (1990). Urban areas. In M.J. Rotheram-Borus, J. Bradley, & N. Oblensky (Eds.) (1990), *Planning to live: Evaluating and treating suicidal adolescents in community settings* (pp. 151-167). Norman, OK: National Resource Center for Youth Services, the University of Oklahoma.

Abramson, L.Y., Alloy, L.B., Hankin, B.L., Clements, C.M., Zhu, L., Hogan, M., & Whitehouse, W. (2000). Optimistic cognitive styles and invulnerablility to depression. In Jane Gillham (Ed.), *The science of optimism and hope* (pp. 75-98). Philadelphia, PA: Templeton Foundation Press.

Abramson, L.Y., Metalsky, G.I., & Alloy, L.B. (1989). Hopelessness depression: A theory-based subtype of depression. *Psychological Review, 96,* 358-372.

Ackerman, D. (1997). *A slender thread: Rediscovering hope at the heart of crisis.* New York: Random House.

Advisory Group on Youth Suicide Prevention (2003). *Acting on what we know: Preventing youth suicide in First Nations.* Ottawa, ON: Health Canada, First Nations and Inuit Health Branch.

Ajdacic-Gross, V., Killias, M., Hepp, U., Gadola, E., Bopp, M., Loubec, C., Schnyder, U., Gutzwiller, F., & Rossler, W. (2006). Changing times: A longitudinal analysis of international firearm suicide data. *American Journal of Public Health, 96*(10), 1752-1755.

Alexander, D.A., Klein, S., Gray, N.M., Dewar, I.G., & Eagles, J.M. (2000). Suicide by patients: Questionnaire study of its effect on consultant psychiatrists *British Medical Journal, 320,* 1571-1574.

Allen, K., Shykoff, B.E., & Izzo, J.L. Jr. (2001). Pet ownership, but not ACE inhibitor therapy, blunts home blood pressure responses to mental stress. *Hypertension, 38*(4), 815-820.

Allgood, S.M., Parham, K.B., Salts, C.J., & Smith, T.A. (1995). The association between pretreatment change and unplanned termination in family therapy. *The American Journal of Family Therapy, 23,* 277-290.

Allgulander, C. (2000). Psychiatric aspects of suicidal behaviour: Anxiety disorders. In K. Hawton & K. van Heeringen (Eds.), *International handbook of suicide and attempted suicide* (pp. 179-192). Chichester, UK: Wiley.

Ambrose, J. (1996). Assessing and treating suicidal adolescents in context—The family: Part of the problem, part of the solution. Handout for workshop presented at the Canadian Association for Suicide Prevention Conference, Toronto, Ontario, Canada, October 16-19.

Ambrose, J., Ball, P.B., & Fiske, H. (2001). Suicide, family, and the caregiver. Presented at the Canadian Association for Suicide Prevention Conference, St. John's, Newfoundland, Canada, October 24-27.

American Academy of Pediatrics, Committee on Adolescents (2000). Suicide and suicide attempts in adolescents (RE9928). Retrieved July 11, 2002, from http://www.aap.org/policy/re9928.html.

American Foundation for Suicide Prevention and Centers for Disease Control and Prevention (2001). *Reporting on suicide: Recommendations for the media.* New York: Centers for Disease Control and Prevention.

American Psychiatric Association (1994). *Diagnostic and statistical manual of mental disorders* (4th ed.). Washington, DC: Author.

Angst, J., Angst, F., Gerber-Werder, R., & Gamma, A. (2005). Suicide in 406 mood-disorder patients with and without long-term medication: A 40 to 44 years' follow-up. *Archives of Suicide Research, 9,* 279-300.

Appleby, L. (2000). Prevention of suicide in psychiatric patients. In K. Hawton & K. van Heeringen (Eds.), *International handbook of suicide and attempted suicide* (pp. 617-630). Chichester, UK: Wiley.

Appleby, L., Amos, T., Doyle, U., Tomenson, B., & Woodman, M. (1996). General practitioners and young suicides. *British Journal of Pyschiatry, 168,* 330-333.

Apter, A. & Freudenstein, O. (2000). Adolescent suicidal behaviour: Psychiatric populations. In K. Hawton & K. van Heeringen (Eds.), *International handbook of suicide and attempted suicide* (pp. 261-273). Chichester, UK: Wiley.

Arensman, E. & Kerkhof, A. (2004). Negative life events and non-fatal suicidal behavior. In D. DeLeo, U. Bille-Brahe, A. Kerkhof, & A. Schmidtke (Eds.), *Suicidal behaviour: Theories and research findings* (pp. 93-109). Cambridge, MA: Hogrefe & Huber.

Ash, E. (2007). Puppets, parachutes, and Pandora's box: Solution-focused therapy in action. Presented at the Solution-Focused Brief Therapy Association Conference, Toronto, November 3-4.

Asay, T.P. & Lambert, M.J. (1999). The empirical case for the common factors in therapy: Quantitative findings. In M.A. Hubble, B.L. Duncan, & S.D. Miller (Eds.), The heart and soul of change: What works in therapy (pp. 33-55). Washington, DC: American Psychological Association.

Ashworth, J. (2001). *Practice principles: A guide for mental health clinicians working with suicidal children and youth.* Vancouver, BC: Ministry of Children and Family Development/University of British Columbia. Retrieved from http://www.mheccu.ubc.ca/publications/youth.htm.

Austen, P. (2000). Must we "bake sale" our way to suicide prevention? Presented at the Canadian Association for Suicide Prevention Annual Conference, Vancouver, British Columbia, Canada, October 11-14.

Austen, P. (2003). *Community capacity building and mobilization in youth mental health promotion: The story of the community of West Carleton. How the community helper program developed from a community's experience of youth sui-*

cide. Ottawa, ON: Health Canada. Retrieved October 20, 2005, from http://www.communitylifelines.ca/resources.htm.

Aykroyd, P. (2003). Creating balance. Presented at the Canadian Bar Association Conference, Montreal, Quebec, Canada, August 16-19.

Bachelor, A. (1991). Comparison and relationship to outcome of diverse dimensions of the helping alliance as seen by client and therapist. *Psychotherapy, 28,* 534-549.

Ball, P.B. (2003a, May 1). Message posted to the Survivor Advocates Listserv. Retrieved from: http://www.SurvivorAdvocates@yahoogroups.com.

Ball, P.B. (2003b). Survivors—partners in suicide prevention. Presented at the Canadian Association for Suicide Prevention Conference, Iqlauit, Nunavut, Canada, May 15-18.

Ball, P.B. (2005a). Resetting our sails: Suicide survivors and posttraumatic growth. Presented at the Canadian Association for Suicide Prevention conference, Ottawa, Ontario, Canada, October 16-19.

Ball, P.B. (2005b). Survivor-researcher partnerships. Presented at the Canadian Association for Suicide Prevention Pre-conference Research Day, Ottawa, Ontario, Canada, October 16.

Ball, P.B. & White, J. (2005). Wonderings and wanderings: Ongoing conversations about suicide prevention. *Visions: B.C.'s Mental Health and Addictions Journal, 2*(7), 4-5.

Barber, C. (2005). Fatal connection: The link between guns and suicide. *Advancing Suicide Prevention, 1*(2), 25-26.

Bavelas, J.B. (2006). Research on psychotherapy: A variety of methods. Presented at the Department of Psychology, Free University of Brussels, Brussels, Belgium, March 22.

Bavelas, J.B., McGee, D., Phillips, B., & Routledge, R. (2000). Microanalysis of communication in psychotherapy. *Human Systems: The Journal of Systemic Consultation and Management, 11*(1), 47-66.

Beasley, C.M.J., Dornseif, B.E., Bosomworth, J.C., Sayler, M.E., Rampey, A.H.J., Heiligenstein, J.H., et al. (1991). Fluoxetine and suicide: A meta-analysis of controlled trials of treatment for depression. *British Medical Journal, 303,* 685-692.

Beautrais, A. (2004). Global perspectives of suicide prevention strategies. In J.F. Connolly & J.Scott (Eds.), *Suicide prevention: What you can do. Proceedings of the Irish Association of Suicidology ninth annual conference* (pp. 44-50). Castlebar, Ireland: IAS.

Beautrais, A. (2006). Complexity of suicide—Suicide prevention: What we know and don't know. Presented at the Canadian Association for Suicide Prevention Annual Conference, Toronto, Ontario, Canada, October 25 27.

Beck, A.T., Brown, G.K., Berchik, R.J., Stewart, B.L., & Steer, R.A. (1990). Relationship between hopelessness and ultimate suicide: A replication with suicidal inpatients. *American Journal of Psychiatry, 147,* 190-195.

Beck, A.T., Kovacs, M., & Weissman, A. (1975). Hopelessness and suicidal behavior: An overview. *Journal of the American Medical Association, 234*, 1146-1149.

Beck, A.T., Rush, A.J., Shaw, B.F., & Emery, G. (1979). *Cognitive therapy of depression*. New York: Guilford.

Berg, I.K. (1989). Solution-focused brief therapy. Workshop, Ontario Institute for Studies in Education, Toronto, Ontario, Canada.

Berg, I.K. (1992). A wolf in disguise is not a grandmother. *Journal of Systemic Therapies, 13*(1), 13-14.

Berg, I.K. (1994). *Family based services: A solution-focused approach*. New York: Norton.

Berg, I.K. (2004). *"I'm glad to be alive . . .": Working with a suicidal youth*. (Videotape). Milwaukee, WI: Brief Family Therapy Center.

Berg, I.K. & de Shazer, S. (1993). Making numbers talk: Language in therapy. In S. Friedman (Ed.), *The new language of change: Constructive collaboration in psychotherapy* (pp. 5-24). New York: Guilford.

Berg, I.K. & de Shazer, S. (1994). *A tap on the shoulder: Six useful questions in building solutions*. (Audiotape). Milwaukee, WI: Brief Family Therapy Center.

Berg, I.K. & Dolan, Y. (2001). *Tales of solutions: A collection of hope-inspiring stories*. New York: Norton.

Berg, I.K. & Miller, S.D. (1992). *Working with the problem drinker: A solution-focused approach*. New York: Norton.

Berg, I.K. & Reuss, N.H. (1998). *Solutions step by step: A substance abuse treatment manual*. New York: Norton.

Berg, I.K. & Steiner, T. (2003). *Children's solution work*. New York: Norton.

Berman, A.L. (2005). The end of the food chain. *NEWSlink, 32*(3), 3.

Berman, A.L, Jobes, D.A., & Silverman, M.M. (2005). *Adolescent suicide: Assessment and intervention* (2nd ed.). Washington, DC: American Psychological Association.

Bernagie, K. (2004). Suicidal and aggressive behavior: Commonalities and differences. Presented at the European Symposium on Suicide and Suicidal Behaviour: Research, Prevention, Treatment and Hope, Copenhagen, Denmark, August 25-28.

Bertolino, B. (1999). *Therapy with troubled teenagers: Rewriting young lives in progress*. New York: Wiley.

Bertolino, B. & O'Hanlon, W.H. (2002). *Collaborative, competency-based counselling and therapy*. Boston: Allyn & Bacon.

Bertolino, B. & Schultheis, G. (2002). *The therapist's notebook for families: Solution-oriented exercises for working with children, adolescents, and families*. Binghamton, NY: The Haworth Press.

Bertolote, J.M., Fleischmann, A., DeLeo, D., & Wasserman, D. (2004). Psychiatric diagnoses and suicide: Revisiting the evidence. *Crisis, 25*(4), 147-155.

Bille-Brahe, U. & Jensen, B. (2004). The importance of social support. In D. DeLeo, U. Bille-Brahe, A. Kerkhof, & A. Schmidtke (Eds.), *Suicidal Behaviour: Theories and research findings* (pp. 197-208.). Cambridge, MA: Hogrefe & Huber.

Bluehouse, P. & Zion, J. (1993). Hozhooji Naat'aanii: The Navaho Justice and Harmony Ceremony. *The Mediation Quarterly, 10*(4), 328-339.

Bohart, A. & Tallman, S. (1999). The client as a common factor: Clients as self-healers. In M. Hubble, B. Duncan, & S. Miller (Eds.), *The heart and soul of change: The role of common factors across the helping professions* (pp. 91-131). Washington, DC: American Psychological Association.

Bolton, I. (1983). *My son, my son*. Atlanta, GA: Link Counseling Centre.

Boorstein, S. (1995). *It's easier than you think: The Buddhist way to happiness*. New York: Harper Collins.

Boronovalova, M.A., Lejuez, C.W., Daughters, S.B., Rosenthal, M.Z., & Lynch, T.R. (2005). Impulsivity as a common process across borderline personality disorder and substance use disorders. *Clinical Psychology Review, 25*, 790-812.

Bornstein, K. (1994). *Gender outlaw: On men, women, and the rest of us*. New York: Routledge.

Bostwick, J.M. (2006). Do SSRIs cause suicide in children? The evidence is underwhelming. *Journal of Clinical Psychology: In Session, 62*(2), 235-241.

Brain, K.L., Haines, J., & Williams, C.L. (2002). The psychophysiology of repetitive self-mutilation. *Archives of Suicide Research, 6*, 199-210.

Brent, D., Baugher, M., Brimaher, B., Kolko, D., & Bridge, J. (2000). Compliance with recommendations to remove firearms in families participating in a clinical trial for adolescent depression. *Journal of the American Academy of Child and Adolescent Psychiatry, 32*, 521-529.

Brent, D., Poling, K., McKain, B., & Slaughter, M. (1993). A psychoeducational program for families of affectively ill children and adolescents. *Journal of the American Academy of Child and Adolescent Psychiatry, 32*, 770-774.

Breton, J.J., Boyer, R., Bilodeau, H., Raymond, S., Joubert, N., & Nantel, M.A. (1998). *Review of evaluative research on suicide intervention and prevention programs for young people in Canada: Theoretical context and results*. Ottawa, ON: Health Canada.

Bridges, F.S. (2004). Gun control law (Bill C-17), suicide, and homicide in Canada. *Psychological Reports, 94*(3, pt.1), 819-826.

Brief Family Therapy Centre (n.d.). Handout on story construction. Milwaukee, WS: BFTC.

Bright Mind (2006). *Advancing Suicide Prevention, II*(I), 13-15.

Brown, G.K., Ten Have, T., Henriques, G.R., Xie, S.X., Hollander, J.E., & Beck, A.T. (2005). Cognitive therapy for the prevention of suicide attempts: A randomized controlled trial. *Journal of the American Medical Association, 294*(55), 563-570.

Brown, J.B. (2001). *Patient-centred collaboration: Core practices*. Ottawa, ON: Health Canada.

Brown, M.Z. (2006). Linehan's theory of suicidal behaviour: Theory, research, and dialectical behavior therapy. In T.E. Ellis (Ed.), *Cognition and suicide* (pp. 91-117). Washington, DC: American Psychological Association.

Butler, W.R. & Powers, K.V. (1996). Solution-focused grief therapy. In S. Miller, M.A. Hubble, & B.L. Duncan (Eds.), *Handbook of solution-focused brief therapy* (pp. 228-247). San Francisco: Jossey-Bass.

Buxton, B. (2004). *Damaged angels.* Toronto: Knopf.

Callahan, J. (1997). Correlates and predictors of grief in suicide survivors. In J.L. McIntosh (Ed.), *The legacy of suicide: Proceedings of the American Association of Suicidology Conference, Memphis* (pp. 40-41). Washington, DC: AAS.

Callcott, A. (2003). Solution-focused assessment and interventions with suicidal or self harming patients. *Journal of Primary Care Mental Health, 7*(3), 75-77.

Campbell, F., Cataldie, L., McIntosh, J., & Millet, K. (2004). An active postvention program. *Crisis, 25*(1), 30-32.

Camus, A. (1983). Return to Tipasa. In *The myth of Sisyphus and other essays* (pp. 193-204). New York: Vintage International. (Original work published 1955).

Canadian Association for Suicide Prevention (n.d.). *Media guidelines.* Edmonton, AB: Author.

Canadian Association for Suicide Prevention (2005). *Blueprint for a Canadian National Strategy on Suicide Prevention.* Edmonton, AB: Author.

Cantor, C. (2000). Suicide in the Western world. In K. Hawton and K. vanHeeringen (Eds.), *The international handbook of suicide and attemptedsuicide* (pp. 9-28). Chichester, UK: Wiley.

Cantwell, P. & Holmes, S. (1994). Social construction: A paradigm shift for systemic therapy and training. *Australia and New Zealand Journal of Family Therapy, 15*(1), 17-26.

Carroll, L., Gilroy, P.J., & Ryan, J. (2002). Counseling transgendered, transsexual, or gender-variant clients. *Journal of Counseling and Development, 80*(Spring), 131-139.

Carson, R.E. (2002, March). The X-ercise factor: Turning pain into pleasure. Presented at the Southern Coastal International Conference on Addictions and Mental Health, Jekyll Island, Georgia, March 6-10.

Center for Suicide Prevention (2003). *Suicide among Canada's Aboriginal peoples.* SIEC alert number 53. Calgary, AB: Author. Retrieved March 5, 2004, from http://www.suicideinfo.ca/csp/assets/Alert52.pdf.

Chandler, M.J. & Lalonde, C. (1998). Cultural continuity as a hedge against suicide in Canada's First Nations. *Transcultural Psychiatry, 35*(2), 191-219.

Chandler, M.J. & Lalonde, C. (2000). Cultural continuity as a protective factor against suicides in First Nations youth. *Lifenotes, 5*(1), 10-11.

Chang, E.C. & Sanna, L.J. (2001). Optimism, pessimism, and negative affectivity in middle-aged adults: A test of a cognitive-affective model of psychological adjustment. *Psychology and Aging, 16,* 524-531.

Chang, J. (1998). Children's stories, children's solutions: Social constructionist therapy for children and their families. In M.F. Hoyt (Ed.), *The handbook of constructive therapies* (pp. 251-275). San Francisco: Jossey-Bass.

Chang, J. (1999). Collaborative therapies with young children and their families: Developmental, pragmatic, and procedural issues. *Journal of Systemic Therapies, 18*(2), 44-64.

Chevalier, A.J. (1996). *On the counsellor's path: A guide to teaching brief solution-focused therapy.* Oakland, CA: New Harbinger.

Chiarelli, L., Davidson, S., Hutchinson, T., Manion, I., Shapiro, N., & Stewart, E. (2000). Youth in the know: Promoting mental health with a safety net. Presented at Suicide Intervention and Prevention in Adolescents, University of Toronto/Hospital for Sick Children, Toronto, Ontario, Canada, April 26.

Chiles, J.A. & Strosahl, K. (1995). *The suicidal patient: Principles of assessment, treatment, and case management.* Washington, DC: American Psychiatric Press.

Chiles, J.A. & Strosahl, K. (2005). *Clinical manual for assessment and treatment of suicidal patients.* Washington, DC: American Psychiatric Publishing.

Chopin, E., Kerkhof, A., & Arensman, E. (2004). Psychological dimensions of attempted suicide: Theories and data. In D. DeLeo, U. Bille-Brahe, A. Kerkhof, & A. Schmidtke (Eds.), *Suicidal behaviour: Theories and research findings* (pp. 41-60). Cambridge, MA: Hogrefe & Huber.

Clark, D., Donovan, M., & Painter, M. (2003). Co-creating alternative group cultures: Conversations about solution-focused brief therapy. Presented at the Solution-Focused Brief Therapy Association Conference, Loma Linda, California, Nov.ember 2-3.

Clark, D.C. & Goebel-Fabbri, A.E. (1999). Lifetime risk of suicide in major affective disorders. In D.G. Jacobs (Ed.), *The Harvard Medical School guide to suicide assessment and intervention* (pp. 270-286). San Francisco: Jossey-Bass.

Clark, S. (2001). Bereavement after suicide—How far have we come and where do we go from here? *Crisis, 22,* 102-108.

Clark, S. & Goldney, R. (1995). Grief reactions and recovery in a support group for people bereaved by suicide. *Crisis, 16*(1), 27-33.

Clark, S. & Goldney, R. (2000). The impact of suicide on relatives and friends. In K. Hawton & K. van Heeringen (Eds.), *International handbook of suicide and attempted suicide* (pp. 466-484). Chichester, UK: Wiley.

Cohen, L. (1992). Anthem. On *The future.* New York: Sony.

Cole, C.M., O'Boyle, M., Emory, L., & Meyyer, W.J. (1997). Comorbidity of gender dysphoria and other major psychiatric diagnoses. *Archives of Sexual Behavior, 26,* 13-26.

Comtois, K.A. & Linehan, M.M. (2006). Psychosocial treatments of suicidal behaviors: A practice-friendly review. *Journal of Clinical Psychology: In Session, 62*(2), 161-170.

Congdon, P. (1996). Suicide and parasuicide in London: A small area study. *Urban Studies, 33,* 137-158.

Conner, K.R., Meldrum, S., Wieczorek, W.F., Duberstein, P.R., & Welte, J.W. (2004). The association of irritability and impulsivity with suicidal ideation among 15- to 20-year-old males. *Suicide and Life-Threatening Behavior, 34*(4), 363-373.

Connors, E.A. (1996). The healing path: Suicide and self-destructive behavior in North American native people. In A. Leenaars & D. Lester (Eds.), *Suicide and the unconscious* (pp. 259-272). London: Jason Aronson.

Cooper, G. (2006). Exercising for mental health, Clinician's Digest. *Psychotherapy Networker 30*(1), 21.

Cooper, S., Darmody, M., & Dolan, Y. (2003). Impressions of hope and its influence: An international e-mail trialogue. *Journal of Systemic Therapies, 22*(3), 67-78.

Corcoran, J. (2002). Developmental adaptations of solution-focused brief therapy. *Brief Treatment and Crisis Intervention, 2*(4), 301-313.

Couture, S.J. & Sutherland, O.A. (2004). Investigating change: Compatible research and practice. *Journal of Systemic Therapies, 23*(2), 3-17.

Cross, T.L. (1998). Understanding family resiliency from a relational world view. In H.I. McCubbin, E.A. Thompson, A.I. Thompson, & J.E. Fromer (Eds.), *Resiliency in Native American and immigrant families* (pp. 143-157). Thousand Oaks, CA: Sage.

Daigle, M.S. (2005). Suicide prevention through means restriction: Assessing the risk of substitution: A critical review and synthesis. *Accident Analysis and Prevention, 37*(4), 625-632.

de Groot, M.H., de Keijser, J., & Neeleman, J. (2006). Grief shortly after suicide and natural death: A comparative study among spouses and first-degree relatives. *Suicide and Life-Threatening Behavior, 36*(4), 418-432.

De Jong, P. & Berg, I.K. (2002). *Interviewing for solutions* (2nd ed.). New York: Brooks/Cole.

De Jong, P. & Berg, I.K. (2007). *Interviewing for solutions* (3rd ed.). Belmont, CA: Wadsworth.

de Man, A.F. (1991). Community support and suicide ideation: An evaluation of two programs. Unpublished research. Sherbrooke, QE: Suicide Intervention Center (CIS).

de Shazer, S. (1984). The death of resistance. *Family Process, 23,* 79-93.

de Shazer, S. (1985). *Keys to solution in brief therapy.* New York: Norton.

de Shazer, S. (1988a). *Clues: Investigating solutions in brief therapy.* New York: Norton.

de Shazer, S. (1988b). Utilization: The foundation of solutions. In J.K. Zeig & S.R. Lankton (Eds.), *Developing Ericksonian therapy: State of the art.* New York: Brunner/Mazel.

de Shazer, S. (1991a). Foreword. In Y. Dolan, *Resolving sexual abuse: Solution-focused therapy and Ericksonian hypnosis for adult survivors.* New York: Norton.

de Shazer, S. (1991b). *Putting difference to work.* New York: Norton.

de Shazer, S. (1994). *Words were originally magic.* New York: Norton.

de Shazer, S. (1998). *The right path or the other path: Working with a teenage substance misuser.* (Videotape). Milwaukee, WS: Brief Family Therapy Centre.

de Shazer, S. (2004). *I want to want to.* Videotape. Milwaukee, WI: Brief Family Therapy Center.

de Shazer, S., Berg, I.K., & Miller, G. (1995). Solution-focused brief therapy: Advanced supervision seminar, Brief Therapy Center, Milwaukee, Wisconsin, November 3-5.

de Shazer, S., Dolan, Y., Korman, H., McCollum, E., Trepper, T., & Berg, I.K. (2007). *More than miracles: The state of the art of solution-focused brief therapy.* Binghamton, NY: The Haworth Press.

Dear, G. (2001). Further comments on the nomenclature for suicide-related thoughts and behaviour. *Suicide and Life-Threatening Behaviour, 31,* 234-235.

Dechant, H. (2005, Oct.). Aboriginal youth suicide prevention strategy—Alberta Children and Youth Initiative. Presented at the Canadian Association for Suicide Prevention Conference, Ottawa, Ontario, Canada, October 16-19.

DeLeo, D., Burgis, S., Bertolote, J.M., Kerkhof, A., & Bille-Brahe, U. (2004). Definitions of suicidal behaviour. In D. DeLeo, U. Bille-Brahe, A. Kerkhof, & A. Schmidtke (Eds.), *Suicidal behaviour: Theories and research findings* (pp. 17-39). Cambridge, MA: Hogrefe & Huber.

Denny, D. (2004). Changing models of transsexualism. In U. Leli & J. Drescher (Eds.), *Transgender subjectivities: A clinician's guide* (pp. 25-40). Binghamton, NY: The Haworth Press.

Denton, W.H. & Burwell, S.R. (2006). Systemic couple intervention for depression in women. *Journal of Systemic Therapies, 25*(3), 43-57.

Depression Information Resource and Education Center (DIRECT) (1997). Fact sheets on depression. Retrieved from http://www.fhs.mcmaster.ca/direct.

Dobbs, D. (2006). Turning off depression. *Scientific American Mind, 17*(4), 26-31.

Dolan, Y. (1991). *Resolving sexual abuse: Solution-focused therapy and Ericksonian hypnosis for adult survivors.* New York: Norton.

Dolan, Y. (1994). Solution-focused therapy with sexual abuse survivors–Handout. Workshop, Hincks Institute, Toronto, Ontario, Canada, April 6-7.

Dolan, Y. (2002). The pragmatics of hope. Presented at the Brief Therapy Network Conference, Toronto, Ontario, Canada, April 25-26.

Dolan, Y. (2006). Implicit ways to communicate hope during conversation. Workshop handout, Western Canadian Solution-Focused Conference, Vancouver, British Columbia, Canada, April 26-28.

Donaldson, D., Spirito, A., & Overholser, J. (2003). Treatment of adolescent suicide attempters. In A. Spirito & J. Overholser (Eds.), *Evaluating and treating adolescent suicide attempters: From research to practice* (pp. 295-321). San Diego: Academic Press.

Drye, R.C., Goulding, R.L., & Goulding, M.E. (1973). No-suicide decisions: Patient monitoring of suicide risk. *American Journal of Psychiatry, 130,* 171-174.

Dulit, E. (1995). Immediately after the suicide attempt. In J.K. Zimmerman & G.M. Asnis (Eds.), *Treatment approaches with suicidal adolescents* (pp. 91-105). New York: Wiley.

Duncan, B., Hubble, M., & Miller, S. (1997). *Psychotherapy with "impossible" cases: The efficient treatment of therapy veterans.* New York: Norton.

Duncan, B. & Miller, S. (Eds.) (2000). *The heroic CLIENT: Doing client-directed, outcome-informed therapy.* San Francisco: Jossey-Bass.

Duncan, B.L. & Miller, S.D. (2005). Treatment manuals do not improve outcomes. Retrieved May, 15, 2006, from http://www.talkingcure.com/reference.

Duncan, B.L., Miller, S.D., Sparks, J.A., Claud, D.A., Reynolds, L.R., Brown, J., & Johnson, L.D. (2003). The session rating scale: Preliminary psychometric properties of a "working" alliance measure. *Journal of Brief Therapy, 3*(1), 3-12.

Dunne-Maxim, K. (2000). Students against destructive decisions. Presented at the American Association of Suicidology Conference, Los Angeles, California, April 12-15.

Duvall, J. & Rockman, P. (1996). Living a wonderful life: A conversation with Yvonne Dolan. *Journal of Systemic Therapies, 15*(3), 82-92.

Eagles, J.M., Carson, D.P., Begg, A., & Naji, S.A. (2003). Suicide prevention: A study of patients' views. *British Journal of Psychiatry, 182,* 261-265.

Edmunds, A. (1994). Creating and implementing support groups. Presented at the Canadian Association for Suicide Prevention Conference, Iqaluit, Northwest Territories, Canada, May 12-15.

Edmunds, A. (1998). My story: Thoughts of a survivor. In A.A. Leenaars, S. Wenckstern, I. Sakinofsky, R.J. Dyck, M.J. Kral, & R.C. Bland (Eds.), *Suicide in Canada* (pp. 369-375). Toronto: University of Toronto Press.

Edmunds, A. (2000). Rituals as a way of remembering and healing. Presented at the Canadian Association for Suicide Prevention Conference, Vancouver, British Columbia, Canada, October 11-14.

Edmunds, H. (2006). The experience of men's grief: A video and print presentation. Presented at the Canadian Association for Suicide Prevention Conference, Toronto, Ontario, Canada, October 25-29.

Egel, L. (1999). On the need for a new term for suicide. *Suicide and Life-Threatening Behavior, 29,* 393-394.

Eisen, A. (1995). *Good advice for a happy life: A book of quotations.* Kansas City, MO: Andrews and McMeel.

Ekins, R. & King, D. (1997). Blending genders: Contributions to the emerging field of transgender studies. *The International Journal of Transgenderism, 1*(1). Retrieved from http://www.symposion.com/ijt/.

Eliot, T.S. (1969). Ash-Wednesday. In *The complete poems and plays of T.S. Eliot.* London: Faber and Faber. (Original work published 1930).

Ellenbogen, S. & Gratton, F. (2001). Do they suffer more? Reflections on research comparing suicide survivors to other survivors. *Suicide and Life-Threatening Behavior, 31,* 83-90.

Ellis, T.E. (2000). Therapies for suicidal patients: Common threads. Presented at the American Association of Suicidology Conference, Santa Fe, New Mexico, April 22-26.

Ellis, T.E. & Newman, C.F. (1996). *Choosing to live: How to defeat suicide through cognitive therapy*. Oakland, CA: New Harbinger.

Esposito-Smythers, C., McClung, T.J., & Fairlie, A.M. (2006). Adolescent perceptions of a suicide prevention group on an inpatient unit. *Archives of Suicide Research, 10*, 265-276.

Evans, W., Smith, M., Hill, G., Albers, E., & Neufeld, J. (1966). Rural adolescent views of risk and protective factors associated with suicide. *Crisis Intervention, 3*, 1-12.

Eyler, A.E. & Wright, K. (1997). Gender identification and sexual orientation among genetic females with gender-blended self-perception in childhood and adolescence. *The International Journal of Transgenderism, 1*(1). Retrieved from http://www.symposion.com/ijt./.

Favazza, A. (1989). Why patients mutilate themselves. *Hospital and Community Psychiatry, 40*, 137-145.

Favazza, A. (1996). *Bodies under siege* (2nd ed.). Baltimore: Johns Hopkins University Press.

Feinberg, L. (1998). *Transliberation: Beyond pink or blue*. Boston: Beacon Press.

Figley, C.R. (Ed.) (1995). Compassion fatigue: Coping with secondary traumatic stress disorder in those who treat the traumatized. New York: Brunner/Mazel.

Fiske, H. (1993). *A psychoeducational group program for parents of suicidal adolescents*. Presented at the International Association of Suicide Prevention Conference, Montreal, Quebec, Canada, May 31-June 2.

Fiske, H. (1995). Solution-focused brief therapy in suicide prevention. Presented at the International Association of Suicide Prevention Conference, Venice, Italy, June 4-8.

Fiske, H. (1997). Solution-focused brief therapy in suicide prevention. Presented at the American Association of Suicidology Annual Conference, Memphis, Tennessee, April 23-27.

Fiske, H. (1998a). Applications of solution-focused therapy in suicide prevention. In D. Deleo, A. Schmidtke, & R.F.W. Diekstra (Eds.), *Suicide prevention: A holistic approach* (pp. 185-197). Dordrecht, the Netherlands: Kluwer.

Fiske, H. (1998b). Including parents of suicidal adolescents in the treatment process (summary). Presented at the American Association of Suicidology Annual Conference, Bethesda, MD, April 15-18.

Fiske, H. (2000). Utilizing approaches that fit with adolescent development and priorities. A Y2K special: Three skills building workshops. Presented at the American Association of Suicidology Annual Conference, Los Angeles, California, April 12-15.

Fiske, H. (2001). Clinicians' round table: Sonya—treating a suicidal 13-year-old. *Lifenotes, 6*(1), 11-12.

Fiske, H. (2002). Reasons for living: Ideas for intervention. Presented at the American Association of Suicidology Annual Conference, Bethesda, Maryland, April 10-13.

Fiske, H. (2003). Reasons for living via the telephone. Presented at the American Association of Suicidology Annual Conference, Santa Fe, New Mexico, April 22-26.

Fiske, H. (2004a). Eliciting and using suicidal callers' reasons for living. Presented at the American Association of Suicidology Annual Conference, Miami, Florida, April 14-17.

Fiske, H. (2004b). Living with a suicidal person: What families can do. In J.F. Connolly & J. Scott (Eds.), *Suicide prevention: What you can do. Proceedings of the Irish Association of Suicidology ninth annual conference* (pp. 130-135). Castlebar, Ireland: IAS.

Fiske, H., Ball, D., Edmunds, H., & Hill, A. (2003). Men's experiences as survivors of suicide. Presented at the Canadian Association of Suicide Prevention conference, Iqaluit, Northwest Territories, Canada, May 15-18.

Fiske, H. & "James" (2002). Working with a suicidal transgendered client: Treatment issues. Presented at the 13th Annual Conference of the Canadian Association for Suicide Prevention, Saint John, New Brunswick, Canada, October 20-23.

Fiske, H. & "James" (2003). Treating transgendered clients: Suicide risk. Poster presented at the Annual Conference of the American Association of Suicidology, Santa Fe, New Mexico, April 22-26.

Fiske, H. & Zalter, B. (2005). Solution-focused approaches to bereavement. Presented at the Solution-Focused Brief Therapy Association Conference, Fort Lauderdale, Florida, November 3-5.

Frankl, V.E. (1997). *Man's search for ultimate meaning.* New York: Insight Books.

Franklin, C., Corcoran, J., Nowicki, J., & Streeter, C.L. (1997). Using client self-anchored scales to measure outcomes in solution-focused therapy. *Journal of Systemic Therapies, 16*(3), 246-265.

Frederickson, B.L. (2000). Cultivating positive emotions to optimize health and well-being. *Prevention and Treatment, 3*, article 0001a. Retrieved February 20, 2003, from http://www.journals.apa.org/prevention/volume3/pre0030001a.html.

Frederickson, B.L. (2001). The role of positive emotions in positive psychology: The broaden-and-build theory of positive emotions. *American Psychologist, 56,* 218-226.

Frederickson, B.L. & Joiner, T. (2002). Positive emotions trigger upward spirals toward emotional well-being. *Psychological Science, 13,* 172-175.

Freedman, J. & Combs, G. (1997). Lists. In C. Smith & D. Nylund (Eds.), *Narrative therapies with children and adolescents* (pp.147-161). New York: Guilford.

Freud, S. (1959). On psychotherapy. In E. Jones (Ed.), *Collected papers,* (Vol. 1, pp. 249-263). Joan Riviere, trans. New York: Basic Books. (Original work published 1904).

Furst, J. & Huffine, C.L. (1991). Assessing vulnerability to suicide. *Suicide and Life-Threatening Behavior, 21,* 329-344.

Gallagher, D. & Korman, H. (2006). Some "new" ideas in the treatment of substance abuse with a focus on "relapse." Presented at the Solution-Focused Brief Therapy Association Conference, Denver, Colorado, November 2-4.

Garrison, C.Z., McKeown, R.E., Valois, R.F., & Vincent, M.L. (1993). Aggression, substance use, and suicidal behaviors in high school students. *American Journal of Public Health, 83,* 179-184.

Gassmann, D. & Grawe, K. (2006). General change mechanisms: The relation between problem activation and resource activation in successful and unsuccessful therapeutic interactions. *Clinical Psychology and Psychotherapy, 13,* 1-11.

Geller, J., Brown, K.E., Zaitsoff, S.L., Goodrich, S., & Hastings, F. (2003). Collaborative versus directive interventions in the treatment of eating disorders: Implications for care providers. *Professional Psychology: Research and Practice, 34,* 406-413.

George, E., Iveson, C., & Ratner, H. (1999). *Problem to solutions: Brief therapy with individuals and families,* (Rev. ed.). London: Brief Therapy Press.

Ghul, R. (2005). Introducing solution-focused thinking: A half-day workshop. In T. Nelson (Ed.), *Education and training in Solution-Focused Brief Therapy* (pp. 169-174). Binghamton, NY: The Haworth Press.

Gibbons, R.D., Hur, K., Bhaumik, D.K., & Mann, J.J. (2005). The relationship between antidepressant medication use and rate of suicide. *Archives of General Psychiatry, 62,* 165-172.

Gingerich, W.J. & Eisengart, S. (2000). Solution-focused brief therapy: A review of the outcome research. *Family Process, 39,* 477-498.

Goldfried, M.R. & Wolfe, B.E. (1999). Toward a more clinically valid approach to therapy research. *Journal of Consulting and Clinical Psychology, 66*(1), 143-150.

Goldman, S. & Beardslee, W.R. (1999). Suicide in children and adolescents. In D.G. Jacobs (Ed.), *The Harvard Medical School guide to suicide assessment and intervention* (pp. 417-442). San Francisco: Jossey-Bass.

Goldney, R.D. (2000). Prediction of suicide and attempted suicide. In K. Hawton & K. van Heeringen (Eds.), *International handbook of suicide and attempted suicide* (pp. 585-595.). Chichester, UK: Wiley.

Goldney, R.D. (2005). Suicide prevention: A pragmatic review of recent studies. *Crisis, 26*(3), 128-140.

Gordon, D. & Meyers-Anderson, M. (1981). *Phoenix: Therapeutic patterns of Milton H. Erickson.* Cupertino, CA: Meta.

Gould, M.S., Marrocco, F.A., Kleinman, M., Thomas, J.G., Mostkoff, K., Cote, J., & Davies, M. (2005). Evaluating iatrogenic risk of youth screening programs: A randomized controlled trial. *Journal of the American Medical Association, 293*(13), 1635-1643.

Grad, O., Clark, S., Dyregrov, K., & Andriessen, K. (2004). What helps and what hinders the process of surviving the suicide of somebody close? *Crisis, 25*(3), 134-139.

Greenberg, R.P., Constantino, M.J., & Bruce, N. (2006). Are patient expectations still relevant for psychotherapy process and outcome? *Clinical Psychology Review, 26,* 657-678.

Greene, G.J., Lee, M.-Y., & Trask, R. (1996). Client strengths and crisis intervention: A solution-focused approach. *Crisis Intervention and Time-Limited Treatment, 3*(1), 43-63.

Greene G.J., Lee, M.L., Trask, R. & Rheinscheld, J. (2000). How to work with clients' strengths in crisis intervention: A solution-focused approach. In A.R. Roberts (Ed.), *Crisis intervention handbook: Assessment, treatment, and research* (2nd ed., pp. 31-55). New York: Oxford University Press.

Greenhill, L.L. & Waslick, B. (1997). Management of suicidal behaviour in children and adolescents. *Psychiatric Clinics of North America, 20,* 641-666.

Group for the Advancement of Psychiatry, Committee on Adolescence (1996). *Adolescent suicide.* Washington, DC: American Psychiatric Press.

Handron, D.S., Dosser, D.A. Jr., McCammon, S.L., & Powell, J.Y. (1998). "Wraparound"—The wave of the future: Theoretical and professional practice implications for children and families with complex needs. *Journal of Family Nursing, 4,* 65-86.

Harry, J. (1994). Parasuicide, gender, and gender deviance. In G. Remafedi (Ed.), *Death by denial: Studies of suicide in gay and lesbian teenagers* (pp. 69-88). Boston: Alyson.

Hawkes, D., Marsh, T.I., & Wilgosh, R. (1998). *Solution-focused therapy: A handbook for health care professionals.* Boston: Butterworth-Heinemann.

Hawkins, M.T. & Miller, R.J. (2003). Cognitive vulnerability and resilience to depressed mood. *Australian Journal of Psychology, 55,* 176-183.

Hawton, K. (2000). General hospital management of suicide attempters. In K. Hawton & K. van Heeringen (Eds.), *The international handbook of suicide and attempted suicide* (pp. 518-537). Chichester, UK: Wiley.

Hawton, K., Rodham, K., & Evans, E. (2006). *By their own young hand: Deliberate self-harm and suicidal ideas in adolescence.* London: Jessica Kingsley Publishers.

Hawton, K. & van Heeringen, K. (2000). Future perspectives. In K. Hawton & K. van Heeringen (Eds.), *International handbook of suicide and attempted suicide* (pp. 713-724). Chichester, UK: Wiley.

Hazell, P. (2000). Treatment strategies for adolescent suicide attempters. In K. Hawton & K. van Heeringen (Eds.), *International handbook of suicide and attempted suicide* (pp. 539-554). Chichester, UK: Wiley.

Healy, D. (2003). Lines of evidence on the risks of suicide with selective serotonin reuptake inhibitors. *Psychotherapy and Psychosomatics, 72,* 71-79.

Heard, H.L. (2000). Psychotherapeutic approaches to suicidal ideation and behaviour. In K. Hawton & K. van Heeringen (Eds.), *International handbook of suicide and attempted suicide* (pp. 503-518). Chichester, UK: Wiley.

Heisel, M.J. & Flett. G.L. (2000). Meaning in life and the prevention of suicide ideation. Presented at the American Association of Suicidology Annual Conference, Los Angeles, California, April 12-15.

Henden, J. (2005). Preventing suicide using a solution-focused approach. *The Journal of Primary Care Mental Health, 8* (3), 81-88

Hendin, H., Maltsberger, J.T., Haas, A.P., Szanto, K., & Rabinowicz, H. (2004). Desperation and other affective states in suicidal patients. *Suicide and Life-Threatening Behavior 34*(4), 386-394.

Herman, J. (1992). *Trauma and recovery: The aftermath of violence.* New York: Basic Books.

Hjelmeland, H. & Hawton, K. (2004). Intentional aspects of non-fatal suicidal behaviour. In D. DeLeo, U. Bille-Brahe, A. Kerkhof, & A. Schmidtke (Eds.), *Suicidal behaviour: Theories and research findings* (pp. 66-78). Cambridge, MA: Hogrefe & Huber.

Hill, A. (2000). Suicide in the legal profession. *It takes a village: Ontario Suicide Prevention Network Newsletter, 3*(1), 1-2.

Hill, A., Fox, F., Campbell, F., & Fiske, H. (2004). Men's experience of grief after suicide loss. Presented at the American Association of Suicidology Conference, Miami, Florida, April 14-17.

Hirsch, J.K. & Conner, K.R. (2006). Dispositional and explanatory style optimism as potential moderators of the relationship between hopelessness and suicidal ideation. *Suicide and Life-Threatening Behavior, 36*(6), 661-669.

Hoff, L.A. (2001). *People in crisis: Clinical and public health perspectives* (5th ed.). San Francisco: Jossey-Bass.

Hoffman, A. (1995). *Practical magic.* New York: Berkley Books.

Holman, G. & Lorig, K. (2000). Patients as partners in managing chronic disease. *British Medical Journal, 72*(34), 526-527.

Hopson, L. & Kim, J. (2005). A solution-focused approach to crisis intervention with adolescents. *Journal of Evidence-Based Social Work, 1*(2-3), 93-110.

Howard, K., Kopta, M., Krause, M., & Orlinsky, D. (1986). The dose-response relationship in psychotherapy. *American Psychologist, 41,* 149-164.

Hoyt, M.F. (1996). Solution-building and language games: A conversation with Steve de Shazer [and Insoo Kim Berg]. In M.F. Hoyt (Ed.), *Constructive Therapies 2* (pp. 60-86). New York: Guilford.

Hoyt, M.F. & Berg, I.K. (1998). Solution-focused couple therapy: Helping couples construct self-fulfilling realities. In Michael Hoyt (Ed.), *The handbook of constructive therapies* (pp. 314-340). San Francisco: Jossey-Bass.

Hoyt, M.F., Miller, S.D., Held, B.S., & Matthews, W.J. (2001). A conversation about constructivism; or, If four colleagues talked in New York, would anyone hear it? *Journal of Systemic Therapies, 20*(1), 78-94.

Humphreys, H. (2002). *The lost garden.* Toronto: HarperCollins.

Idlout, L. & Kral, M.J. (2005). *Katujjiqatigiit: Community models of successful suicide prevention in Nunavut.* Presented at the Canadian Association for Suicide Prevention Conference, Ottawa, Ontario, Canada, October 16-19.

Irwin, C. (1998). *Conquering the beast within: How I fought depression and won . . . and how you can, too.* Toronto: Random House Canada.

Isaacson, G. (2000). Suicide prevention: A medical breakthrough. *Acta Psychiatrica Scandinavica, 102,* 113-117.

Isen, A.M. (2002). Positive affect and decision-making. In M. Lewis and J.M. Haviland-Jones (Eds.), *Handbook of emotions* (2nd ed., pp. 417-435). New York: Guilford.

Iveson, C. (2002). Solution-focused brief therapy. *Advances in Psychiatric Treatment, 8,* 149-157.

Iveson (2003). Solution-focused couple therapy. In B. O'Connell & S. Palmer (Eds.), *Handbook of solution-focused brief therapy* (pp. 62-73). London, UK: Sage.

Jamison, K.R. (1995). *An unquiet mind: A memoir of moods and madness.* New York: Knopf.

Janoff-Bulman, R. (1992). *Shattered assumptions: Toward a new psychology of trauma.* New York: Free Press.

Janoff-Bulman, R. (1999). Rebuilding shattered assumptions after traumatic life events: Coping processes and outcomes. In C.R. Snyder (Ed.), *Coping: The psychology of what works* (pp. 305-323). New York: Oxford.

Jenkins, R. & Singh, B. (2000). General population strategies of suicide prevention. In K. Hawton & K. van Heeringen (Eds.), *International handbook of suicide and attempted suicide* (pp. 597-616). Chichester, UK: Wiley.

Jennings, G.L.R., Reid, C.M., Christy, I., Jennings, J., Anderson, W.P., & Dart, A. (1998). Animals and cardiovascular health. In C.C. Wilson & D.C. Turner (Eds.), *Companion animals in human health* (pp. 161-171). Thousand Oaks: Sage.

Jobes, D.A. (1995). The psychodynamic treatment of adolescent suicide attempters. In J. Zimmerman & G.M. Asnis (Eds.), *Treatment approaches with suicidal adolescents* (pp.137-154). New York: Wiley.

Jobes, D.A. (2006). *Managing suicidal risk: A collaborative approach.* New York: Guilford.

Jobes, D.A. & Nelson, K.N. (2006). Shneidman's contributions to the understanding of suicidal thinking. In T.E. Ellis (Ed.), *Cognition and suicide* (pp. 29-49). Washington, DC: American Psychological Association.

Jobes, D.A., Wong, S.A., Conrad, A., Drozod, J.F., & Neal-Walden, T. (2005). The collaborative assessment and management of suicidality vs. treatment as usual: A retrospective study with suicidal outpatients. *Suicide and Life-Threatening Behavior, 35,* 483-497.

Johnson, A., Cooper, J., & Kapur, N. (2006). Exploring the relationship between area characteristics and self-harm. *Crisis, 27*(2), 88-91.

Johnson, C.E. & Goldman, J. (1996). Taking safety home: A solution-focused approach with domestic violence. In M.F. Hoyt (Ed.), *Constructive therapies 2* (pp. 184-196). New York: Guilford.

Johnson, L.D. (1995). *Psychotherapy in the age of accountability*. New York: Norton.

Johnson, L.D. & Miller, S.D. (1994). Modification of depression risk factors: A solution-focused approach. *Psychotherapy Theory Research Practice and Training, 31*, 244-253.

Johnson, L.D., Miller, S.D., & Duncan, B.L. (2000). Session rating scale (SRS V. 3.0). Retrieved June 2, 2004, from http://www.talkingcure.com/bookstore.asp ?id=106.

Johnson, L.N., Nelson, T.S., & Allgood, S.M. (1998). Noticing pre-treatment change and therapy outcome: An initial study. *The American Journal of Family Therapy, 26*, 159-168.

Joiner, T.E. (2005). *Why people die by suicide*. Cambridge, MA: Harvard University Press.

Joiner, T.E., Pettit, J.W., Perez, M., Burns, A.B., Gencoz, T., Gencoz, F., et al. (2001). Can positive emotion influence problem-solving attitudes among suicidal adults? *Professional psychology: Research and Practice, 32*, 507-512.

Joiner, T.E., Rudd, M.D., & Rajab, M.H. (1999). Agreement between self- and clinician- rated symptoms in a clinical sample of young adults: Explaining discrepancies. *Journal of Consulting and Clinical Psychology, 67*(2), 171-176.

Jordan, J.R. (2001). Is suicide bereavement different? A reassessment of the literature. *Suicide and Life-Threatening Behavior, 31,* 91-102,

Jordan, J.R. & McMenamy, J. (2004). Interventions for suicide survivors: A review of the literature. *Suicide and Life-Threatening Behavior, 34*(4), 337-349.

Jureidini, J.N., Doecke, C.J., Mansfield, P., Haby, M., Menkes, D., & Tonkin, A. (2004). Efficacy and safety of antidepressants for children and adolescents. *British Medical Journal, 328*, 879-883.

Kast, V. (1994/1991). *Joy, inspiration, and hope*. D. Whitcher, trans. New York: Fromm International.

Katt, M., Kinch, P., Boone, M., & Minore, B. (1998). Coping with northern aboriginal youths' suicides. In A. Leenaars, I. Sakinofsky, R.J. Dyck, M.J. Kral, & R.C. Bland (Eds.), *Suicide in Canada* (pp. 212-226). Toronto: University of Toronto Press.

Kazdin, A.E. (1999). The meanings and measurement of clinical significance. *Journal of Consulting and Clinical Psychology, 67*(3), 332-339.

Kazdin, A.E., & Nock, M.K. (2003). Delineating mechanisms of change in child and adolescent therapy: Methodological issues and research recommendations. *Journal of Child Psychology and Psychiatry, 44*, 1116-1129.

Keeley, H.S., Corcoran, P., & Bille-Brahe, U. (2004). Addiction and suicidal behaviour: Questions and answers in the EPSIS. In D. DeLeo, U. Bille-Brahe, A.
Kerkhof, & A. Schmidtke (Eds.), *Suicidal behaviour: Theories and research
findings* (pp. 165-184). Cambridge, MA: Hogrefe & Huber.

Kerkhof, A. (2000). Attempted suicide: Patterns and trends. In K. Hawton & K. van
Heeringen (Eds.), *International handbook of suicide and attempted suicide* (pp.
49-64). Chichester, UK: Wiley.

Kerkhof, A. & Arensman, E. (2004). Repetition of attempted suicide: Frequent, but
hard to predict. In D. DeLeo, U. Bille-Brahe, A. Kerkhof, & A. Schmidtke
(Eds.), *Suicidal Behaviour: Theories and research findings* (pp. 111-124). Cambridge, MA: Hogrefe & Huber.

Kidd, S.A. (2006). Risk and resilience among homeless youth. Presented at Suicide
Study Rounds, the Arthur Sommer Rotenberg Chair in Suicide Studies, Toronto,
Ontario, Canada, April 10.

Kidd, S.A. & Kral, M.J. (2002). Suicide and prostitution among street youth: Qualitative analysis. *Adolescence, 37,* 411-430.

Kids' Help Phone (1994). *Counselling young people by phone: A Kids Help Phone
handbook for professional and volunteer counsellors.* Toronto: Kids Help
Phone.

Killias, M., van Kesteren, J., & Rindlisbacher, M. (2001). Guns, violent crime, and
suicide in 21 countries. *Canadian Journal of Criminology, 43,* 429-448.

King, C.A., Kramer, A., Preuss, L., Kerr, D.C.R., Weisse, L., & Venkataraman
(2006). Youth nomimated support team for suicidal adolescents (version 1): A
randomized clinical trial. *Journal of Consulting and Clinical Psychology, 74*(1),
199-206.

King, T. (1990). Introduction. In T. King (Ed.), *All my relations: An anthology of
contemporary native fiction.* Toronto: McClelland & Stewart.

King, T. (2003). The truth about stories: A native narrative. Toronto: Anansi.

Kirmayer, L., Fletcher, C., & Boothroyd, L.J. (1998). Suicide among the Inuit of
Canada. In A.A. Leenaars, S. Wenckstern, I. Sakinofsky, R.J. Dyck, M.J. Kral,
& R.C. Bland (Eds.), *Suicide in Canada* (pp. 189-211). Toronto: University of
Toronto Press.

Knekt, P. & Lindfors, O. (Eds.) (2004). A randomized trial of the effects of four
forms of psychotherapy on depressive and anxiety disorders: Design, methods,
and results on the effectiveness of short-term dynamic psychotherapy and solution-focused therapy during a one-year follow-up. *Studies in Social Security and
Health, 77.* Helsinki, Finland: KELA The Social Insurance Institution.

Korhonen, M.I. (2006). *Basic counselling skills: Inuit voices, modern methods.* Ottawa: The Ajunnginiq Centre of the National Aboriginal Health Organization.

Korman, H. (2005). Comment on the Solution-Focused Listserv, www.sikt.nu.

Korman, H. (2006). Plenary presentation. Solution-Focused Brief Therapy Association Conference, Denver, Colorado, November 2-4.

Kral, M.J. (2003). Unikkaartuit: *Meanings of well-being, sadness, suicide and change in two Inuit communities*. Final Report to the National Health Research and Development Programs, Health Canada. Ottawa: Health Canada.

Kreider, J.W. (1998). Solution-focused ideas for briefer therapy with longer-term clients. In M.F. Hoyt (Ed.), *The handbook of constructive therapies* (pp. 341-357). San Francisco: Jossey-Bass.

Kronkite, K. (1994). *On the edge of darkness: Conversations about conquering depression*. New York: Doubleday.

Kruesi, M., Grossman, J., Pennington, J., Woodward, P., Duda, D., & Hirsch, J. (1999). Suicide and violence prevention: Parent education in the emergency department. *Journal of the American Academy of Child and Adolescent Psychiatry, 38,* 250-255.

Kuehl, B.P., Barnard, C.P., & Nelson, T.S. (1998). Making the genogram solution based. In T. Nelson & T. Trepper (Eds.), *101 more interventions in family therapy*. Binghamton, NY: The Haworth Press.

La Cerva, V. (1999). *Worldwords: Global reflections to awaken the spirit*. Cordova, TN: HEAL Foundation Press.

Lam, R.W. & Tam, E.M. (2000). Effects of light therapy on suicidal ideation in patients with winter depression. *Journal of Clinical Psychiatry, 61*(1), 30-32.

Lamarre, J. (2003). The pearl in the oyster: The trouble that builds something marvellous. Presented at the Solution-Focused Brief Therapy Association Conference, Loma Linda, California, November 2-3.

Lambert, M.J. (1992). Implications of outcome research for psychotherapy integration. In J.C. Norcross & M.R. Goldfried (Eds.), *Handbook of psychotherapy integration* (pp. 94-129). New York: Basic.

Lambert, M. (2004) (Ed.). *Bergin and Garfield's handbook of psychotherapy and behaviour change* (5th ed.). New York: Wiley.

Lambert, M.J., Hansen, M.J., Unphress, V., Lunnen, K., Okiishi, J., Burlingame, G. et al. (1996). *Administration and scoring manual for the Outcome Questionnaire (OQ 45.2)*. Washington, DC: American Professional Credentialing Services.

Lambert, M.J., Okiishi, J.C., Finch, A.E., and Johnson, L.D. (1998). Outcome assessment: From conceptualization to implementation. *Professional Psychology: Research and Practice, 29,* 63-70.

Lamott, A. (1999). *Traveling mercies*. New York: Anchor Books.

Langer, E.J. (1989). *Mindfulness*. Reading, MA: Addison-Wesley.

Langer, E. (1997). *The power of mindful learning*. Reading, MA: Addison-Wesley.

Laszloffy, T. (2000). Awesome allies: Tapping the wisdom of an adolescent's peers. *Psychotherapy Networker,* January/February, 71-77.

Latham, A.E. & Prigerson, H.G. (2004). Suicidality and bereavement: Complicated grief as psychiatric disorder presenting greatest risk for suicidality. *Suicide and Life-Threatening Behavior, 34*(4), 350-363.

Lawlor, D.A. & Hopker, G.W. (2001). The effectiveness of exercise as anintervention in the management of depression: Systematic review and meta-regression of randomised controlled trials. *British Medical Journal, 322,* 763-767.

Lawson, D. (1994). Identifying pretreatment change. *Journal of Counselling and Development, 72,* 244-248.

Lee, M.Y., Greene, G.J., Mentzer, R.A., Pinnell, S., & Niles, D. (2001). Solution-focused brief therapy and the treatment of depression: A pilot study. *Journal of Brief Therapy, 1,* 33-49.

Leenaars, A.A. (2006a). Psychotherapy with suicidal people: The commonalities. *Archives of Suicide Research, 10,* 305-322.

Leenaars, A.A. (2006b). Suicide among indigenous peoples: Introduction and a call to action. *Archives of Suicide Research, 10,* 103-115.

Leenaars, A.A., Wenckstern, S., Sakinofsky, I., Dyck, R.J., Kral, M.J., & Bland, R.C. (Eds.) (1998). Preface. In A.A. Leenaars, S. Wenckstern, I. Sakinofsky, R.J. Dyck, M.J. Kral, & R.C. Bland (Eds.), *Suicide in Canada.* Toronto: University of Toronto Press.

Leichensring, F. & Leibing, E. (2003). The effectiveness of psychodynamic therapy and cognitive behaviour therapy in the treatment of personality disorders. *American Journal of Psychiatry, 160,* 123-1232.

Lester, D. (2000). *Why people kill themselves: A 2000 summary of research on suicide.* Springfield, IL: Charles Thomas.

Lethem, J. (2003). Using solution-focused therapy with women. In B. O'Connell and S. Palmer (Eds.), *Handbook of Solution-Focused Therapy* (pp. 118-128). London: Sage.

Letofsky, K. (1998). Trauma and suicide bereavement. Presented at "Helping Suicide Survivors," Conference sponsored by Council on Adolescent Suicide Prevention in Peel, Mississauga, Ontario, Canada, November 6.

Lev, A.I. (2004). *Transgender emergence: Therapeutic guidelines for working with gender-variant people and their families.* Binghamton, NY: The Haworth Press.

Levy, S. & Fletcher, E. (1998). Kamatsiaqtut, Baffin Crisis Line: Community ownership of support in a small town. In A.A. Leenaars, S. Wenckstern, I. Sakinofsky, R.J. Dyck, M.J. Kral, & R.C. Bland (Eds.), *Suicide in Canada* (pp. 353-366). Toronto: University of Toronto Press.

Levy, S., Idlout, L., Toomasie, L., Borg, C., Kunuk, C., & the Nunavut Embrace Life Council (2005). Embrace Life Council model—Partnerships for Life. Presented at the Canadian Association for Suicide Prevention Conference, Ottawa, Ontario, Canada, October 16-19.

Lewins, F. (1995). *Transsexualism in society: A sociology of male-to-female transsexuals.* Melbourne: Macmillan Education Australia.

Linehan, M.M. (1993a). *Cognitive-behavioural treatment of borderline personality disorder.* New York: Guilford.

Linehan, M.M. (1993b). *Skills training manual for treating borderline personality disorder.* New York: Guilford.

Linehan, M.M. (1998). Is anything effective for reducing suicidal behaviour? or, Treatment of suicidal behaviors: The good news and the bad news. Presented at the American Association of Suicidology Annual Conference, Bethesda, Maryland, April 15-18.

Linehan, M. M. (1999a). On creating a life worth living when suicide seems like the only option. (Dublin Award presentation). Presented at the American Association of Suicidology Annual Conference, Houston, Texas, April 16-18.

Linehan, M.M. (1999b). Standard protocol for assessing and treating suicidal behaviors for patients in treatment. In D.G. Jacobs (Ed.), The *Harvard Medical School guide to suicide assessment and intervention* (pp. 146-187). San Francisco: Jossey-Bass.

Linehan, M. (2004). Treating the suicidal person: An update on the science. Presented at the American Association of Suicidology Annual Conference, Miami, Florida, April 14-17.

Linehan, M.M., Goodstein, J.L., Nielsen, S.L., & Chiles, J.A. (1983). Reasons for staying alive when you are thinking of killing yourself: the reasons for living inventory. *Journal of Consulting and Clinical Psychology, 51,* 276-286.

Linehan, M.M., Rizvi, S.L., Welch, S.S., & Page, B. (2000). Psychiatric aspects of suicidal behavior: Personality disorders. In K. Hawton & K. van Heeringen (Eds.), *The international handbook of suicide and attempted suicide* (pp. 147-178). Chichester, UK: Wiley.

Links, P.S. (2004). Evidence-based practices: Researching crisis services using qualitative and quantitative methods. Presented at the Canadian Association for Suicide Prevention Conference, Edmonton, Alberta, Canada, October 20-23.

Links, P.S., Bergmans, Y., & Cook, M. (2003). Psychotherapeutic interventions to prevent repeated suicidal behavior. *Brief Treatment and Crisis Intervention, 3*(4), 445-464.

Links, P.S. & Rourke, S. (2000) Affective lability and suicidal behavior. Presented at the Canadian Association for Suicide Prevention Conference, Vancouver, British Columbia, Canada, October 11-14.

Littrell, J.M. (1998). *Brief counselling in action.* New York: Norton.

Lönnqvist, J.K. (2000). Psychiatric aspects of suicidal behaviour: Depression. In K. Hawton & K. van Heeringen (Eds.), *International handbook of suicide and attempted suicide* (pp. 107-120). Chichester, UK: Wiley.

Luby, J.L., Heffelfinger, A.K., Makrotsky, C., Brown, K.M., Hessler, M.J., Wallis, J.M., & Spitznagel, E.L. (2003). The clinical picture of depression in preschool children. *Journal of the American Academy of Child and Adolescent Psychiatry, 42*(3), 340-348.

Luoma, J.B., Martin, C.E., & Pearson, J.L. (2002). Contact with mental health and primary care providers before suicide: A review of the evidence. *American Journal of Psychiatry, 159,* 909-916.

MacDonald, A. (1995). Brief therapy in adult psychiatry. *Journal of Family Therapy, 16,* 415-426.

MacDonald, A. (1997). Brief therapy in adult psychiatry—Further outcomes. *Journal of Family Therapy, 19,* 213-222.

MacDonald, A. (2003). Research in solution-focused brief therapy. In B. O'Connell & S. Palmer (Eds.), *Handbook of solution-focused therapy* (pp. 12-24). London: Sage.

MacDonald, A. (2005). Brief therapy in adult psychiatry: Results from 15 years of practice. *Journal of Family Therapy, 27*(1), 65-75.

MacDonald, A. (2007). *Solution-focused therapy: Theory, research, and practice.* London: Sage.

MacLeod, A.K. & Moore, R. (2000). Positive thinking revisited: Positive cognitions, well-being and mental health. *Clinical Psychology and Psychotherapy, 7*(1), 1-10.

MacLeod, A.K., Pankhania, B., Lee, M., & Mitchell, D. (1997). Brief communication: Parasuicide, depression and the anticipation of positive and negative future experiences. *Psychological Medicine, 27,* 973-977.

MacLeod, A.K., Rose, G.S., & Williams, J.M.G. (1993). Components of hopelessness about the future and parasuicide. *Cognitive Therapy and Research, 17*(5), 441-455.

MacLeod, A.K. & Salaminiou, E. (2001), Reduced positive future-thinking in depression: Cognitive and affective factors. *Cognition and emotion, 15*(1), 99-107.

MacLeod, W. (1986). Stuffed team members. *Dulwich Centre Review.* Adelaide, Australia: Dulwich Centre.

Maine, S., Shute, R., & Martin, G. (2001). Educating parents about youth suicide: Knowledge, response to suicidal statements, attitude and intention to help. *Suicide and Life-Threatening Behavior, 31*(3), 320-333.

Maione, P.V. & Chenail, R.J. (2000). Qualitative inquiry in psychotherapy: Research on the common factors. In M.A. Hubble, B.L. Duncan, & S.D. Miller (Eds.), *The heart and soul of change: What works in therapy* (pp. 57-88). Washington, DC: American Psychological Association.

Malinen, T. (2004). The wisdom of not knowing—A conversation with Harlene Anderson. *Journal of Systemic Therapies, 23*(2), 68-77.

Malinen, T., Cooper, S., & Dolan, Y. (2003). Lighting the smallest candle: A conversation with Yvonne Dolan. *The Brief Therapy Network News,* Spring, 3-7. Retrieved January 30, 2004, from http://www.brieftherapynetwork.com/yvonne .htm.

Malone, K.M. (2000). Protective factors against suicide acts in a major depression: Reasons for living. *American Journal of Psychiatry, 157,* 1084-1088.

Maltsberger, J.T. & Buie, D.H. (1974). Countertransference hate in the treatment of suicidal patients. *Archives of General Psychiatry, 30,* 625-633.

Mann, J.J., Apter, A., Bertolote, J., Beautrais, A., Currier, D., Haas, A., Hegerl, U., Lonnqvist, J., Malone, K., Marusic, A., Mehlum, L., Patton, G., Phillips, M., Rutz, W., Rihmer, Z., Schmidtke, A., Shaffer, A., Silverman, M., Takahashi, Y., Varnik, A., Wasserman, D., Yip, P., & Hendin, H. (2005). Suicide prevention strategies: A systematic review. *Journal of the American Medical Association, 294*(16), 2064-2074.

March, J.S. & Curry, J.F. (1996). Predicting the outcome of treatment. *Journal of Abnormal Psychology, 26*(1), 39-51.

Marlatt, G.A. & Gordon, J.R. (1989). *Relapse prevention.* New York: Guilford.

Mars, J. (Ed.) (2002). *Zen.* Kansas City: Ariel Books.

Masecar, D. (1998). Suicide prevention in rural communities: "Designing a way forward." In A.A. Leenaars, S. Wenckstern, I. Sakinofsky, R.J. Dyck, M.J. Kral, & R.C. Bland (Eds.), *Suicide in Canada* (pp. 242-255). Toronto: University of Toronto Press.

Masecar, D. (1999). Before the first decade: Children and suicide. Presented at the Canadian Association of Suicide Prevention Conference, Halifax, Nova Scotia, Canada, October 13-16.

Masecar, D. (2006). *Niagara region suicide prevention strategy.* St. Catherines, ON: Niagara Region Suicide Prevention Coalition. Retrieved November 30, 2006, from http://www.communitylifelines.ca/Projects.htm.

Masten, A.S. (2001). Ordinary magic: Resilience processes in development. *American Psychologist, 56*(3), 227-238.

May, P.A. (2003). A brief overview of the history of suicide epidemiology and research among American Indians. Presented at the American Association of Suicide Prevention Annual Conference, Santa Fe, New Mexico, April 22-26.

May, P.A., Serna, P., Hurt, L., & DeBruyn, L. (2005). Outcome evaluation of a public health approach to suicide prevention in an American Indian Tribal Nation. *American Journal of Public Health, 95*(7), 238-244.

McGee, D., DelVento, A., & Bavelas, J. (2005). An interactional model of questions as therapeutic interventions. *Journal of Marital and Family Therapy, 31*(4), 371-384.

McGlothin, J.M. (2006). Assessing perturbation and suicide in families. *The Family Journal, 14*(2), 129-134.

McIntosh, J.L. (1997). Suicide's aftermath: Development of a curriculum. In J.L. McIntosh (Ed.), *The legacy of suicide: Proceedings of the American Association of Suicide Conference, Memphis, TN* (p. 48). Washington, DC: AAS.

McIntosh, J.L., Allbright, S., & Jones, F.A. (2002). Therapist survivors: An AAS survey. Poster presented at American Association of Suicidology Conference, Bethesda, Maryland, April 10-13.

McKeel, A.J. (1996). A clinician's guide to research on solution-focused brief therapy. In S. Miller, M. Hubble, & B. Duncan (Eds.), *Handbook of solution-focused brief therapy.* San Francisco: Jossey-Bass.

McKeel, A.J. (1999). A selected review of research of solution-focused brief therapy, 1-13. Retrieved June 13, 2003, from http://www.solutions.doc.co.uk /McKeel.htm.

Metcalf, L. (1997). *Parenting toward solutions; How parents can use skills they already have to raise responsible, loving kids.* Englewood Cliffs, NJ: Prentice-Hall.

Metcalf, L. (1998). *Solution-focused group therapy.* New York: The Free Press.

Michel, K. & Valach, L. (2001). Suicide as goal-directed action. In K. van Heeringen (Ed.), *Understanding suicidal behavior* (pp. 230-254). New York: Wiley.

Miller, G. (1997). *Becoming miracle workers: Language and meaning in brief therapy*. Hawthorne, NY: Aldine de Gruyter.

Miller, G., Gessner, M., & Korman, H. (2006). Impractical conversation about ideas, language, and meaning. Workshop presented at the 2006 Conference on Solution-Focused Practices, Denver, Colorado, November 2-4.

Miller, M., Azrael, D., & Hemenway, D. (2006). Belief in the inevitability of suicide: Results from a national survey. *Suicide and Life-Threatening Behavior, 36*(1), 1-11.

Miller, M.C. (1999). Suicide prevention contracts: Advantages, disadvantages, and an alternative approach. In D.G. Jacobs (Ed.), *The Harvard Medical School guide to suicide assessment and intervention* (pp. 463-481). San Francisco: Jossey-Bass.

Miller, S.D., Duncan, B.L., Sorrell, B., & Brown, G.S. (2004). The Partners for Change outcome management system. *Journal of Clinical Psychology: In Session, 60*. Retrieved May 16, 2006, from http://www.talkingcure.com/documents/LambertInSessionProof.pdf.

Milner, J. & O'Byrne (2002). *Brief counselling: Narratives and solutions*. New York: Palgrave.

Milton, J. (1990). Book XI, The argument, paradise lost. In *The Complete English Poems* (Rev. ed., p. 401, line 139). New York: Random House.

Mishara, B.L. (1998). Childhood conceptions of death and suicide: Empirical investigations and implications for suicide prevention. In D. Deleo, A. Schmidtke, & R.F.W. Diekstra (Eds.), *Suicide prevention: A holistic approach* (pp. 111-119). Dordrecht, the Netherlands: Kluwer.

Mishara, B.L., Houle, J., & LaVoie, B. (2005). Comparison of the effects of four suicide prevention programs for family and friends of high-risk suicidal men who did not seek help themselves. *Suicide and Life-Threatening Behavior, 35*(3), 329-342.

Mishara, B.L. & Weisstub, D.N. (2005). Ethical and legal issues in suicide research. *International Journal of Law and Psychiatry, 28*(1), 23-41.

Mitchell, A.M., Kim, Y., Prigerson, H.G., & Mortimer-Stepehens, M.K. (2004). Complicated grief in survivors of suicide. *Crisis, 25*(1), 12-18.

Mitchell, A.M., Kim, Y., Prigerson, H.G., & Mortimer-Stephens, M.K. (2005). Complicated grief and suicidal ideation in adult survivors of suicide. *Suicide and Life-Threatening Behavior, 35*(5), 498-506.

Montgomery, S.A. (1997). Suicide and antidepressants. *Annals of the New York Academy of Sciences, 286*, 329-336.

Morris, T. (2002). A husband's story. In J. Nunes & S. Simmie (Eds.), *Beyond crazy: Journeys through mental illness* (pp.135-139). Toronto: McClelland & Stewart.

Morrissette, P.J. (1992). Engagement strategies with reluctant homeless young people. *Psychotherapy, 29,* 447-451.

Morrissette, P.J. & McIntyre, S. (1989). Homeless youth in residential care. *Social Casework, 20,* 165-188.

Motto, J.A. & Bostrom, A.G. (2001). A randomized controlled trial of postcrisis suicide prevention. *Psychiatric Services, 52,* 828-833.

Muehlenkamp, J. (2003). Differences between self-injurious behavior and suicide attempts. Presented at the American Association of Suicidology Annual Conference, Santa Fe, New Mexico, April 22-26.

Murphy, G.E. (2000). Psychiatric aspects of suicidal behaviour: Substance abuse. In K. Hawton & K. van Heeringen (Eds.), *International handbook of suicide and attempted suicide* (pp. 107-120). Chichester, UK: Wiley.

Murphy, J.J. & Duncan, B.L. (1997). *Brief interventions for school problems: Collaborating for practical solutions.* New York: Guilford.

Mussell, B. (1997). Considering preventive measures: Balancing community supports and constraints. Presented at the Canadian Association for Suicide Prevention Conference, Thunder Bay, Ontario, Canada, October 29-31.

Myers, M.F. & Fine, C. (2006). *Touched by suicide: Hope and healing after loss.* New York: Gotham/Penguin.

Neeleman, J., Wilson-Jones, C., & Wessely, S. (2001). Ethnic density and deliberate self-harm: A small area study in southeast London. *Journal of Epidemiology and Community Health, 55,* 85-90.

Nelson, T. (Ed.) (2005). *Education and training in solution-focused brief therapy.* Binghamton, NY: The Haworth Press.

Newman, S.C. & Thompson, A.H. (2003). A population-based study of the association between pathological gambling and attempted suicide. *Suicide and Life-Threatening Behavior, 33*(1), 80-87.

Nietzsche, F.W. (1997). *Beyond good and evil.* H. Zimmern, trans. New York: Courier. (Original work published 1886.)

Nock, M.J. & M.K. Prinstein (2005). Contextual features and behavioral functions of self-mutilation among adolescents. *Journal of Abnormal Psychology, 114*(1), 140-146.

Nolen-Hoeksma, S. (2000). Growth and resilience among bereaved people. In J.E. Gillham (Ed.), *The science of optimism and hope* (pp. 107-127). Philadelphia: Templeton Foundation Press.

O'Brien, P.J. (2006). Creating compassion and connection in the work place. *Journal of Systemic Therapies, 25*(1), 16-36.

O'Carroll, P.W., Berman, A.L., Maris, R.W., Moscicki, E.K., Tanney, B.L., & Silverman, M.M. (1996). Beyond the Tower of Babel: A nomenclature for suicidology. *Suicide and Life-Threatening Behaviour, 26,* 237 252.

O'Connell, B. (2001). *Solution-focused stress counselling.* London: Continuum.

Odendaal, J.S.J. (2000). Animal-assisted therapy: Magic or medicine? *Journal of psychosomatic research, 49,* 275-280.

O'Hanlon, W.H. (1993). Take two people and call me in the morning: Brief solution-oriented therapy with depression. In S. Friedman (Ed.), *The new language of change: Constructive collaboration in psychotherapy* (pp. 50-85). New York: Guilford.

O'Leary, P. (1997). *The gift.* New York: Tor.

Olfson, M., Marcus, S., Pincus, H., Zito, J., Thompson, J., & Zarin, D. (1998). Antidepressant prescribing practices of outpatient psychiatrists. *Archives of General Psychiatry, 55,* 310-316.

Olfson, M., Shaffer, D., Marcus, S.C., & Greenberg, T. (2003). Relationship between antidepressant medication treatment and suicide in adolescents. *Archives of General Psychiatry, 60,* 978-982.

Omer, H. (1996). Three styles of constructive therapy. In M.F. Hoyt (Ed.), *Constructive Therapies 2* (pp. 319-333). New York: Guilford.

Omer, H. (1998). Using therapeutic splits to construct empathic narratives. In M.F. Hoyt (Ed.), *The handbook of constructive therapies* (pp. 414-427). San Francisco: Jossey-Bass.

Ontario Suicide Prevention Network (2005). Suicide prevention is everybody's business. Press release for Suicide Prevention Week. Retrieved February 1, 2007, from http://www.ontariosuicidepreventionnetwork.ca/Newsletters_and_Documents/WSPW_2005_PR.pdf.

Orbach, I. (1988). *Children who don't want to live: Understanding and treating the suicidal child.* San Francisco: Jossey-Bass.

Osborn, C.J. (1999). Solution-focused strategies with "involuntary" clients: Practical applications for the school and clinical setting. *Journal of Humanistic Education and Development, 37,* 169-181.

Overholser, J.C. & Spirito, A. (2003). Precursors to adolescent suicide attempts. In A. Spirito & J.C. Overholser (Eds.), *Evaluating and treating adolescent suicide attempters: From research to practice* (pp. 19-40). San Diego: Academic Press.

Parker, G., Gibson, N., Brotchie, H., Heruc, G., Rees, A-M., & Hadsi-Pavlovic, D. (2006). Omega-3 fatty acids and mood disorders. *American Journal of Psychiatry, 163*(6), 1098-1102.

Parry, A. & Doan, R.E. (1994). *Story re-visions: Narrative therapy in the postmodern world.* New York: Guilford.

Patton, M. & Meara, N. (1982). The analysis of language in psychological treatment. In R. Russell (Ed.), *Spoken interaction in psychotherapy* (pp. 101-131). New York: Irvington.

Paul, H. (2004). Issues and controversies surrounding recent texts on empirically-based psychotherapy: A meta-review. *Brief Treatment and Crisis Intervention, 4*(4), 389-399.

Paulson, B.P. & Everall, R.D. (2006). Suicidal adolescents: Helpful aspects of psychotherapy. *Archives of Suicide Research, 7,* 309-321.

Pearlman, L.A. & Saaktvine, K.W. (1995). *Trauma and the* THERAPIST*: Countertransference and vicarious traumatisation in psychotherapy with incest survivors.* New York: Norton.

Pearsall, D. (2001). Child and youth suicide. Presented at the Ontario Suicide Prevention Network Conference, Sudbury, Ontario, Canada, June 13-14.

Perez-Smith, A., Spirito, A., & Boergers, J. (2002). Neighborhood predictors of hopelessness among adolescent suicide attempters: Preliminary investigation. *Suicide and Life-Threatening Behavior, 32*(2), 139-145.

Perret-Catipovic, M. (1999). Suicide prevention in adolescents and young adults: The Geneva University Hospitals' Program. *Crisis, 20*(1), 36-40.

Perry, J.C., Banon, E., & Ianni, R. (1999). Effectiveness of psychotherapy for personality disorders. *American Journal of Psychiatry, 156,* 1312-1321.

Pfeffer, C.R. (1986). *The suicidal child.* New York: Guilford.

Pfeffer, C.R. (2000). Suicidal behaviour in children: An emphasis on developmental influences. In K. Hawton & K. van Heeringen (Eds.), *International handbook of suicide and attempted suicide* (pp. 237-248). Chichester, UK: Wiley.

Pfeffer, C.R. (2006). The most vulnerable among us: Our children. *Advancing Suicide Prevention, II*(I), 1.

Pfuhlmann, B. & Schmidtke, A. (2002). Pathological gambling and suicidal behavior. *Archives of Suicide Research, 6,* 257-267

Phillips, S.U. (1973). Some sources of social variability in the regulation of talk. *Language in Society, 5,* 81.

Pichot, T. (2007). Looking beyond depression. In T. Nelson and F. Thomas (Eds.), *Handbook of solution-focused brief therapy: Clinical applications* (pp. 117-135). Binghamton, NY: The Haworth Press.

Pichot, T. & Coulter, M. (2007). *Animal-assisted solution-focused therapy: Partnering with animals to create miracles.* Binghamton, NY: The Haworth Press.

Pichot, T. & Dolan, Y. (2003). *Solution-focused brief therapy: Its effective use in agency settings.* Binghamton, NY: The Haworth Press.

Platt, S. & Hawton, K. (2000). Suicidal behaviour and the labour market. In K. Hawton & K. van Heeringen (Eds.), *International handbook of suicide and attempted suicide* (pp. 309-384). Chichester, UK: Wiley.

Popadiuk, N. (2005). Family support: SAFER's Concerned Other Program. *Visions: BC's Mental Health and Addictions Journal, 2*(7), 37-38.

Prochaska, J.O. (1999). How do people change, and how can we change to help many more people? In M. Hubble, B. Duncan, & S. Miller (Eds.), *The heart and soul of change: The role of common factors across the helping professions* (pp. 227-255). Washington, DC: American Psychological Association.

Prochaska, J.O., DiClemente, C.C., & Norcross, J. (1992). In search of how people change: Applications to addictive behaviors. *American Psychologist 47,* 1102-1114.

Quinnett, P. (2000). *Counselling suicidal people: A therapy of hope.* Spokane, WA: QPR Press. Retrieved September 30, 2006, from http://www.qprinstitute.com/counselingbook.htm.

Quinnett, P. (2005). Letter to the editor: A response to Ron Bonner's review of "Autopsy of a Suicidal Mind." *Newslink, 32*(3), 4.

Ramsay, G. (1996). *Transsexuals: Candid answers to private questions*. Freedom, CA: The Crossing Press.

Rando, T.A. (1996). Complications in mourning traumatic death. In K.J. Doka (Ed.), *Living with grief after sudden loss: Suicide, homicide, accident, heart attack, stroke* (pp. 139-159). Washington, DC: Hospice Foundation of America.

Reeve, C. (1998). *Still me*. New York: Ballantine.

Reeve, C. (2002). *Nothing is impossible*. London: Century/Random House.

Reid, W.J. (1998). Promises, promises: Don't rely on patients' no-suicide/no-violence "contracts." *Journal of Practical Psychiatry and Behavioral Health, 4*(5), 316-318.

Reimer, W.L. & Chatwin, A. (2006). Effectiveness of solution-focused brief therapy for affective and relationship problems in a private practice context. *Journal of Systemic Therapies, 25*(1), 52-67.

Renberg, E.S., Lindgren, S., & Osterberg, I. (2004). Sexual abuse and suicidal behaviour. In D. DeLeo, U. Bille-Brahe, A. Kerkhof, & A. Schmidtke (Eds.), *Suicidal Behaviour: Theories and research findings* (pp. 185-195). Cambridge, MA: Hogrefe & Huber.

Research Committee of the Solution-Focused Brief Therapy Association (2005). Research Pre-conference Day. Presented at the Solution-Focused Brief Therapy Association Conference, Fort Lauderdale, Florida, November 3-5.

Research Committee of the Solution-Focused Brief Therapy Association (2005). *Solution-Focused Therapy Treatment Manual for Working with Individuals*, Revison October 2006. Logan, UT: Solution-Focused Brief Therapy Association.

Roberts, A.R. (2000). An overview of crisis theory and crisis intervention. In A.R. Roberts (Ed.), *Crisis Intervention Handbook* (2nd ed., pp. 3-30). New York: Oxford University Press.

Roberts, A.R. (2002). Assessment, crisis intervention, and trauma treatment: The integrative ACT intervention model *Brief Treatment and Crisis Intervention, 2*(1), 1-21.

Roberts, A.R. & Ottens, A.J. (2005). The seven-stage crisis intervention model: A road map to goal attainment, problem solving, and crisis resolution. *Brief Treatment and Crisis Intervention, 5*(4), 329-340.

Rosenberg, B. (2000). Mandated clients and solution-focused therapy: "It's not my miracle." *Journal of Systemic Therapies, 19*(1), 90-99.

Ross, R. (1992). *Dancing with a ghost: Exploring Indian reality*. Toronto: Reed Books.

Ross, R. (1996). *Returning to the teachings: Exploring aboriginal justice*. Toronto: Penguin.

Rotheram-Borus, M.J., Piacentini, J., Cantwell, C., Beline, T.R., & Sone, J. (2000). The impact of an emergency room intervention for adolescent female suicide attempters. *Journal of Counseling and Clinical Psychology, 68*(6), 1081-1093.

Rotheram-Borus, M.J., Piacentini, J., Van Rossem, R., Graae, F., Cantwell, C., Castro-Bianco, C., Miller, S., & Feldman, J. (1996). Enhancing treatment adherence with a specialized emergency room program for adolescent suicide attempters. *American Academy of Child and Adolescent Psychiatry, 35*(5), 654-663.

Royal Commission on Aboriginal Peoples (1995). *Choosing life: Special report on suicide among aboriginal people.* Ottawa: Ministry of Supply and Services Canada.

Rudd, M.D. (1997). What's in a name. . . . *Suicide and Life-Threatening Behaviour, 27,* 326-327.

Rudd, M.D. (2004). Rethinking hopelessness and suicide risk. Presented at the American Association of Suicidology Conference, Miami, Florida, April 14-17.

Rudd, M.D. (2006). *Science and suicide prevention: Contributions, challenges, and controversies.* Presented at the Canadian Association for Suicide Prevention Conference, Toronto, Ontario, Canada, October 25-27.

Rudd, M.D., Berman, A.L., Joiner, T.E., Nock, M.K., Silverman, M.M., Mandrusiak, M., Van Orden, K.A., & Witte, T. (2006). Warning signs for suicide: Theory, research, and clinical applications. *Suicide and Life-Threatening Behavior, 36*(3), 255-262.

Rudd, M.D. & Joiner, T.E. (1998). An integrative conceptual framework for treating suicidal behavior in adolescents. *Journal of Adolescence, 21*(4), 489-498.

Rudd, M.D., Joiner, T., & Rajab, M. H. (2001). *Treating suicidal behaviour: An effective, time-limited approach.* New York: Guilford.

Rudd, M.D., Mandrusiak, M., & Joiner, T.E. (2006). The case against no-suicide contracts: The commitment to treatment statement as a practice alternative. *Journal of Clinical Psychology, 62*(2), 243-251.

Rudd, M.D., Mandrusiak, M., Joiner, T.E., Berman, A.L., Van Orden, K.A., & Hollar, D. (2006). The emotional impact and ease of recall of warning signs for suicide. *Suicide and Life-Threatening Behavior, 36*(3), 288-295.

Ruescu, D. (2004). Aggression-related genes in suicidal behavior: An intermediate phenotype strategy in the search for genetic susceptibility. Presented at the European Symposium on Suicide and Suicidal Behaviour: Research, Prevention, Treatment and Hope, Copenhagen, Denmark, August 25-28.

Rutter, M. (1987). Psychosocial resilience and protective mechanisms. *American Association of Orthopsychiatry, 57*(3), 316-331.

Rutter, M. (2001). Psychosocial adversity: Risk, resilience and recovery. In J.M. Richman & M.W. Fraser (Eds.), *The context of youth violence: Resilience, risk and protection* (pp. 13-41). Westport, CT: Praeger.

Ryncarson, E.K. (2001). *Retelling violent death.* Philadelphia: Brunner-Routledge.

Saaktvine, K.W. & Pearlman, L.A. (1996). *Transforming the pain: A workbook on vicarious traumatization.* New York: Norton.

Sackett, D.L., Strauss, S.E., Richardson, W.S., Rosenberg, W., & Haynes, R.B. (2000). *Evidence-based medicine: How to practice and teach EBM.* London: Churchill Livingstone.

Sakinofsky, I. (1998). The epidemiology of suicide in Canada. In A. Leenaars, I. Sakinofsky, R.J. Dyck, M.J. Kral, & R.C. Bland (Eds.), *Suicide in Canada* (pp. 37-66). Toronto: University of Toronto Press.

Sakinofsky, I. (2000). Repetition of suicidal behaviour. In K. Hawton & K. van Heeringen (Eds.), *The international handbook of suicide and attempted suicide* (pp. 385-404). New York: Wiley.

Santa Minna, E.E. & Gallop, R.M. (1998). Childhood sexual and physical abuse and adult self-harm and suicidal behaviour: A literature review. *Canadian Journal of Psychiatry, 43,* 793-800.

Satcher, D. (2001). Preface. *National Strategy for Suicide Prevention: Goals and objectives for action.* Rockville, MD: U.S. Department of Health and Human Services, Public Health Service.

Saunders, D. (2004). Evaluating ESTs: Nothing more than psychotherapy's power in technique's 'clothing.' *Psynopsis,* Spring, p. 13.

Schools and suicide (2006). *Advancing Suicide Prevention, II*(I), 17-26.

Segal, Z.V., Williams, J.M., & Teasdale, J.D. (2002). *Mindfulness-based cognitive therapy for depression: A new approach for preventing relapse.* New York: Guilford.

Selekman, M. (1993). *Pathways to change: Brief therapy solutions with difficult adolescents.* New York: Guilford.

Selekman, M. (1997). *Solution-focused therapy with children: Harnessing family strengths for systemic change.* New York: Guilford.

Seligman, M.E.P. (1991). *Learned optimism.* New York: Knopf.

Shakespeare, W. (1954). The tragedy of Romeo and Juliet. In R. Hosley (Ed.), *The Yale Shakespeare.* New Haven, CT: Yale University Press. (Original work published 1599.)

Sharry, J., Darmody, M., & Madden, B. (2002). A solution-focused approach to working with suicidal clients. *British Journal of Guidance and Counselling, 30*(4), 383-399.

Sharry, J., Madden, B., & Darmody, M. (2003). *Becoming a solution detective: Identifying your clients' strengths in practical brief therapy.* Binghamton, NY: The Haworth Press.

Sheehan, M. (2005). *La prevention du suicide: Est-elle la responsabilité de tous?(Vers une stratégie nationale de prevention du suicide).* Presented at the Canadian Association for Suicide Prevention Conference, Ottawa, Ontario, Canada, October 16-19. Retrieved February 1, 2007, from http://www.ontario suicidepreventionnetwork.ca/Newsletters_and_Documents/Sheehan.

Shilts, L. & Reiter, M.D. (2000). Integrating externalization and scaling questions: Using "visual" scaling to amplify children's voices. *Journal of Systemic Therapies, 19*(1), 82-89.

Shneidman, E.S. (1973). *Deaths of man.* New York: Penguin.

Shneidman, E.S. (1985). *The definition of suicide.* New York: Wiley.

Shneidman, E.S. (1993). *Suicide as psychache: A clinical approach to self-destructive behaviour.* Northvale, NJ: Jason Aronson.

Shneidman, E.S. (2005). How I read. *Suicide and Life-Threatening Behavior, 35*(2), 117-120.

Simon, J. & Nelson, T. (2007). *Solution-focused brief practice with long-term clients in mental health services: I am more than my label.* Binghamton, NY: The Haworth Press.

Sinclair, M. (1998). Keynote presentation at the Canadian Association of Suicide Prevention Annual Conference, Winnipeg, Manitoba, Canada, October 21-24.

Smith, E.C. & Grawe, K. (2005). Which therapeutic mechanisms work when? A step toward the formulation of empirically validated guidelines for therapists; session-to-session decisions. *Clinical Psychology and Psychotherapy, 12,* 112-123.

Snyder, C.R. (2000). The hope mandala: Coping with the loss of a loved one. In J.E. Gillham (Ed.), *The science of optimism and hope* (pp. 129-142). Philadelphia: Templeton Foundation Press.

Snyder, C.R., Cheavens, J.S., & Michael, S.T. (1999). Hoping. In C.R. Snyder (Ed.), *Coping: The psychology of what works* (pp. 215-231). New York: Oxford.

Snyder, C.R., Michael, S.T., & Cheavens, J.S. (2000). Hope as a psychotherapeutic foundation of common factors, placebos, and expectancies. In M.A. Hubble, B.S. Duncan, & S.D. Miller (Eds.), *The heart and soul of change: What works in psychotherapy* (pp. 129-200). Washington, DC: American Psychological Association.

Softas-Niall, L. & Francis, P.C. (1998a). A solution-focused approach to a family with a suicidal member. *The Family Journal: Counselling and Therapy for Couples and Families, 6*(3), 227-230.

Softas-Niall, L. & Francis, P.C. (1998b). A solution-focused approach to suicide assessment and intervention with families. *The Family Journal: Counselling and Therapy for Couples and Families, 6,* 64-66.

Solomon, A. (2001). *The noonday demon: An atlas of depression.* New York: Touchstone.

Sommer-Rotenberg, D. (2005). Suicide and language. *Visions: B.C.'s Mental Health and Addictions Journal, 2*(7), 16-17.

Sparks, J. (1997). Voices of experience: Inviting former clients to rejoin the therapy process as consultants. *Journal of Systemic Therapies, 16*(4), 367-375.

Sparks, J. & Duncan, B.L. (2001). Clients as resources. In B. Duncan & J. Sparks (Eds.), *Heroic clients, heroic agencies: Partners for change* (pp. 132-138). Fort Lauderdale, FL: Nova Southeastern University.

Spicce, J., Duberstein, P.R., Conner, K.R., Eberly, S.W., & Conwell, Y. (2004). Perceived social support and suicide. Poster presented at the American Association of Suicidology Conference, Miami, Florida, April 14-17.

Spielberg, S. (Producer/Director) (1993). *Schindler's List*. United States: Universal Studios.

Stanford, E.J., Goetz, R.R., & Bloom, J.D. (1994). The no harm contract in the emergency room assessment of suicidal risk. *Journal of Clinical Psychiatry, 55*(8), 344-348.

Steiner, T. (2005). *Eagle and a mouse: Treatment of a fearful boy*. Videotape. Milwaukee, WS: Brief Family Therapy Centre.

Stellrecht, N.E., Gordon, K.H., Van Orden, K., Witte, T.K., Wingate, L.R., Cukrowicz, K.C., Butler, M., Schmidt, N.B., Fitzpatrick, K.K., & Joiner, T.E. (2006). Clinical applications of the interpersonal-psychological theory of attempted and completed suicide. *Journal of Clinical Psychology, 62*(2), 211-222.

Strong, T.E. (2002). Constructive curiosities. *Journal of Systemic Therapies, 21*(1), 77-90.

Strosahl, K. (1999). Cognitive and behavioural management of the suicidal patient. Presented at the Banff Conference on Behavioural Science, Banff, Alberta, Canada, March 14-17.

Strosahl, K., Chiles, J.A., & Linehan, M. (1992). Prediction of suicide intent in hospitalized parasuicides: reasons for living, hopelessness and depression. *Comprehensive Psychiatry, 33*, 366-373.

Styron, W. (1992). *Darkness visible*. New York: Vintage Books.

Tallman, K. & Bohart, A. (1999). The client as a common factor: Clients as self healers. In M. Hubble, B. Duncan, & S. Miller (Eds.), *The heart and soul of change: What works in therapy* (pp. 91-132). Washington, DC: American Psychological Association.

Talmon, M. (1990). *Single-session therapy*. San Francisco: Jossey-Bass.

Task Force Report on Promotion and Dissemination of Psychological Practices (1993). Training in and dissemination of empirically-validated psychological treatment: Report and recommendations. *The Clinical Psychologist, 48*, 2-23.

Taylor, L. (2005). A thumbnail map for solution-focused brief therapy. In T.S. Nelson (Ed.), *Education and training in solution-focused brief therapy* (pp. 27-33). Binghamton, NY: The Haworth Press.

Taylor, L. & Fiske, H. (2005). Tapping into hope. In S. Cooper and J. Duval (Eds.), *Catching the winds of change: Proceedings of the Brief Therapy Network Annual Conference* (pp. 82-87). Toronto: The Brief Therapy Network.

Taylor, L., Gallagher, D., Campbell, J., Nelson, T., & Fiske, H. (2005). SFBTA Summer Clinical Intensive Training, Cochrane, Alberta, Canada, June 16-19.

Tedeschi, R., Park, C., & Calhoun, L. (Eds.) (1998). *Posttraumatic growth: Positive change in the aftermath of crisis*. Nahwah, NJ: Lawrence Erlbaum Associates.

Thayer, R. (2003). *Calm energy: How people regulate mood with diet and exercise*. New York: Oxford University Press.

Thyer, B.A. (2004). What is evidence-based practice? *Brief Treatment and Crisis Intervention, 4*(2), 167-176.

Tkachuk, G.A. & Martin, G.L. (1999). Exercise therapy for patients with psychiatric disorders: Research and clinical implications. *Professional Psychology: Research and Practice, 30,* 275-282.

Tohn, S.L. & Oshlag, J. (1996). Solution-focused therapy with mandated clients: Cooperating with the uncooperative. In S. Miller, M. Hubble, & B. Duncan (Eds.), *Handbook of solution-focused brief therapy.* San Francisco: Jossey-Bass.

Tomori, C. & Bavelas, J.B. (2007). Using microanalysis of communication to compare solution-focused and client-centered therapies. *Journal of Family Psychotherapy, 18*(3), 25-43.

Trautman, P.D. (1989). Specific treatment modalities for adolescent suicide attempters. In M.R. Feinleib (Ed.), *Report of the secretary's task force on youth suicide: Volume 3: Practice and interventions in youth suicide* (pp. 253-263). Washington, DC: U.S. Government Printing Office.

Trautman, P. (2000). The keys to the pharmacy: Integrating solution-focused brief therapy and psychopharmacological treatment. *Journal of Systemic Therapies, 19*(1), 100-110.

Triantafillou, N. (n.d.). When is change really real—An excerpt from a conversation I had on the Internet. Retrieved April 2, 2005, from http://www.brieftherapynetwork.com/howto.html#change.

Trovato, F. (1998). Immigrant suicide in Canada. In A.A. Leenaars, S. Wenckstern, I. Sakinofsky, R.J. Dyck, M.J. Kral, & R.C. Bland (Eds.), *Suicide in Canada* (pp. 85-107). Toronto: University of Toronto Press.

Turnell, A. & Edwards, S. (1999). *Signs of safety: A solution- and safety-oriented approach to child protection casework.* New York: Norton.

Ungar, M. (2004). *Nurturing hidden resilience in troubled youth.* Toronto: University of Toronto Press.

van der Kolk, B.A., Greenberg, M.S., Orr, S.P., & Pittman, R.K. (1989). Endogenous opioids and stress induced analgesia in posttraumatic stress disorder. *Psychopharmacology Bulletin, 25,* 108-119.

Van Heeringen, C., Jannes, C., Buylaert, W., & Henderick, H. (1998). Risk factors for non-compliance with outpatient aftercare: Implications for the management of attempted suicide patients. In D. De Leo, A. Schmidtke, & R.F.W. Diekstra (Eds.), *Suicide prevention: A holistic approach* (pp. 211-218). Dordrecht, the Netherlands: Kluwer.

Van Orden, K.A., Joiner, T.E., Hollar, D., Rudd, M.D., Mandrusiak, M., & Silverman, M.M. (2006). A test of the effectiveness of a list of suicide warning signs for the public. *Suicide and Life-Threatening Behavior, 36*(3), 272-287.

VanDenBerg, John & Grealish, Mary E. (1996). Individualized services and supports through the wraparound process: Philosophy and procedures. *Journal of Child and Family Studies, 5*(1), 7-21.

Vaughn, K., Young, B.C., Webster, D.C., & Thomas, M.R. (1996). Solution-focused work in the hospital: A continuum-of-care model for inpatient treatment. In S. Miller, M.A. Hubble, & B.L. Duncan (Eds.), *Handbook of solution-focused brief therapy*, (pp. 91-127). San Francisco: Jossey-Bass.

Vieland, V., Whittle, B., Garland, A., Hicks, R., & Shaffer, D. (1991). The impact of curriculum-based suicide-prevention programs for teenagers: An 18-month follow-up. *Journal of the American Academy of Child and Adolescent Psychiatry, 30,* 811-815.

von Kibed, M.V. & de Shazer, S. (2003). Plenary Parts I & II: "A conversation on Wittgenstein." Presented at the Conference on Solution-Focused Practices 2003, first annual conference of the Solution-Focused Brief Therapy Association, Loma Linda, California, November 2-3.

Wade, A. (1997). Small acts of living: Everyday resistance to violence and other forms of oppression. *Contemporary Family Therapy: An International Journal, 19,* 23-29.

Wade, A. (2004). *Social responses to victims of violence: A brief summary of recent research.* Handout for "Violence, language and responsibility," workshop presented at the Western Conference on Solution-Focused Brief Therapy, Vancouver, BC, April 26-28, 2006.

Wade, A. (2006a). Response-based practice with victims of violent crime. Presented at the Western Conference on Solution-Focused Brief Therapy, Vancouver, British Columbia, Canada, April 26-28.

Wade, A. (2006b). Violence, language and responsibility. Presented at the Western Conference on Solution-Focused Brief Therapy, Vancouver, British Columbia, Canada, April 26-28.

Walsh, B.W. (2002). Understanding, managing and treating self-injury. Pre-conference workshop presented at the American Association of Suicidology Annual Conference, Bethesda, Maryland, April 10.

Walsh, B.W. (2005). *Treating self-injury.* New York: Guilford

Walsh, B.W. & Rosen, P.M. (1988). *Self-mutilation: Theory, research and treatment.* New York: Guilford.

Walter, J.L. & Peller, J.E. (1992). *Becoming solution-focused in brief therapy.* New York: Brunner-Mazel.

Walter, J.L. & Peller, J.E. (1994). "On track" in solution-focused brief therapy. In Michael F. Hoyt (Ed.), *Constructive therapies* (pp. 111-125). New York: Guilford.

Warren, B.E., Blumenstein, R., & Walker, L. (1998). Appendix: The empowerment of a community. In D. Denny (Ed.), *Current concepts in transgender identity* (pp. 427-430). New York: Garland Publishing.

Webb, W. (1999). *Solutioning: Solution-focused interventions for counselors.* Philadelphia, PA: Taylor & Francis.

Weiner-Davis, M., deShazer, S., & Gingerich, W.J. (1987). Building on pretreatment change to construct the therapeutic solution: An exploratory study. *Journal of Marital and Family Therapy, 13,* 359-363.

Wernecke, U., Turner, T., & Priebe, S. (2006). Complementary medicines in psychiatry: Review of effectiveness and safety. *British Journal of Psychiatry, 188,* 109-121.

What's in a Name? (2006). *NEWSlink, 32*(4), 10.

White J. (2004). *Preventing suicide in youth: Taking action with imperfect knowledge.* Vancouver, BC: University of British Columbia. Retrieved April 30, 2005, from http://www.sfu.ca/publications/documents/RR_9_05_finalreport.pdf.

White, J. & Jodoin, N. (1998). *"Before the fact" interventions: A manual of best practices in youth suicide prevention.* Vancouver, BC: Suicide Information and Resource Centre of British Columbia.

White, J. & Jodoin, N. (2004). *Aboriginal youth: A manual of promising suicide prevention strategies.* Calgary, AB: Center for Suicide Prevention.

White, M. (1991). Deconstruction and therapy. *Dulwich Centre Newsletter, 3,* 1-22. (Reprinted in S. Gilligan & R. Price [Eds.], *Therapeutic conversations* [pp. 22-61]. New York: Norton, 1993.)

White, M. (1996). *Narrative therapy workshop.* Toronto: Brief Therapy Centers International.

White, M. & Epston, D. (1990). *Narrative means to therapeutic ends.* New York: Norton.

Wieman, C. (2006). Addressing suicide in aboriginal communities: Advancing the research agenda. Presented at the Canadian Association for Suicide Prevention Conference, Toronto, Ontario, Canada, October 25-27.

Wiesel, E. (2006). *Night.* M. Wiesel, trans. New York: Douglas & McIntyre. (Original work published 1958.)

Wingate, L.R., Burns, A.B., Gordon, K.H., Perez, M., Walker, R.L., Williams, F.M., & Joiner, T.E. (2006). Suicide and positive cognitions: Positive psychology applied to the understanding and treatment of suicidal behaviour. In T.E. Ellis (Ed.), *Cognition and suicide* (pp. 29-49). Washington, DC: American Psychological Association.

Wittgenstein, L. (1968). *Philosophical investigations* (3rd ed.). G.E.M. Anscombe, trans. New York: MacMillan.

Wittgenstein, L. (1980). *Culture and value.* G.H. von Wright, Ed. P. Finch, trans. Chicago: University of Chicago Press.

Wolfsdorf, B.A., Freeman, J., D'Eramo, K., Overholser, J., & Spirito, A. (2005). Mood states: Depression, anger, and anxiety. In A. Spirito & J.C. Overholser (Eds.), *Evaluating and treating adolescent suicide attempters: From research to practice* (pp. 53-88). San Diego: Academic Press.

Worden, J.W. (2002). *Grief counseling and grief therapy* (3rd ed.). New York: Springer.

World Health Organization (1993). *The ICD-10 classification of mental and behavioural disorders: Diagnostic criteria for research.* Geneva, Switzerland: World Health Organization.

World Health Organization (2000). *Preventing suicide: A resource for media professionals.* Geneva, Switzerland: Author.

Wright, J. & Patenaude, S. (1998). Crisis intervention: Distress-Centre model. In A.A. Leenaars, S. Wenckstern, I. Sakinofsky, R.J. Dyck, M.J. Kral, & R.C. Bland (Eds.), *Suicide in Canada* (pp. 325-341). Toronto: University of Toronto Press.

Yapko, M.D. (2006). Treating depression systemically: A guest commentary. *Journal of Systemic Therapy, 25*(3), 73-77.

Yeager, K.R. (2002). Crisis intervention with mentally ill chemical abusers: Application of brief solution-focused therapy and strengths perspective. *Brief Treatment and Crisis Intervention, 2*(3), 197-216.

Yeager, K.R. & Gregoire, T.K. (2000). Crisis intervention application of brief solution-focused therapy in addictions. In A.R. Roberts (Ed.), *Crisis Intervention Handbook: Assessment, treatment, and research* (pp. 275-306). New York: Oxford University Press.

Young People In Crisis: A film and training program (1990). Presented by Youth Suicide Prevention and the American Association of Suicidology in consultation with the Harvard Medical School. Cambridge, MA: Youth Suicide Prevention.

Young-Eisendrath, P. (1996). *The resilient spirit.* Cambridge, MA: Perseus.

Zalter, B. & Ash, E. (2006). Solution-focused brief therapy in action. Presented at the Solution-Focused Brief Therapy Association conference, Denver, Colorado, November 2-4.

Zanarini, M.C., Frankenburg, F.R., Hennen, J., & Silk, K.R. (2003). The longitudinal course of borderline psychopathology: 6-year prospective follow-up of the phenomenology of borderline personality disorder. *American Journal of Psychiatry, 160,* 274-283.

Zimmerman, J.K. (1995). Treating suicidal adolescents: Is it really worth it? In J.K. Zimmerman & G.M. Asnis (Eds.), *Treatment approaches with suicidal adolescents* (pp. 3-16). New York: Wiley.

Zimmerman, J.K., Asnis, G.M., & Schwartz, B.J. (1995). Enhancing outpatient treatment compliance: A multifamily psychoeducational intake group. In J.K. Zimmerman & G.M. Asnis (Eds.), *Treatment approaches with suicidal adolescents* (pp. 106-134). New York: Wiley.

Zlotnick, C., Mattia, J.I., & Zimmerman, J.K. (1999). Clinical correlations of self-mutilation in a sample of general psychiatric patients. *Journal of Nervous and Mental Disease, 187,* 296-301.

Index

Printed in the United States
by Baker & Taylor Publisher Services

Printed in the United States
by Baker & Taylor Publisher Services